T0372039

Evidence-Based Practice with Emotionally Troubled Children and Adolescents

Evidence-Based Practice with Emotionally Troubled Children and Adolescents

Morley D. Glicken, DSW
Department of Social Work
Arizona State University West, Phoenix, Arizona

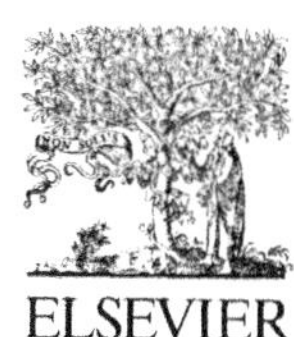

AMSTERDAM • BOSTON • HEIDELBERG • LONDON •
NEW YORK • OXFORD • PARIS • SAN DIEGO •
SAN FRANCISCO • SYDNEY • TOKYO
Academic Press is an imprint of Elsevier

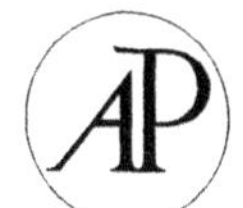

Academic Press is an imprint of Elsevier
The Boulevard, Langford Lane, Kidlington, Oxford OX5 1GB, UK
525 B Street, Suite 1900, San Diego, California 92101-4495, USA
32 Jamestown Road, London NW1 7BY, UK

First edition 2009

British Library Cataloguing in Publication Data
A catalogue record for this book is available from the British

Library of Congress Cataloguing in Publication Data
A catalogue record for this book is available from the Library of Congress

ISBN 978-0-12-374523-1

For information on all Academic Press publications
visit our website at www.elsevierdirect.com

Typeset by Thomson Digital, Noida, India

Printed and bound in the United Kingdom

Transferred to Digital Printing, 2010

Evidence-Based Practice with Emotionally Troubled Children and Adolescents

Morley D. Glicken, DSW

Table of Contents

This book is dedicated to my daughter Amy Jennifer Glicken
who taught me everything I know about children and who is,
as an adult, all any father could ask for

Preface

Over the years I've thought about the many children I've worked with during my time as a school social worker. Fresh from my MSW degree and not knowing much about the helping process, I used common sense helping approaches that I'd learned from watching my father deal with union members who came to our house on weekends with serious problems brought about by alcoholism that I would later realize were very much like what we did in social work. The men who came to our house were men whose burned out lives was a reminder to me that boredom and lack of recognition in the workplace destroy the will to live meaningful lives. My father was always kind, generous, and supportive. My mother did the same thing in her daily coffee and tea sessions with our neighbor ladies. You might say that I grew up in a social work home where the helping process was simple yet effective.

Although the children I saw in the school system had some troubled behavior, it never crossed my mind that they had serious emotional difficulties. Instead, I saw them as children coping with over-worked parents who were doing the best they could. I felt that forming a partnership with parents, children, and the schools would make kids better, and it did. I never used play therapy in the orthodox sense but strove to help children see what was good about them. I used cognitive therapy, which I was just learning in the 1960s with success, and brought to our suburban Chicago community an Adlarian group from Chicago to do a wonderful form of parent effectiveness training that worked so well that each week we would have hundreds of parents attending.

Over the years I've met a few of my clients. They are doing well. I can't say that for certain about everyone I worked with, but I have a sense that many have done well, and that the little help I provided got a number of children over emotional bumps at important moments in their lives. I never thought of my kids as having a diagnosis. They were having problems, to be sure, but they were all open to change. And they loved coming to sessions, many of which were done in groups and consisted of joke telling and anything to loosen the emotional constraints that parents had sometimes placed on them. It was a glorious experience and certainly the best time in my life.

Imagine then my concern to see so much in the literature about early childhood schizophrenia, bi-polar disorder, and the heavy reliance on medications for children who are, it seems to me, no different than the children I worked with in the 1960s. Having written a number of books before this one, I was surprised to see so little in the literature about childhood problems, particularly effective treatment for abused and neglected children. Rather than developing a concise framework to assess and treat children, we were, it seemed to me, using an adult model of assessment and treatment that seemed unlikely to help and fairly likely to hurt children if, for no other reason than by misdiagnosing them and using medications with troublesome side effects.

Furthermore, it seemed to me that rather than giving children room to grow and develop in their own unique ways we were restricting normal development by making the word "normal" increasingly limited and narrow. The growing literature, on the interference with normal male development in youth by creating diagnostic categories for boys who we all know needs a bit of space and support to develop well, is just one of many examples. The over-attentive parents who shelter children from obstacles that might be necessary for healthy development, or what has been called the millennium children who grow up lacking preparation for life challenges or independence, is yet another trend that troubles me.

Consequently, my second book on evidence-based practice is written in hopes of bringing some common sense back to the treatment of children by finding and evaluating best evidence. It's the type of book I would have wanted to read and use when I worked with children. Hopefully, you the reader, will find it helpful in your work with the children of America who deserve the best help we can offer. And I hope, as I do in all my books, that in reading this book you will remember the many children among us who suffer because of the abuse and neglect of their bodies and their spirit. Their anguish should motivate us to open our hearts and minds to new ideas, to new treatment approaches and, in Bertrand Russell's words, to have "unbearable sympathy for the suffering of others."

Morley D. Glicken, DSW

Acknowledgement

I want to thank the staff at Elsevier, particularly my editors, Mica Haley and Renske van Dijk for their support, encouragement, and help with this book. Writing about children is a gift for an older writer and working with Elsevier has been a joy.

Two of my wonderful MSW students, Joan Bourke and Meghan Anaya helped with chapters in this book on ADHD and cyber bullying, respectively. Teaching is a privilege and having such great students to work with is more than any educator can ask for.

Thanks to my colleague at Arizona State University West Department of Social Work for her insightful comments about evidence-based practice in Chapter 1 of the book.

Thanks also to the wonderful people at Sage, Allyn and Bacon/Longman, and Rowman and Littlefield for their permission to use material from several of my prior books. The addition of that material enriches this book and I appreciate their kind help.

Finally, I want to thank the children I've worked with over the years who provided the motivation to write this book. Their desire to change and their hard work to cope with difficult life problems are, as always, an inspiration to me.

About the Author

Dr. Morley D. Glicken is the former Dean of the Worden School of Social Service in San Antonio; the founding director of the Master of Social Work Department at California State University, San Bernardino; the past Director of the Master of Social Work Program at the University of Alabama; and the former Executive Director of Jewish Family Service of Greater Tucson. He has also held faculty positions in social work at the University of Kansas and Arizona State University. He currently teaches in the Department of Social Work at Arizona State University West in Phoenix, Arizona.

Dr. Glicken received his BA degree in social work with a minor in psychology from the University of North Dakota and holds an MSW degree from the University of Washington and the MPA and DSW degrees from the University of Utah. He is a member of Phi Kappa Phi Honorary Fraternity.

Dr. Glicken published two books for Allyn and Bacon/Longman Publishers in 2002: *The Role of the Helping Professions in the Treatment of Victims and Perpetrators of Crime* (with Dale Sechrest), and *A Simple Guide to Social Research;* and two additional books for Allyn and Bacon/Longman in 2003: *Violent Young Children, and Understanding and Using the Strengths Perspective.* He published *Improving the Effectiveness of the Helping Professions: An Evidence-Based Approach to Practice* in 2004 for Sage Publications and *Working with Troubled Men: A Practitioner's Guide* for Lawrence Erlbaum Publishers in Spring 2005. In 2006 he published *Life Lessons from Resilient People,* and *Social Work in the 21st Century: An Introduction to Social Problems, Social Welfare Organizations, and the Profession of Social Work,* both published by Sage Publications. In 2008 he published *A Guide to Writing for Human Service Professionals* for Rowman and Littlefield Publishers. In 2009 Rowman and Littlefield will publish his book *Evidence Based Practice with Older Adults: A Psychosocial Perspective.* His intro to social work book, *Social Work in the 21st Century: An Introduction to Social Problems, Social Welfare Organizations, and the Profession of Social Work,* will be published as a second edition in 2009 by Sage Publications.

Dr. Glicken has published over 50 articles in professional journals and has written extensively on personnel issues for Dow Jones, the publisher of the *Wall Street Journal.* He has held clinical social work licenses in Alabama and Kansas and is a member of the Academy of Certified Social Workers. He is currently

Professor Emeritus in Social Work at California State University, San Bernardino, and Director of the Institute for Personal Growth: A Research, Treatment, and Training Institute in Prescott, Arizona offering management consulting and research services to public and private agencies. More information about Dr. Glicken may be obtained on his website: www.morleyglicken.com, and he may be contacted by e-mail at: mglicken@msn.com.

Part One
The Current State of Practice with Children and Adolescents

Part One
The Current State of Practice with Children and Adolescents

1 The Current State of Assessment, Diagnosis, and Treatment of Children and Adolescents with Social and Emotional Problems

At a time when increasing numbers of children are being diagnosed and treated for emotional problems, the unsettling thought of misdiagnosing children who need help but are not being served because of racial and gender issues, and treatment of large numbers of children who are, in reality, responding in normal ways to maturational and social changes has begun to capture a great deal of attention in the popular and professional literature.

Unlike most adults, young children are often unable or unwilling to talk about their symptoms, leaving mental health professionals to rely on observation and information from parents and teachers, which may be incorrect or biased. Because children develop so quickly, what may look like attention deficit disorder in January may seem like something else or perhaps nothing at all in the summer. So subjective is the process of evaluating the problems encountered by children that the trial and error search for a diagnosis and treatment often ends with serious errors. Also, adult diagnoses are often used in lieu of diagnostic categories for children (US Department of Health and Human Services, 2000).

The Surgeon General's Report (US Department of Health and Human Services, 2000) suggests that many human service professionals prefer not to use a diagnosis with children because "[m]any of the symptoms, such as outbursts of aggression, difficulty in paying attention, fearfulness or shyness, difficulties in understanding language, food fads, or distress of a child when habitual behaviors are interfered with, are normal in young children and may occur sporadically throughout childhood" (Chapter 3).

Contrary to the current practice of assigning a diagnosis indicating serious emotional problems using adult diagnostic categories, the Surgeon General's Report (US Department of Health and Human Services, 2000) wisely cautions clinicians about the use of adult diagnostic categories by noting that:

> *Well-trained clinicians overcome this problem by determining whether a given symptom is occurring with an unexpected frequency, lasting for an unexpected length of time, or is occurring at an unexpected point in development. Clinicians with less experience may either over-diagnose normal behavior as a disorder or miss a diagnosis by failing to recognize abnormal behavior. Inaccurate diagnoses are more likely in children with mild forms of a disorder (Chapter 3).*

Yet the problem of misdiagnosing children seems more serious than ever, with new and increasingly arcane diagnostic categories developing that suggest the existence of very large numbers of American children with emotional problems. Some commonly diagnosed mental disorders in younger children include attention deficit hyperactivity disorder (ADHD), depression, anxiety, and oppositional defiant disorder (ODD). The DSM-IV (American Psychiatric Association, 1994) says that ODD exists if a child demonstrates four of eight of the following behavior patterns: "(a) often loses temper; (b) often argues with adults; (c) is often touchy or easily annoyed by others; (d) and is often spiteful or vindictive." (p. 93). These behaviors are characteristic of many children and adolescents and would not, in and of themselves, give most children an accurate diagnosis of oppositional defiant disorder.

Attention deficit disorder is perhaps the most common diagnosis used with children. Questions used to determine ADHD, such as "Does the child have difficulty in sustaining attention, following instructions, listening, organizing tasks? Does he or she fidget, squirm, impulsively interrupt, leave the classroom?" are such common behaviors, particularly in boys, that one might ask why attention disorder is a diagnosis given to boys at a rate twice that of girls when the rates, medically speaking, are the same.

More troubling is the finding regarding serious mental disorders. Carey (2007) reports that the number of American children and adolescents treated for bi-polar disorder increased 40-fold from 1994 to 2003, and has certainly risen further since 2003. According to Carey, in studies of doctors in private or group practice in New York, Maryland and Madrid, the numbers of visits in which doctors recorded diagnoses of bi-polar disorder increased from 20 000 in 1994 to 800 000 in 2003, about one percent of the population under age 20. Carey (2007, p. 1) also notes that:

> *According to government surveys at least six million American children have difficulties that are diagnosed as serious mental disorders, a number that has tripled since the early 1990s even though one of the largest continuing surveys of mental illness in children, tracking 4500 children ages 9 to 13, found no cases of full-blown bi-polar disorder and only a few children with the mild flights of excessive energy that could be considered nascent bi-polar disorder. Moreover, the symptoms diagnosed as serious emotional problems in children often bare little resemblance to those in adults. Instead, children's moods often flip on and off throughout the day, and their upswings often look more like extreme agitation than bi-polar disorder.*

In an interview with Judith Rapoport, chief of child psychiatry at the National Institute of Mental Health, Dess (2000) asked if childhood onset schizophrenia is on the increase. Rapoport responded that in 8 years, NIMH had identified only 55 cases of early childhood schizophrenia and notes that they are looking hard to find other cases to provide additional information on the early physical and emotional markers of schizophrenia, a disease usually associated with late adolescence.

However, in studies reported by the Medical College of Wisconsin (2003) the reported the use of certain psychotropic medications in 2–4-year-olds rose three-fold between 1991 and 1995. One of the reasons for this increase, according to the report, may the growing acceptance and misuse of psychotropic medications with children. The mounting pressure for children to conform to social standards of good behavior may also contribute to this increase. School administrators play a critical role in determining which children are seen as having emotional problems in need of treatment. However, as the above report argues, "it is not their responsibility, nor do they have the training, to recommend or mandate the use of medications as a solution to behavior problems" (p. 1).

Coyle (2000) reports that the use of psychotropic medications in very young children in two Medicaid programs and a managed care organization suggests that 1–1.5% of all children 2–4-years old enrolled in these programs are currently receiving stimulants, antidepressants, or antipsychotic medications. According to Coyle (2000), since there is no empirical evidence to support psychotropic drug treatment in very young children and there are valid concerns that such treatment could have serious negative side effects on the developing brain, he suggests that limited reimbursements for mental health services to children by many state Medicaid programs "are now increasingly subjected to quick and inexpensive pharmacologic fixes as opposed to informed, multimodal therapy associated with optimal outcomes. These disturbing prescription practices suggest a growing crisis in mental health services to children and demand more thorough investigation" (p. 1).

These concerns are compounded by continuing problems providing needed services to troubled groups of children because of race, gender, and ethnicity. The US Department of Health and Human Services (2000) indicates that Black and Hispanic youths comprise 32% of the general population but approximately 60% of the youth within detention and secure settings. Research by Cross et al. (1989) suggest that African American youth are less likely to receive treatment prior to coming into the system, and when identified in the community are more likely than their Caucasian counterparts to be referred to juvenile justice as opposed to mental health settings.

According to Puzzanchera et al. (2003), rates of incarceration among females are increasing at a faster rate than for males. Odgers et al. (2005) believe that girls within correctional settings "are often more likely than boys to suffer from a number of disorders, including: depression, anxiety and PTSD and (that those problems) increase exponentially for girls within juvenile justice settings; leading some to suggest that a gender paradox exists whereby girls at the most extreme end of the continuum with respect to behavioral and mental health profiles are filtered into correctional settings" (p. 28).

O'Neill (2000) describes an educational crisis for boys in which glaring discrepancies exist in reading, writing, and math scores at grades three and six, suggesting that boys will do badly in high school and higher education. In discussing male under-performance, O'Neill (2000) writes, "We have created a monster which is very difficult to escape from. There is nobody who is going to stand on a platform and start talking about the problems that face young boys, especially if it means criticizing the kind of education policies that got us into this position in the first place" (p. 54). O'Neill believes that those policies have worked against the best interests of boys by creating an educational system in which the primary focus is on the achievement and learning styles of girls, creating an atmosphere in which boys think no one cares about them.

The end result of educational discrepancies affecting boys is that women receive an average of 57% of the bachelor's degrees and 58% of all master's degrees in the United States or, 133 women are getting B.A.s for every 100 men, a number that will increase to 142 women per 100 men by 2010, according to the US Education Department. If current trends continue, there will be 156 women per 100 men earning degrees by 2020 (Conlin, 2003). The discrepancy in male educational achievement raises the issue of an economic imbalance that could create, "societal upheavals, altering family finances, social policies, and work-family practices" (Conlin, 2003, p. 77).

According to Conlin, men are dropping out of the work force, abandoning children, and removing themselves from community involvement. Since 1964, the rate of decline of men voting in presidential elections is twice that of the rate of women. More women now vote than men. As the decrease in men with comparable credentials and earning power continues, increasing numbers of women will, in all probability, never marry. Currently, 30% of all African American women 40–44 years of age have never been married (Conlin, 2003, p. 77). As women pull further ahead of men, the lack of availability of suitable men will reduce the probability of forming families.

In further concerns about the way boys are dealt with, Forbes (2003) suggests that boys are experiencing a severe crisis, which hampers their development and can be harmful to others. Forbes blames this crisis on restrictive male norms which:

> *... pressures male youths to prove their masculinity through stoic inexpressiveness and control, avoidance of qualities considered to be feminine, homophobia, competition, domination, and aggression. Influential and highly visible institutions, such as the government and the media, tend to favor male values such as aggression as a means to solve problems. Equally problematic is that male youths often grow up without adequate emotional and conceptual tools that enable them to distance themselves from the norm and become conscious of their own development. Recent incidents of school violence are examples of the destructive effects of boys caught up in the norm. Schools contribute to gender formation and the making of masculinities but do so in an unreflective, inchoate way (p. 146).*

In another area of practice with children and adolescents, predictions of serious reactions to traumas by children and adolescents often turn out to be incorrect.

Gist and Devilly (2001) indicate that the immediate predictions of PTSD in victims of the World Trade Center bombings turned out to be almost 70% higher than actually occurred 4 months after the event. Predictions of PTSD by school personnel turned out to be much higher than were determined after time permitted natural healing.

Attempts to help children who experience traumatic events (school shootings, acts of violence and terrorist acts) by using debriefing (van Emmerik et al., 2002), have been shown to be unhelpful. Debriefing is a type of crisis intervention in a very abbreviated form with information provided to group members about typical reactions to traumas, what to look for if group members experience any of these symptoms, and who to see if additional help is needed. Gist and Devilly (2001) write "... immediate debriefing has yielded null or paradoxical outcomes" (p. 742) because the approaches used in debriefing are often those "kinds of practical help learned better from grandmothers than from graduate training" (p. 742). The authors report that while still high, the estimates of PTSD after the 9/11 bombing dropped by almost two-thirds within 4 months of the tragedy and conclude that "[t]hese findings underscore the counterproductive nature of offering a prophylaxis with no demonstrable effect, but demonstrated potential to complicate natural resolution, in a population in which limited case-conversion can be anticipated, strong natural supports exist, and spontaneous resolution is prevalent" (p. 742).

Many of the children diagnosed with mental disorders are treated with medications that may or may not help but that certainly have side effects including weight gain and suicidal ideations. The Surgeon Generals report on mental health issues and children notes that there are only studies of the effectiveness of six classes of medication for use with children: the psychostimulants (Greenhill et al., 1998), the mood stabilizers and antimanic agents (Ryan et al., 1999), the selective serotonin reuptake inhibitors (SSRIs) (Emslie et al., 1999), antidepressants (Geller et al., 1998), antipsychotic agents (Campbell et al., 1999), and other miscellaneous agents (Riddle et al., 1998). The report goes on to say that only two classes of medication were found to be effective with children: SSRIs for childhood/adolescent obsessive–compulsive disorder, and the psychostimulants for ADHD. For many other disorders and medications, information from rigorously controlled trials is sparse or altogether absent.

While these data might be explained by a lack of good research on children, the tendency to increasingly view many children as having emotional problems and the focus on using medication to treat child emotional problems, often very early in life, seems clear. To offer best evidence of the amount, diagnostic confusion, and non-drug treatment for problems experienced by children and adolescents using evidence-based practice guidelines seems vital in this moment of infancy in the diagnosis and treatment of children. Let us begin by looking at estimates of the numbers of children and adolescents diagnosed with a variety of common to severe emotional problems.

1.1. THE NUMBERS OF CHILDREN AND ADOLESCENTS ESTIMATED TO HAVE EMOTIONAL DIFFICULTIES

1.1.1. *Anxiety Disorders*

Anxiety disorders are among the most common of childhood disorders. According to the US Department of Health and Human Services (2000), as many as 13 of every 100 young people have an anxiety disorder. Anxiety disorders include: (1) Phobias, which are unrealistic and overwhelming fears of objects or situations; (2) generalized anxiety disorder, which causes children to demonstrate a pattern of excessive, unrealistic worry that cannot be attributed to any recent experience; (3) panic disorder, which causes terrifying "panic attacks," including physical symptoms such as a rapid heartbeat and dizziness; (4) obsessive–compulsive disorder, which causes children to become "trapped" in a pattern of repeated thoughts and behaviors, such as counting or hand washing; and (5) post-traumatic stress disorder, which causes a pattern of flashbacks and other symptoms and occurs in children who have experienced a psychologically distressing event, such as abuse, being a victim or witness of violence, or exposure to other types of trauma such as wars or natural disasters.

1.1.2. *Severe Depression*

The National Institutes of Health (1999) indicates that two out of every 100 children may have major depression, and as many as eight out of every 100 adolescents may be affected. The disorder is marked by changes in: (1) emotions, whereby children often feel sad, cry, or feel worthless; (2) motivation, in which children lose interest in play activities, or their schoolwork declines; (3) physical well-being, in which children may experience changes in appetite or sleeping patterns and may have vague physical complaints; and (4) thoughts, during which children believe they are ugly, unable to do anything right, or that the world or life is hopeless.

1.1.3. *Bi-Polar Disorder*

Children and adolescents who demonstrate exaggerated mood swings which range from extreme highs (excitedness or manic phases) to extreme lows (depression) may have bi-polar disorder (sometimes called manic depression). Periods of moderate mood occur between the extreme highs and lows. During manic phases, children or adolescents may talk nonstop, need very little sleep, and show unusually poor judgment. At the low end of the mood swing, children experience severe depression. Bi-polar mood swings can recur throughout life. Adults with bi-polar disorder (about one in 100) often experienced their first symptoms during their teenage years (National Institutes of Health, 2001).

1.1.4. *Attention–Deficit/Hyperactivity Disorder*

Young people with attention–deficit/hyperactivity disorder are unable to focus their attention and are often impulsive and easily distracted. Attention–deficit/hyperactivity disorder occurs in up to five of every 100 children (US Department of Health and Human Services, 1999). Most of children with this disorder have great difficulty in remaining still, taking turns, and keeping quiet. Symptoms must be evident in at least two settings, such as home and school, in order for attention–deficit/hyperactivity disorder to be diagnosed.

1.1.5. *Conduct Disorder*

Youths with conduct disorders usually have little concern for others and repeatedly violate the basic rights of others and the rules of society. Conduct disorder causes children and adolescents to act out their feelings or impulses in destructive ways. The offenses these children and adolescents commit often grow more serious over time. Such offenses may include lying, theft, aggression, truancy, the setting of fires, and vandalism. Current research has yielded varying estimates of the number of young people with this disorder, ranging from one to four of every 100 children between nine to 17 years of age (US Department of Health and Human Services, 1999).

1.1.6. *Eating Disorders*

Children or adolescents who are intensely afraid of gaining weight and do not believe that they are underweight may have eating disorders. Eating disorders can be life threatening. Young people with anorexia nervosa, for example, have difficulty maintaining a minimum healthy body weight. Anorexia affects one in every 100–200 adolescent girls and a much smaller number of boys (National Institutes of Health, 1999).

Youngsters with bulimia nervosa feel compelled to binge (eat huge amounts of food in one sitting). After a binge, in order to prevent weight gain, they rid their bodies of the food by vomiting, abusing laxatives, taking enemas, or exercising obsessively. Reported rates of bulimia vary from one to three of every 100 young people (National Institutes of Health, 1999).

Obesity affects 20% or more of American children (Department of Agriculture, 1998). Childhood obesity is likely to persist into adult life and puts individuals at risk for stroke, hypertension, diabetes and other chronic diseases. It is also in childhood where eating habits are formed for a lifetime. Recent concerns about childhood diabetes suggest that obesity is at a crisis stage for American children.

1.1.7. *Autism*

Children with autism have problems interacting and communicating with others. Autism appears before the third birthday, causing children to act inappropriately, often repeating behaviors over long periods of time. For example, some children bang their heads, rock, or spin objects. Symptoms of autism range from mild to severe. Children with autism may have a very limited awareness of others and are at increased risk for other mental disorders. Studies suggest that autism affects 10–12 of every 10 000 children (US Department of Health and Human Services, 1999).

1.1.8. Schizophrenia

Young people with schizophrenia have psychotic periods which may involve hallucinations, withdrawal from others, and loss of contact with reality. Other symptoms include delusional or disordered thoughts and an inability to experience pleasure. Schizophrenia occurs in about five of every 1000 children (National Institutes of Health, 1997).

1.2. WHAT DOES THIS DATA SUGGEST?

In future chapters we will explore studies that suggest contradictory data and disagreement about the use of best evidence. Certainly, however, children and adolescents suffer from a host of emotional problems that if left untreated could result in serious psychosocial problems in later life. To make certain that clinicians use the best evidence available from the research literature when working with children and adolescents, this book on evidence-based practice will consider best evidence from the research literature for the assessment, diagnosis and treatment of common and more serious emotional problems in children and adolescents, including ADHD; bi-polar disorder; anxiety and depression; eating disorders; autism; Asperger's Syndrome; substance abuse; social isolation; underachievement; sexual acting out; oppositional defiant and conduct disorders; childhood schizophrenia; gender issues; prolonged grief; gang involvement; and a number of other problems experienced by children and adolescents.

Because concrete research evidence is often not used as the basis for practice with children and adolescents, and the next edition of the DSM series, which promises more information about children is not due until 2011, this book provides a timely guide for practitioners, students, mental health professionals, and parents to a research-oriented approach for understanding and helping children experiencing emotional difficulties and their families.

1.3. CASE STUDY: MENTAL ILLNESS OR A SEVERE REACTION TO STRESS?

James Becker is a 17-year-old high school student who suddenly began showing symptoms of mental illness and was diagnosed with schizophrenia, undifferentiated type (DSM-IV Code# 295.90, APA, 1994, p. 289). James had no prior history of mental illness and no one in the immediate family had experienced mental illness. James was under a great deal of pressure in an attempt to get admitted to a nationally recognized tier one college. His grades and his performance in interviews would determine whether he would be accepted into a prestigious college, the key to a successful life for a working class adolescent with parents who were very ambitious for him to succeed. James began to experience a feeling of gross disorganization and a strange sense of aloofness from others, described by his friends as severe withdrawal and flat affect. The symptoms grew progressively worse and on the advice of his school counselor James was sent to a private psychiatrist where the diagnosis of schizophrenia, undifferentiated type was given. James was not considered a danger to himself or to others but was unable to continue with his studies. He was placed on anti-psychotic medication and was seen in a day program in the community where psycho-educational treatment was offered. As his symptoms worsened, he was sent to a private inpatient facility specializing in the care of the mentally ill where he stayed for almost 4 months. His symptoms included mild hallucinations, social withdrawal and isolation, and some delusional thinking in which he described a presence that was about to kill him.

After 3 months in the group facility with a general deterioration in his symptoms, James began to show significant signs of improvement. He was able to attend counseling sessions and contribute to the discussion. He interacted well with others and spoke about returning to school. His medication was reduced in strength, and the improvement in his condition continued. Six months after the sudden onset of symptoms, he was able to return to school with no other signs of schizophrenia a year and a half after onset.

1.4. DISCUSSION

The psychiatrist who initially treated James and who followed him after he returned to school said that the original diagnosis was now amended to add that it was a single episode of schizophrenia, undifferentiated type, now in full remission (AMA, 1994, p. 279). Like many diseases, schizophrenia may have an initial acute phase followed by a complete return to normal functioning. The cause of the single episode is difficult to determine. James was asked to comment on his experience:

> *"I don't think I was psychotic. One day I was walking home from school and I suddenly had the most ominous feeling that I was going to die. It had never happened to me before and it was very frightening. I withdrew from people. Some days I couldn't talk. I was very certain that someone was going to kill me, but I was aware and conscious of everything taking place around me. I don't think I had any hallucinations but maybe I did. It was more that I felt a presence nearby and that it would do me great harm. Maybe I was overstressed from school pressure, but I don't think so. One minute I was fine*

and the next minute I was scared out of my wits. It took many months for the fear to go away and for me to be able to talk to anyone. When I began to get better, it seemed to happen all by itself. It was like a cloud lifted and suddenly I was well again. I doubt if the medication helped and I'm certain that therapy didn't help at all. There were some very kind professionals who were really nice to me, and many wonderful patients who sat with me when I was really frightened, but while I don't think I was psychotic, at the same time I can't tell you why this happened or why I improved. I really don't think it will ever happen to me again, but if it does, I certainly have a better handle on what to do about it."

Commenting further on James' experience, his psychiatrist said that James was one of many students he had worked with who'd had a spontaneous remission from mental illness. He said:

"We still don't know enough about brain chemistry or the reasons for the sudden onset of symptoms of schizophrenia. I'm of the opinion that a combination of life stressors and bio-chemical conditions interact with one another to cause symptoms which appear to be psychotic. When you talk to patients who have immediate remissions, you hear stories very similar to the one James told. I'm increasingly convinced that like any opportunistic disease, schizophrenia attacks when the body is least capable of resisting. James was under extreme pressure to do well in his interviews with prestigious colleges. His father was very ambitious for James and had placed considerable pressure on James to succeed. His schoolwork took him away from any social life, and while he was not abusing drugs, he was using a combination of sleeping pills and Xanax to cope with anxiety. Perhaps this all contributed to his illness and maybe it didn't. We have a lot to learn about psychosis, but optimism is something we should all have. Many people like James come out of psychotic episodes, are just fine afterwards, and never have another psychotic experience. The worst part of the problem is the social stigma. I don't know how many letters I had to write on his behalf before several prestigious colleges would seriously consider his application. He's a healthy, intelligent young man but the stigma of this one experience will very likely follow him throughout his life. He's already been rejected by several top colleges that showed so much interest in him before his illness. The real tragedy of mental illness often takes place after the patient is cured. It's an illness full of social stigma which endlessly and needlessly harms people who have every reason to tell the world that they're just fine now."

1.5. SUMMARY

This introductory chapter discusses the debate among clinicians regarding the actual numbers of youth with accurate diagnoses of emotional problems. The chapter also discusses concerns in the literature with the use of unproven psychotropic medications with very young children, their possible side effects and the lack of research evidence that medication is a better treatment than a variety of psychosocial interventions. The chapter ends with a case study showing the difficulty inherent in diagnosing youth whose behavior is still developing.

1.6. QUESTIONS FROM THE CHAPTER

1. The author says that we have gone way overboard in diagnosing emotional problems in children and adolescents and then cites some very high numbers by the US Government. Who do you believe and why?
2. The use of medication for children should be carefully monitored but don't you think there are children who benefit from medication including children who are highly agitated, depressed, or hyperactive?
3. The author talks about how he never diagnosed children he saw as a school social worker and how most of them were, in a broad sense of the word, normal. But, do you think times have changed and that more and more children have to cope with very difficult life situations that were uncommon 40 years ago? What might some of them be?
4. How would you explain that more boys are diagnosed with ADHD than girls while studies suggest that both genders should have the same amount of ADHD?
5. Many of the children who end up in juvenile corrections facilities come from families that live in poverty. If we eliminated poverty would this also substantially reduce the number of youth in the juvenile justice system?

References

Campbell, M., Rapoport, J. L., & Simpson, G. M. (1999). Antipsychotics in children and adolescents. *Journal of American Academy of Child and Adolescent Psychiatry, 38*, 537–545.

Carey, B. (September 4, 2007). *Bipolar Illness Soars as a Diagnosis for the Young.* http://www.nytimes.com/2007/09/04/health/04psych.html?_r=1&th=&oref=slogin&emc=th&pagewanted=print

Conlin, M. (2003, May 26). The new gender gap. *Business Week, 3834*, 74–81. (No volume listed).

Coyle, J. T. (February 23, 2000). Psychotropic drug use in very young children. *The Journal of American Medical Association, 283*(8). http://www.contac.org/contaclibrary/children19.htm

Cross, T., Bazron, B., Dennis, K., & Isaacs, M. (1989). *Towards a culturally competent system of care: A monograph on effective services for minority children who are severely emotionally disturbed.* Washington, DC: Georgetown University Child Development Center/CASSP Technical Assistance Center.

Dess, N. K. (July/August, 2000). When mental illness strikes children. *Psychology Today. Interviews Judith Rapoport, chief of child psychiatry at the National Institute of Mental Health. Prevalence of mental illness; Information on obsessive–compulsive disorder (OCD); Why OCD exist; What should parents, teacher and significant others watch for an OCD.*

Emslie, G. J., Walkup, J. T., Pliszka, S. R., & Ernest, M. (1999). Nontricyclic antidepressants: Current trends in children and adolescents. *Journal of the American Academy of Child and Adolescent Psychiatry, 38*, 517–528.

Forbes, D. (2003). Turn the wheel: Integral school counseling for male adolescents. *Journal of Counseling & Development, 81*, 142–150.

Geller, B., Cooper, T. B., Sun, K., Zimerman, B., Frazier, J., Williams, M., & Heath, J. (1998). Double-blind and placebo-controlled study of lithium for adolescent bipolar disorders with secondary substance dependency. *Journal of the American Academy of Child and Adolescent Psychiatry, 37*, 171–178.

Greenhill, L., Abikoff, H., Arnold, L., Cantwell, D., Conners, C. K., Cooper, T., Crowley, K., Elliot, G., Davies, M., Halperin, J., Hechtman, L., Hinshaw, S., Jensen, P., Klein, R., Lerner, M., March, J., MacBurnett, K., Pelham, W., Severe, J., Sharma, V., Swanson, J., Vallano, G., Vitiello, B., Wigal, T., & Zametkin, A. (1998). *Psychopharmacological treatment manual, NIMH multimodal treatment study of children with attention deficit hyperactivity disorder (MTA Study)*. New York: Psychopharmacology Subcommittee of the MTA Steering Committee.

Medical College of Wisconsin. (2003). *Children, mental illness and medicines*. http://healthlink.mcw.edu/article/954384940.html

National Institutes of Health. (1997). *Press Release: Progressive Brain Changes Detected in Childhood Onset Schizophrenia*. Retrieved May 11, 2008, from http://mentalhealth.samhsa.gov/publications/allpubs/CA-0006/default.asp

National Institutes of Health. (1999). *Brief Notes on the Mental Health of Children and adolescents*. Retrieved September 5, 2001, from the World Wide Web. http://mentalhealth.samhsa.gov/publications/allpubs/CA-0006/default.asp

National Institutes of Health. (2001). *Fact Sheet: Going to Extremes, Bipolar Disorder*. Bethesda, MD: National Institutes of Health. Retrieved from the Internet May 12, 2006 at http://mentalhealth.samhsa.gov/publications/allpubs/CA-0006/default.asp

O'Neill, T. (December 4, 2000). Boys' problems don't matter. *Newsmagazine* (Alberta Edition), *29*(15), pp. 54–56.

Odgers, C. L., Burnette, M. A., Chauhan, M. S., Moretti, M. M., & Reppucci, D. (Feb. 2005). Misdiagnosing the problem: Mental health profiles of incarcerated juveniles. *The Canadian and Adolescent Psychiatry Review, 1*(14), 26–29.

Puzzanchera, C., Stahl A. L., Finnegan, T. A., Tierney, N., & Snyder, H. N. (2003). Juvenile Court Statistics 1998. Washington, DC: *Office of Juvenile Justice and Delinquency Prevention*.

Riddle, M. A., Subramaniam, G., & Walkup, J. T. (1998). Efficacy of psychiatric medications in children and adolescents: A review of controlled studies. *Psychiatric Clinics of North America: Annual of Drug Therapy, 5*, 269–285.

Ryan, N. D., Bhatara, V. S., & Perel, J. M. (1999). Mood stabilizers in children and adolescents. *Journal of American Academy of Child and Adolescent Psychiatry, 38*, 529–536.

US Department of Agriculture; Center for Nutrition Policy and Promotion. (October 27, 1998). *Childhood obesity: Causes and prevention Symposium Proceedings*. http://www.google.com/search?q=cache:_Bca9PTT_r0J:www.usda.gov/cnpp/Seminars/obesity.PDF+child+obesity&hl=en&gl=us&ct=clnk&cd=7

US Department of Health Human Services. (2000). *Mental Health: A Report of the Surgeon General*. Rockville, MD: US Department of Health and Human Services.

van Emmerik, A. P., Kamphuis, J. H., Hulsbosch, A. M., & Emmelkamp, P. M. (2002). Single session debriefing after psychological trauma: A meta-analysis. *Lancet, 360*(9335), 766–772.

Further reading

Enkin, M., Keirse, M. J. N., Renfrew, M., & Neilson, J. (1995). *A guide to effective care in pregnancy and childbirth* (2nd Ed.). New York: Oxford University Press.

Gist, R., & Devilly, G. J. (2001). Post-trauma debriefing: The road too frequently traveled. *National Institutes of Health. Fact Sheet: Going to Extremes, Bipolar Disorder, 360*(9335), 741, 743.

Munoz, R., Hollon, S., McGrath, E., Rehm, L., & VandenBos, G. (1994). On the AHCPR guidelines: Further considerations for practitioners. *American Psychologist, 49*, 42–61.

Part Two
The Core Beliefs of Evidence-Based Practice

2 Understanding Evidence-Based Practice

2.1. INTRODUCTION

The author wishes to thank Sage Publications for permission to use material from the author's book on evidence-based practice (Glicken, 2005, pp. 3–18).

As all too many parents and younger clients can verify, the current practice of psychotherapy, counseling, and much of our work as helping professionals with children and adolescents often relies on clinical wisdom with little evidence that what we do actually works. Clinical wisdom is often a justification for beliefs and values that bond us as professionals but frequently fail to serve younger clients because many of those beliefs and values may be comforting, but they may also be inherently incorrect. O'Donnell (1997) likens this process of clinical wisdom to making the same mistakes, with growing confidence, over a long number of years. Isaacs (1999) calls clinical wisdom vehemence-based practice, in which one substitutes volumes of clinical experience for evidence, which is "an effective technique for browbeating your more timorous colleagues and for convincing relatives of your ability" (p. 1).

Flaherty (2001) believes there is a "murky mythology" behind certain treatment approaches which causes them to persist and that:

> *Unfounded beliefs of uncertain provenance may be passed down as a kind of clinical lore from professors to students. Clinical shibboleths can remain unexamined for decades because they stem from such respected authorities as time-honored textbooks, renowned experts, or well-publicized but flawed studies in major journals (p. 1).*

Flaherty goes on to note that even when sound countervailing information becomes available, clinicians still hold on to myths. More onerous yet, Flaherty points out that we may perpetuate myths "by indulging the mistaken beliefs of patients or by making stereotypical assumptions about patients based on age, ethnicity, or gender" (p. 1), concerns in the mental health field that still plague us.

The clinical wisdom approach to practice is based on what the American Medical Association Evidence-Based Practice Working Group (1992) refers to as unsystematic observations from clinical experience, a belief in common sense, a feeling that clinical training and experience are a way of maintaining a certain level of effective practice, and an assumption that there are wise and more experienced clinicians who we can go to when we need help with clients. All of these assumptions are grounded in a paradigm that tends to be subjective, and is often clinician- rather than client-focused.

Aware of the subjective nature of social work practice, Rosen (1994) called on the social work profession to use a more systematic way of providing practice and writes, "Numerous studies indicate that guidelines [for clinical practice] can increase empirically based practice and improve clients' outcomes" (Found in Howard and Jenson, 1999, p. 283). Rosen (1994) continues by suggesting that guidelines for social work practice would also produce better clinical training, cooperative client decision making, improved clinical training in schools of social work, better cost-effective practice, and would compile knowledge about difficult-to-treat conditions, "[because] few of the practice decisions social workers make are empirically rationalized" (Found in Howard and Jenson, 1999, p. 283).

Clinicians often argue that what we do in practice is intuitive, subjective, artful, and based on long years of experience. Psychotherapy, as this argument goes, is something one learns with practice. The responses made to clients and the approaches used during treatment may be so spontaneous and inherently empathic that research paradigms and knowledge-guided practice are not useful in the moment when a response is required. This argument is, of course, a sound one. The moment-to-moment work of the clinical practitioner *is* often guided by experience. However, as Gambrill (1999) points out, we often over-step our boundaries as professionals when we make claims about our professional abilities that we cannot prove. She points to the following statement made in a professional newsletter, and then responds to it:

> ***A Statement made in a social work publication:*** *Professional social workers possess the specialized knowledge necessary for an effective social services delivery system. Social work education provides a unique combination of knowledge, values, skills, and professional ethics, which cannot be obtained through other degree programs or by on-the-job training. Further, social work education adequately equips its individuals with skills to help clients solve problems that bring them to social services departments and human services agencies, (NASW News, p. 14)*
>
> ***Gambrill's Response:*** *These claims all relate to knowledge. To my knowledge, there is no evidence for any of these claims. In fact, there is counterevidence. In Dawes' (1994) review of hundreds of studies, he concluded that there is no evidence that licenses, experience, and training are related to helping clients. If this applies to social work and, given the overlap in helping efforts among social workers, counselors, and psychologists, it is likely that it does, what are the implications? (Gambrill, 1999, p. 341)*

The psychotherapy literature is replete with concepts and assumptions that seem unequivocally subjective and imprecise. Consider, for example, a definition of psychotherapy that says it is a socially acceptable way of receiving help for an emotional problem by a trained professional. One might use the same definition for faith healers, psychics, and others who have both social sanction and exert social influence. Or consider this whimsical definition of psychotherapy as "two people playing together," or a final definition of psychotherapy as a "systematic use of a human relationship for therapeutic purposes." The vagueness of these definitions fail to convey to clients what we do and makes it more than a little difficult for clinical researchers to evaluate the effectiveness of treatment.

As a response to highly subjective and sometimes incorrect approaches to practice, evidence-based practice (EBP) believes that we should consult the research and involve clients in decisions about the best therapeutic approaches to be used, the issues in a client's life that need to be resolved, and the need to form a positive alliance with clients to facilitate change. This requires a cooperative and equal relationship with clients. EBP also suggests that we act in a facilitative way to help clients gather information and rationally and critically process it. This differs from authoritarian approaches that assume the worker knows more about the client than the client does, and that the worker is the sole judge of what is to be done in the helping process.

2.2. DEFINING EVIDENCE-BASED PRACTICE

Sackett et al. (1997) define evidence-based practice as "... the conscientious, explicit, and judicious use of current best evidence in making decisions about the care of individuals" (p. 2). Gambrill (2000, p. 1) defines EBP as a process involving self-directed learning which requires professionals to access information that permits us to: (1) take our collected knowledge and provide questions we can answer; (2) find the best evidence with which to answer questions; (3) analyze the best evidence for its research validity as well as its applicability to the practice questions we have asked; (4) determine if the best evidence we have found can be used with a particular client; (5) consider the client's social and emotional background; (6) make the client a participant in decision-making, and; (7) evaluate the quality of practice with that specific client.

The Council for Training in Evidence-Based Practice (2007) defines EBP as follows: "Making decisions about behavioral health by integrating the best available research evidence with practitioner expertise and the characteristics of those who will be affected, and doing so in a manner that is compatible with the environmental and organizational context" (p. 1).

Gambrill (1999) believes that EBP "requires an atmosphere in which critical appraisal of practice-related claims flourishes, and clients are involved as informed participants" (Gambrill, 1999, p. 345). In describing the importance of evidence-based practice, The User's Guide to Evidence-Based Practice (1992, p. 2420), findings from a workgroup of The American Medical Association writes:

A new paradigm for medical practice is emerging. Evidence-based medicine de-emphasizes intuition, unsystematic clinical experience, and pathophysiologic rationale as sufficient grounds for clinical decision-making, and stresses the examination of evidence from clinical research. Evidence-based medicine requires new skills of the physician, including efficient literature-searching, and the application of formal rules of evidence in evaluating the clinical literature.

Timmermans and Angell (2001) indicate that evidence-based clinical judgment has five important features:

1. It is composed of both research evidence and clinical experience.
2. There is skill involved in reading the literature that requires an ability to synthesize the information and make judgments about the quality of the evidence available.
3. The way in which information is used is a function of the practitioner's level of authority in an organization and his or her level of confidence in the effectiveness of the applied information.
4. Part of the use of EBP is the ability to independently evaluate the information used and to test its validity in the context of one's own practice.
5. Evidence-based clinical judgments are grounded in the western notions of professional conduct and professional roles, and are ultimately guided by a common value system.

Gambrill (1999) points out that one of the most important aspects of EBP is the sharing of information with clients and the cooperative relationship that ensues. She notes that in EBP, clinicians search for relevant research to help in practice decisions and share that information with clients. If no evidence is found to justify a specific treatment regimen, the client is informed and a discussion takes place about how best to approach treatment. This includes the risks and benefits of any treatment approach used. Clients are involved in all treatment decisions and are encouraged to independently search the literature. As Sackett et al. (1997) note, new information is constantly being added to our knowledge base. Informed clinicians and clients may often find elegant treatment approaches that help provide direction where none may have existed before.

Gambrill (1999) believes that the use of EBP can help us "avoid fooling ourselves that we have knowledge when we do not" (p. 342). She indicates that a complete search for effectiveness research will provide the following information relevant for work with all clients, including children and adolescents (Gambrill, 1999, p. 343) first suggested by Enkin et al. (1995):

1. Beneficial forms of care demonstrated by clear evidence from controlled trials.
2. Forms of care likely to be beneficial. (The evidence in favor of these forms of care is not as clear as for those in category one.)
3. Forms of care with a trade-off between beneficial and adverse effects. (Effects must be weighed according to individual circumstances and priorities.)
4. Forms of care of unknown effectiveness. (There are insufficient or inadequate quality data upon which to base a recommendation for practice.)
5. Forms of care unlikely to be beneficial. (The evidence against these forms of care is not as clear as for those in category six.)

6. Forms of care likely to be ineffective or harmful. (Ineffectiveness or harm demonstrated by clear evidence).

Hines (2000) suggests that some fundamental steps are required by EBP to obtain usable information in a literature search. They are: (1) developing a well-formulated clinical question; (2) finding the best possible answers to your questions; (3) determining the validity and reliability of the data found; and (4) testing the information with your client. Hines indicates that a well-formulated clinical question must accurately describe the problem you wish to look for, limit the interventions you think are feasible and acceptable to the client, search for alternative approaches, and indicate the outcomes you wish to achieve with the client. The advantage of EBP, according to Hines, is that it allows the practitioner to develop quality practice guidelines that can be applied to the client, identify appropriate literature that can be shared with the client, communicate with other professionals from a knowledge-guided frame of reference, and continue a process of self-learning that results in the best possible treatment for clients.

Haynes (1998) writes that the goal of evidence-based practice "is to provide the means by which current best evidence from research can be judiciously and conscientiously applied in the prevention, detection, and care of health disorders" (p. 273). Haynes believes that this goal is very ambitious given "how resistant practitioners are to withdrawing established treatments from practice even once their utility has been disproved" (p. 273).

Denton et al. (2002) believe that most of the therapies used to treat depression, among other conditions, have no empirical evidence to prove their effectiveness. The authors suggest that before we select a treatment approach, we should consult empirically validated research studies that indicate the effectiveness of a particular therapeutic approach with a particular individual. The authors describe EBP as the use of treatments with some evidence of effectiveness. They note that EBP requires a complete literature search, the use of formal rules of proof in evaluating the relevant literature, and evidence that the selection of a practice approach is effective with a particular population.

In describing the ease with which EBP can be used, Bailes (2002) writes, "Evidence-based practice is not beyond your capability, even if you do not engage in research. You do not have to perform research; you can read the results of published studies [including] clinical research studies, meta-analyses, and systematic reviews" (p. 1). Bailes also indicates that the Internet permits access to various databases that allow searches to be done quickly and efficiently.

In clarifying the types of data EBP looks for in its attempt to find best practices, Sackett et al. (1996) write, "Evidence based practice . . . involves tracking down the best external evidence with which to answer our clinical questions" (p. 72). The authors note that non-experimental approaches should be avoided because they often result in positive conclusions about treatment efficacy that are false. If randomized trials have not been done, "we must follow the trail to the next best external evidence and work from there" (Sackett et al., 1996, p. 72)

The Council for Training in Evidence-Based Behavioral Practice (2007, pp. 3–4)) notes that EBP requires the following competencies:

1. *Asking questions*: Evidence-based practitioners formulate practical, answerable questions that help in assessment, intervention, prognosis, and evaluation of potential harm to clients, and cost-effectiveness and understand the type of evidence needed to answer each kind of question.
2. *Acquisition of evidence*: Practitioners effectively and efficiently search for the best available evidence to answer their practical questions. They know how to devise a research plan, use systematic reviews, and understand best sources of information.
3. *Critical appraisal*: Evidence-based practitioners critically evaluate best evidence for validity and for applicability to their patient/client, or community. This requires understanding the strengths and weaknesses of different types of evidence and the applicability of evidence to a particular client or client system.
4. *Decision-making and action*: As a collaborative effort, evidence-based practitioners develop action plans that integrate research evidence that take into consideration the client's uniqueness. With the client they engage in a process of decision-making about treatment decisions that realistically evaluates the research evidence and its potential to help the client.
5. Evaluation and dissemination: Evidence-based practitioners continually assess their work with clients, make changes when necessary, share their findings with other professionals and continue an ongoing process of refining their work to meet the highest possible standards of best evidence.

2.3. CONCERNS ABOUT EVIDENCE-BASED PRACTICE FROM THE PRACTICE COMMUNITY

There are a number of concerns about EBP. One major concern is that it is a paradigm that was originally developed in medicine. Psychotherapy is a good deal less precise than medicine and cannot be open to the same scrutiny or the same standards as medicine because it is often a fairly subjective practice. Another concern is that EBP seems to ignore the importance of practice wisdom and the countless years of experience of effective and dedicated practitioners. Many clinicians believe that researchers do not easily evaluate what we do in practice and attempts to determine effectiveness usually result in inconclusive findings. Psychotherapy effectiveness seems to relate to experience, according to Bergin (1971), and lumping inexperienced workers with experienced workers in a research study often results in inconclusive and misleading findings.

Witkin and Harrison (2001) offer another concern about EBP and the problems encountered in reviewing clinical research:

> *Small alterations in the definitions of problems or "interventions" can lead to changes in what is considered best practice. A review of readily accessible online reports of EBP or evidence-based medicine studies (see, for example,*

> *Research Triangle Institute, 2000) shows that various types of "psychosocial" treatments are sometimes aggregated across studies (p. 293).*

The authors suggest that finding the strongest evidence for a particular intervention may require a great deal of research sophistication at a level many clinicians do not posses and may never be interested in possessing. The authors worry that "best evidence" may deny the fact that therapy is a joint effort, and while the therapist may have a certain treatment in mind that shows research promise, it may not be acceptable to the client. They ask, "But what if practice is viewed as a mutual activity in which what is best (not necessarily effective) is co-generated by clients and practitioners? What is the relative value of different sources and types of evidence in this scenario?" (Witkin and Harrison, 2000, p. 295).

In one of the more large-scale evaluations of the effectiveness of psychotherapy, Seligman (1995) found that most clients are well satisfied with the help they receive. Although Seligman found no difference in client satisfaction between short-and long-term treatment one cannot deny that clients remain in treatment because of a need for ongoing support and encouragement. These two factors are not easy to reconcile with scientific notions of treatment effectiveness. Psychotherapy, unlike medicine, does not often result in a cure. Clients may have prolonged periods of relief followed by a return of symptoms and the need for additional treatment. Using that description of psychotherapy, however, few could deny that medical care also results in relief of symptoms followed by the need for additional treatment. Finally, clinicians are trained in a subjective form of help we incorrectly call treatment. It really is not treatment, which implies a medical process, but a more didactic exercise in which two people focus on the client's hurts and try to provide relief. It is, necessarily, a softhearted and empathic approach to healing that exists outside of an objective framework. Findings in empirical studies of effectiveness are, therefore, likely to indicate vague and undramatic results.

Among the suggested benefits of EBP are practice guidelines that describe best practice with certain types of emotional problems. Commenting on the use of evidence-based guidelines for practice, Parry and Richardson (2000) believe that clinicians are often uncertain of their effectiveness because they believe the research underlying practice recommendations often incorrectly generalize findings from a specific population of clients to all clients. The authors believe that clinicians reject "the medical metaphor that psychotherapies can be 'prescribed' in any 'dosage' in response to a 'diagnosis'. There is also a strong belief amongst psychotherapy practitioners that clinical judgments cannot be reduced to algorithmic procedures" (p. 280).

Barker (2001) wonders if practitioners use best evidence in the form of manuals or standardized protocols, and says that the answer is, "rarely, if ever. Rather, the successful therapist tailors therapy to suit the individual needs of the person, or the contextual factors" (p. 22). He defines tailoring therapy as meeting the needs of "often changing characteristics of clients" (p. 22), a description of therapy that makes effectiveness research improbable. Baker goes on to say:

> *The practice of psychotherapy is increasingly compromised by the pressures of economic rationalism and the demands for evidence-based practice. The diversity, which has characterized psychotherapy practice to date, risks being compromised by the narrow bandwidth of therapies which are deemed to fulfill the 'gold standard' validation criteria of the randomized controlled trials. (p. 11)*

Chambless and Ollendick (2001) confirm that attempts to use EBP in manuals and in other disseminated ways often meet with rejection by practitioners for the following reasons:

1. Concerns about effectiveness studies suggest that non-empirically-based research may be rejected as unscientific, but "[n]o matter how large or consistent the body of evidence found for identified empirically supported treatments (ESTs), findings will be dismissed as irrelevant by those with fundamentally different views, and such views characterize a number of practitioners and theorists in the psychotherapy area" (Chambless and Ollendick, 2001, p. 699).
2. Presenting evidence-based information about treatment effectiveness can be problematic since it is difficult to design a manual or report that meets the specific needs of all therapists. Therapists are often unlikely to use such reports or manuals even when provided.
3. ESTs are effective in clinical settings and with a diverse group of clients; however, the studies found to support evidence-based treatment were high in external validity but low on internal validity. Consequently, while the authors found no compelling evidence why ESTs could not be used in agencies by trained clinicians, more research on their use was suggested.
4. Economic problems facing many social agencies suggest that manuals prescribing treatments for specific social and emotional problems will be more of an issue as the economy softens and services for social and emotional problems are curtailed. The authors write: "Whatever the reluctance of some to embrace ESTs, we expect that the economic and societal pressures on practitioners for accountability will encourage continued attention to these treatments" (Chambless and Ollendick, 2001, p. 700).

In discussing the effectiveness of psychotherapy, Kopta et al. (1999) raise the issue of whether research evidence even exists to support the use of EBP in practice, and note that researchers have been unable to find evidence of the superiority of one type of treatment over another. The researchers also worry that the belief system of the researcher, as Robinson et al. (1990) discovered, actually influences the outcomes of effectiveness studies.

Witkin and Harrison (2001) discuss social work and EBP. They conclude that what social workers do may not be open to the same level or type of evaluation as medicine. Social workers act as cultural bridges between systems, individualize the client and his or her problem in ways that may defy classification, and work with oppressed people so that what we do may not fit neatly into organized theories of practice. In response to the use of EBP, the authors write:

> *Sometimes this involves using the logic of EBP with clients when there is credible evidence of some relevant knowledge available. Other times, however,*

> *the most important work is in educating decision makers or those who have control of resources about how irrelevant the best scientific evidence is to the world of people whose experiences brought them into contact with the professionals. (Witkin and Harrison, 2001, p. 295)*

Witkin and Harrison (2001) raise the issue of whether the helping professions should be placed in the same precarious position as medicine when it relates to issues of managed care and write, "Is it a coincidence that EBP is favored by managed care providers pushing practice toward an emphasis on specificity in problem identification and rapid responses to the identified conditions?" (p. 246). The AMA (EBP Working Group, 1992) reinforces this concern when it states that "Economic constraints and counter-productive incentives may compete with the dictates of evidence as determinants of clinical decisions. The relevant literature may not be readily accessible. Time may be insufficient to carefully review the evidence (which may be voluminous) relevant to a pressing clinical problem" (p. 2423).

2.4. RESPONSES TO CRITICISMS OF EVIDENCE-BASED PRACTICE

In response to concerns that managed care may use EBP to lower costs, Sackett et al. (1996) write, "Some fear that evidence based medicine will be hijacked by purchasers and managers to cut the costs of health care. Doctors practicing evidence based medicine will identify and apply the most efficacious interventions to maximize the quality and quantity of life for individual patients; this may raise rather than lower the cost of their care" (p. 71). An editorial in *Mental Health Weekly* (2001) challenges the idea that EBP is being pushed by the health care crisis. The editorial argues that,

> *Tight budgets make adoption of best practices difficult. Their implementation often requires a restructuring of existing services. And once a best practice is implemented, fidelity to its key elements is critical to success. However, methods of ensuring fidelity in real practice settings remain unproven. (2001, Internet).*

The American Medical Association Working Group on Evidence Based Practice (1992) identifies three misinterpretations about EBP that create barriers to its use, and then responds to those misinterpretations in the following statements:

1. *Evidence-based practice ignores clinical experience and clinical intuition.*

> *On the contrary, it is important to expose learners to exceptional clinicians who have a gift for intuitive diagnosis, a talent for precise observation, and excellent judgment in making difficult management decisions. Untested signs and symptoms should not be rejected out of hand. They may prove extremely useful, and ultimately be proved valid through rigorous*

> *testing. The more experienced clinicians can dissect the process they use in diagnosis, and clearly present it to learners, the greater the benefit (p. 2423).*

2. *Understanding of basic investigation and pathology plays no part in evidence-based medicine.*

> *The dearth of adequate evidence demands that clinical problem-solving must rely on an understanding of underlying pathology. Moreover, a good understanding of pathology is necessary for interpreting clinical observations and for appropriate interpretation of evidence (especially in deciding on its generalizability) (p. 2423).*

3. *Evidence-based practice ignores standard aspects of clinical training such history taking.*

> *A careful history and physical examination provides much, and often the best, evidence for diagnosis and directs treatment decisions. The clinical teacher of evidence-based medicine must give considerable attention to teaching the methods of history and diagnosis, with particular attention to which items have demonstrated validity and to strategies, which enhance observer agreement (p. 2423).*

In a review of the most effective practices in psychotherapy, Chambless (2001) notes that one argument used against EBP is that there is no difference in the effectiveness of various forms of psychotherapy and that identifying best practices is therefore unnecessary. However, Chambless found considerable evidence that in the treatment of anxiety disorders and childhood depression, cognitive and behavioral methods were fairly clearly defined and that positive results often resulted from the treatment.

The British Medical Association raises other issues with EBP in an editorial appearing in the July 1998 *British Medical Journal*. The editorial calls into question the implied ease with which good evidence is available in medicine and by implication, whether it is readily available to the helping professional. The editorial notes that most published research in medical journals is too poorly done or not relevant enough to be useful to physicians. In surveys, more than 95% of the published articles in medical journals did not achieve minimum standards of quality or relevance. Clinical practice guidelines are slow to produce, costly, have poor quality, and are difficult to update (p. 6).

By way of response, Strauss and Sackett (1998) report that EBP has been quite successful in general medical and psychiatric settings and that practitioners read the research accurately and make correct decisions. They write, "A general medicine service at a district general hospital affiliated with a university found that 53% of patients admitted to the service received primary treatments that had been validated in randomized controlled trials" (p. 341). The authors also note that three-quarters of the evidence used in the treatment of clients was immediately available through empirically evaluated topic summaries, and the remaining quarter was "identified and applied by asking answerable questions at the time of admission, rapidly finding good evidence, quickly determining its validity and usefulness, swiftly integrating it with clinical expertise and each patient's unique features, and offering it to the patients" (p. 341). Similar results, according to Strauss and Sackett (1998), have been found in studies of a psychiatric hospital (p. 341).

2.5. WHY PRACTITIONERS SOMETIMES RESIST THE USE OF EBP

The following discussion is from Dr. Suzanne Bushfield, Arizona State University West Dept of Social Work, in a personal correspondence (September 25, 2007).

> *Recent developments in Evidence Based Practice (EBP) suggest the need to combine the best "clinical practice" skills used in engaging and assessing the person in his/her situation, and then apply the best evidence-based interventions. In the absence of evidence regarding the specific aspects of the individual client in his/her situation, what should the practitioner do? Too often, we do what we like or what we are used to doing. We use "clinical wisdom" or "trial and error."*
>
> *The discussion on EBP digs at our roots. Flexner raised the question, "are we really professionals?" Despite nearly a century of development of the social work profession, the core arguments remain: do we have empirical evidence as the basis of our work? Other questions include: is practice wisdom evidence? Whose knowledge do we value? Are there other ways of knowing? Has evidence caught up with the reality of our encounters within a rapidly changing environment?*
>
> *Even when one embraces the need for evidence, it seems that empiricism, attempting to clean up the messiness of subjectivity, has it own messiness. How was data obtained, and from whom? Under what circumstances? What about missing data, and do techniques to handle this merely reinforce the status quo, including stereotypes?*
>
> *Some argue that evidence, even when it has its merits, is missing the nuances discovered in an N of 1. While we can easily agree that the snapshot does not capture reality, it is less obvious that videos, attempting to more accurately capture reality, still carry the influence of the videographer's eye. Even more problematic, when we are aware that the camera is running, we may show a different side of ourselves.*
>
> *So how should practitioners greet EBP? With healthy skepticism, and with a willingness to participate in the building of evidence from the ground up. In social work, we are compelled to know both the general and the unique.*

Since little evidence addresses the multiple aspects of person and environment, the multiple dimensions of time – both life course and life events – and little evidence makes sufficient accounting for both the researcher and the setting, as well as the meaning of the research to its participants, I for one, will offer a different kind of skepticism: not the rejection of evidence, but rather the closer scrutiny of the latest and best evidence for its broader and relevant application to the most vulnerable.

There is still strong evidence that clients prefer the caring relationship, time spent, and provision of hope: engagement and caring presence. To the extent that the latest evidence reflects the influence of these variables on client outcomes, I stand ready to embrace it. Even the best evidence based interventions may depend on the ability to engage the client in the intervention. However, engagement and caring may be insufficient, without effective approaches beyond engagement. So, perhaps we need to think of a "both/and" approach. I would like to communicate both that I want to help, that I believe that help is helpful, and that there is evidence that my ways of helping have a great likelihood of working. Are interventions effective in the absence of relationship? Does the evidence suggest that workers are interchangeable widgets which, when performing the appropriate function, can create effective outcomes? I think not. What is needed is more focus on engaging the client in evaluating the evidence for its application to the client's situation. Strengths and empowerment, sometimes missing in the rush toward evidence, are powerful tools. Further, as an ethical practitioner, I want to have sufficient evidence that what I am doing will work, and therefore am compelled to be a critical consumer of new evidence – and refuse to be "left out" of the discussion. This requires me to understand research and statistical analysis, and to search out the best that evidence has to offer.

2.6. IS EVIDENCE-BASED PRACTICE APPLICABLE TO THE HUMAN SERVICES?

Reynolds and Richardson (2000) argue that despite concerns among clinicians that EBP may impede their freedom, new opportunities in practice research suggest that clinician freedom will be enhanced because more options will be available as creative research methodologies suggest new forms of treatment. As new research opportunities develop, the profile of psychotherapy will rise. And while EBP has been called "cookbook practice" and a "new type of authority" that threatens the autonomy of professionals, the possibility exists that research in psychotherapy effectiveness will have the same positive effect that medical research has had on the practice of medicine. In discussing the benefits of practice guidelines, Parry and Richardson (2000) believe that well-done practice guidelines will help clinicians crystallize their thinking about treatment. Published guidelines will also give clients more information, and consequently give them additional power to decide on their own treatment. High quality guidelines help in training new professionals and influence the writing of textbooks that must increasingly contain evidence of best practices. Parry and Richardson (2000, p. 279) provide the following examples of well-done guidelines for professional practice:

1. The American Psychiatric Association has published practice guidelines for eating disorders (APA, 1993a) and for major depressive disorder in adults (APA, 1993b).
2. The Australian and New Zealand College of Psychiatrists ran a quality assurance project which has produced several treatment outlines; for agoraphobia (Quality Assurance Project, 1982a), depressive disorders (1982b), for borderline, narcissistic and histrionic personality disorders (1991b) and for antisocial personality disorders (1991a).
3. The U.S. Agency for Health Care Policy and Research has been influential. For example, their depression in primary care guideline (Agency for Health Care Policy and Research, 1993a, 1993b) was widely discussed (Persons et al., 1996; Munoz et al., 1994). More recently, Schulberg et al. (1998) reviewed research published between 1992 and 1998 to update this guideline.
4. Other guidelines worth exploring include those on the treatment of bipolar disorder (Frances et al., 1996), choice of antidepressants in primary care (North of England Evidence Based Guideline Development Project, 1997) and treatment of obsessive-compulsive disorder (March et al., 1997).

Whether we want to admit it or not, we are in the midst of a health care crisis in America. While it is easy enough to blame managed care for the part of the crisis that relates to the helping professions, we are largely to blame. As Witkin and Harrison (2000) and others have repeatedly noted, the human services professions have not embraced the concept of best practices or the need to function from a knowledge-guided frame of reference. The result is a growing suspicion among health care analysts and providers that what we do is expendable. And as Peebles (2000) writes, "In North America, policymakers have been taking an interest in the scientific evidence underlying the practice of clinical psychology. Demands for accountability have been mounting from both government agencies and managed care companies (Barlow, 1996; Parloff & Elkin, 1992)" (p. 660). When therapy was offered in private or non-profit settings, its effectiveness was of little concern to policy makers. With the advent of huge public sector expenditures for therapeutic services, "the public gained a right and a responsibility to determine who is entitled to receive services, what conditions warrant treatment, and what treatments will be authorized (Parloff, 1979)" (Peebles, 2000, p. 559). This need for accountability, in light of the large cost for therapeutic services, has been growing and mental health providers are "scrambling," in Peebles words, to prove the need and worth of our services to policy makers and to a skeptical public.

Professionals have a body of knowledge that should be based, not on practice wisdom or practice experience, but on the evidence that we are collecting empirical data that supports our interventions. Without such a body of knowledge, we begin to lose our status as professionals and the future of psychotherapy in the United States seems clear: less therapy provided, irrespective of client need; therapy provided by the least highly-trained worker with heavy reliance on self-help groups; psycho-educational materials in the form of reading for clients in lieu of therapy; and the hope that clients will be resilient and wise enough to get better, essentially, by themselves.

2.7. SUMMARY

This chapter discusses the definitions of EBP and some of the criticisms of the approach found in the literature. Among the strongest criticism of EBP is that we fail to have a well-defined literature at present and what we do have is difficult to read and comprehend, and too time-consuming for most practitioners. There is evidence that clinicians do not use manuals that contain best evidence. On the positive side, there is a need to organize best practices and to assure clients and third-party providers that what we do actually works. EBP is an approach that tries to organize a way of providing the best possible service to clients using a knowledge-guided approach to practice and substantial involvement of clients in decision-making to assure that the client-worker relationship is cooperative.

2.8. QUESTIONS FROM THE CHAPTER

1. Do you think it is possible to organize best practice in ways that capture the individual nature of the client? Is not this the problem with EBP, that it cannot individualize what is actually best for a specific client and his or her needs?
2. Why do you think training manuals are so unpopular with clinicians?
3. There is evidence in this chapter that we do not have enough conclusive data accumulated to indicate best evidence with most client problems. Does not this suggest that EBP cannot function adequately until we have considerably more research evidence?
4. EBP originated in medicine. Do you think that medicine and therapy are similar enough to utilize an approach developed for medical practice?
5. Because therapy requires a more highly involved participation by the client than medicine, do you accept Gambrill's criticism that we make statements in the helping professions about what we do and its effectiveness, which are unsupported by the data and create false impressions?

References

Agency for Health Care Policy and Research. (1993a). *Depression in primary care: Detection and diagnosis*. Washington, DC: U.S. Department of Health and Human Services.

Agency for Health Care Policy and Research. (1993b). *Depression in primary care: Treatment of major depression*. Washington, DC: U.S. Department of Health & Human Services.

American Medical Association Working Group on Evidence Based Practice. (1992, November). Evidence-Based Medicine: A New Approach to Teaching the Practice of Medicine. *Journal of the American Medical Association, 4, 268*(17), 2420–2425.

American Psychiatric Association. (1993a). Practice guideline for eating disorders. *American Journal of Psychiatry, 150*, 207–228.

American Psychiatric Association. (1993b). Practice guideline for major depressive disorder in adults. *American Journal of Psychiatry Supplement, 150*(4, Suppl.).

Bailes, B. K. (2002, June). Evidence-based practice guidelines – one way to enhance clinical practice. *AORN Journal* .

Barker, P. (2001). The ripples of knowledge and the boundaries of practice: The problem of evidence in psychotherapy research. *International Journal of Psychotherapy, 6*(1), 11–24.

Barlow, D. H. (1996). Health care policy, psychotherapy research, and the future of psychotherapy.. *American Psychologist, 51*, 1007–1016.

Bergin, A. E. (1971). The evaluation of therapeutic outcomes. In A. E. Bergin, S. & Garfield (Eds.), *Handbook of psychotherapy and behavior change*. New York: John Wiley and Sons, 217-170.

Bushfield, S. (2007, September 25). Arizona State University West Dept. of Social Work, in a personal correspondence.

Chambless, D. L. (2001). Empirically supported psychological interventions: Controversies and evidence. *Annual Review of Psychology*, Chambless http://www.findarticles.com/cf_0/m0961/2001_Annual/73232726/print.html.

Chambless, D. L., & Ollendick, T. H. (2001). Empirically supported psychological interventions: Controversies and evidence. *Annual Review of Psychology, 52*, 685–716.

Dawes, R. M. (1994). *House of cards: Psychology and psychotherapy built on myth*. New York: Free Press.

Denton, W. H., Walsh, S. R., & Daniel, S. S. (2002). Evidence-based practice in family therapy: Adolescent depression as an example. *Journal of Marital and Family Therapy, 28*(1), 39–45.

Enkin, M., Keirse, M. J. N., Renfrew, M., & Neilson, J. (1995). *A guide to effective care in pregnancy and childbirth* (2nd ed.). New York: Oxford University Press.

Editorial. (1998, July 4). Getting evidence into practice. *British Medical Journal, 317*, 6.

Editorial. (2001, August 20). Project to bring evidence-based treatment into real world. *Mental Health Weekly*. http://www.findarticles.com/cf_0/m0BSC/32_11/77610655/print.jhtml.

Evidence-Based Medicine Working Group. (1992). Evidence-based medicine: A new approach to teaching the practice of medicine. *Journal of the American Medical Association, 268*, 2420–2425.

Flaherty, R. J. (2001, September 15). Medical myths: Today's perspectives. *PatientCare*. http://www.findarticles.com/cf_0/m3233/17_35/78547389/print.jhtml.

Frances, A., Docherty, J. P., & Kahn, D. A. (1996). Treatment of bipolar disorder. *The Journal of Clinical Psychiatry, 57*(12a, Suppl.).

Gambrill, E. (2000, October). *Evidence-based practice. A handout to the dean and directors of schools of social work*, Huntington, Beach, CA.

Gambrill, E. (1999). Evidence-based practice: An alternative to authority-based practice. *Journal of Contemporary Human Services, 80*(4), 341–350.

Glicken, M. D. (2005). *Improving the effectiveness of the helping professions: An evidence-based practice approach to treatment*. Thousand Oaks, CA: Sage.

Haynes, B. (1998, July 25). Barriers and bridges to evidence based clinical practice. (Getting Research Findings into Practice, part 4.). *British Medical Journal, 317*, 273–276.

Hines, S. E. (2000, February 29). Enhance your practice with evidence-based medicine. *Patient Care* .

Howard, M. O., & Jenson, J. M. (1999). Clinical practice guidelines: Should social work develop them?. *Research on Social Work Practice, 9*(3), 283–301.

Isaacs, D. (1999, December 18). Seven alternatives to evidence based medicine. *British Medical Journal* .

Kopta, M. S., Lueger, R. J., Saunders, S. M., & Howard, K. I. (1999, Annual). Individual psychotherapy outcome and process research: Challenges leading to greater turmoil or a positive transition?. *Annual Review of Psychology*. http://www.findarticles.com/cf_0/m0961/1999_Annual/54442307/print.jhtml.

March, J. S., Frances, A., Carpenter, D., & Kahn, D. A. (Eds.) (1997). Treatment of Obsessive-Compulsive Disorder. *The Expert Consensus Guideline Series.*

Munoz, R., Hollon, S., McGrath, E., Rehm, L., & VandenBos, G. (1994). On the AHCPR guidelines: Further considerations for practitioners. *American Psychologist, 49*, 42–61.

North of England Evidence Based Guideline Development Project. (1997). *Evidence based clinical practice guideline: the choice of antidepressants for depression in primary care*. Newcastle upon Tyne: Centre for Health Services Research.

O'Donnell, M. (1997). *A skeptic's medical dictionary*. London: BMJ Books.

Parry, G., & Richardson, P. (2000). Developing treatment choice guidelines in psychotherapy. *Journal of Mental Health, 9*(3), 273–282.

Parloff, M. B., & Elkin, I. (1992). The NIMH Treatment of Depression Collaborative Research Program. In D. K. & Freedheim (Ed.), *History of psychotherapy: A century of change* (pp. 442–450). Washington, DC: American Psychological Association.

Parloff, M. B. (1979). Can psychotherapy research guide the policymaker? A little knowledge may be a dangerous thing. *American Psychologist, 34*, 296–306.

Peebles, J. (2000, November). The future of psychotherapy outcome research: Science or political rhetoric?. *Journal of Psychology, 134*(6), 659–670.

Persons, J. B., Thase, M. E., & Crits-Christoph, P. (1996). The role of psychotherapy in the treatment of depression: review of two practice guidelines. *Archives of General Psychiatry, 53*, 283–290.

Quality Assurance Project. (1982a). A treatment outline for agoraphobia. *Australian and New Zealand Journal of Psychiatry, 16*, 25–33.

Quality Assurance Project. (1982b). A treatment outline for depressive disorders. *Australian and New Zealand Journal of Psychiatry, 17*, 129–148.

Quality Assurance Project. (1991a). Treatment outlines for antisocial personality disorders. *Australian and New Zealand Journal of Psychiatry, 25*, 541–547.

Quality Assurance Project. (1991b). Treatment outlines for borderline, narcissistic and histrionic personality disorders. *Australian and New Zealand Journal of Psychiatry, 25*, 392–403.

Research Triangle Institute. (2000). *Assessing "best evidence": Grading the quality of articles and rating the strength of evidence [Online]*. Available: www.rti.org/epc/grading-article.html.

Reynolds, R., & Richardson, P. (2000). Evidence based practice and psychotherapy research. *Journal of Mental Health, 9*(3), 257–267.

Robinson, L. A., Berman, J. S., & Neimeyer, R. A. (1990). Psychotherapy for the treatment of depression: a comprehensive review of controlled outcome research. *Psychological Bulletin, 108*, 30–49.

Rosen, A. (1994). Knowledge use in direct practice. *Social Service Review, 68*, 561–577.

Sackett, D. L., Rosenberg, W. M. C., Muir-Gray, J. A., Haynes, R. B., & Richardson, W. S. (1996, January 13). Evidence based medicine: what it is and what it isn't. *British Medical Journal, 312*, 71–72. http://bmj.com/cgi/content/full/312/7023/71?ijkey=JflK2VHyVI2F6.

Sackett, D. L., Richardson, W. S., Rosenberg, W., & Haynes, R. B. (1997). *Evidence-based medicine: How to practice and teach EMB*. New York: Churchill Livingstone.

Schulberg, H. C., Katon, W., Simon, G. E., & Rush, A. J. (1998). Treating major depression in primary care practice: an update of the Agency for Health Care Policy and Research Practice Guidelines. *Archives of General Psychiatry, 55*, 1121–1127.

Seligman, M. E. P. (1995). The effectiveness of psychotherapy: the consumers report study. *American Psychologist, 50*(12), 965–974.

Strauss, S. E., & Sackett, D. L. (1998, August 1). Using research findings in clinical practice. *British Medical Journal, 317*, 339–342. http://bmj.com/cgi/content/full/317/7154/339.

Timmermans, S., & Angell, A. (2001). Evidence-based medicine, clinical uncertainty, and learning to doctor. *Journal of Health & Social Behavior, 42*(4), 342.

Users' Guides to Evidence-based Medicine. (1992, November) Evidence-Based Medicine: A New Approach to Teaching the Practice of Medicine. *Journal of the American Medical Association, 4, 268*(17), 2420–2425.

Witkin, S. L., & Harrison, W. D. (2001, October). Editorial: Whose evidence and for what purpose?. *Social Work, 46*(4), 293–296.

Further reading

National Association of Social Work Board of Directors. (1999, January). Proposed public policies of NASW. *NASW News, 44*(3), 12–17.

Robinson, L. A., Berman, J. S., & Neimeyer, R. A. (1990). Psychotherapy for the treatment of depression: a comprehensive review of controlled outcome research. *Psychological Bulletin*, *108*, 30–49.
Rosen, A. (1994). Knowledge use in direct practice. *Social Service Review*, *68*, 561–577.
Sackett, D. L., Rosenberg, W. M. C., Muir Gray, J. A., Haynes, R. B., & Richardson, W. S. (1996, January 13). Evidence based medicine: what it is and what it isn't. *British Medical Journal*, *312*, 71–72. http://bmj.com/cgi/content/full/312/7023/71
Sackett, D. L., Richardson, W. S., Rosenberg, W., & Haynes, R. B. (1997). *Evidence-based medicine: How to practice and teach EBM*. New York: Churchill Livingstone.
Schulberg, H. C., Katon, W., Simon, G. E., & Rush, A. J. (1998). Treating major depression in primary care practice: an update of the Agency for Health Care Policy and Research Practice Guidelines. *Archives of General Psychiatry*, *55*, 1121–1127.
Seligman, M. E. P. (1995). The effectiveness of psychotherapy: the consumer reports study. *American Psychologist*, *50*(12), 965–974.
Straus, S. E., & Sackett, D. L. (1998, August 1). Using research findings in clinical practice. *British Medical Journal*, *317*, 339–342. http://bmj.com/cgi/content/full/317/7155/339
Timmermans, S., & Angell, A. (2001). Evidence-based medicine, clinical uncertainty, and learning to doctor. *Journal of Health and Social Behavior*, *42*, 342–359.
Users' Guide to Evidence-Based Medicine. (1992, November 4). Evidence-Based Medicine: A New Approach to Teaching the Practice of Medicine. *Journal of the American Medical Association*, *268*(17), 2420–2425.
Witkin, S. L., & Harrison, W. D. (2001, October). Editorial: Whose evidence and for what purpose? *Social Work*, *46*(4), 293–296.

Further reading

National Association of Social Work Board of Directors. (1999, January). Proposed public policies of NASW. *NASW News*, *44*(1), 12–17.

3 The Importance of Critical Thinking in Evidenced-Based Practice

3.1. INTRODUCTION

The author wishes to thank Sage Publications for permission to use material from the author's book on evidence-based practice (Glicken, 2005, pp. 39–54).

One of the hallmarks of evidence-based practice (EBP) is its focus on critical thinking. Astleitner (2002) defines critical thinking as "a higher-order thinking skill, which mainly consists of evaluating arguments. It is a purposeful, self-regulatory judgment which results in interpretation, analysis, evaluation and inference, as well as explanations of the evidential, conceptual, methodological, or contextual considerations upon which the judgment is based" (p. 53). In discussing what she calls, "ways of knowing," Gambrill (1999), suggests that "[d]ifferent ways of knowing differ in the extent to which they highlight uncertainty and are designed to weed out biases and distortions that may influence assumptions" (p. 341).

This chapter presents several different ways of knowing that will help the reader understand critical arguments concerning clinical research which will hopefully help in distinguishing how much we can rely on the findings of a given research study. The consumer of research should know the researcher's philosophy of science as part of the evaluation of any study. Throughout this chapter, the opposing points of view of a number of authors are provided as they discuss the limitations and counter-limitations of the various ways of gathering and viewing knowledge. Many helping professionals believe that much of what we do is not open to the scientific method and argue that our work is not quantifiable because of its complexity. Other authors believe that research methodologies which are overly controlling severely limit inquiry and are responsible for the lack of practice research, while some authors call this point of view "pseudo-science," and say that this type of thinking is responsible for the lack of empirical research in the field. A discussion of several well-accepted beliefs in the helping professions will be challenged so that the use of critical thinking might be better understood. A progression of logical questions about a research article will also be offered to show the practical use of critical thinking in evaluating best evidence. The author is indebted to Gambrill (1999) for her work on critical thinking.

3.2. WAYS OF KNOWING

3.2.1. *Theory Building Through Observation*

The use of observation as an approach to gathering knowledge is also called "logical positivism" and suggests that all we need to know about a research issue can be learned through observation. It is a theory-free approach since observation precedes theory. A way of understanding logical positivism in psychotherapy is the belief that by working with a client over time, we can understand the client's behavior and then construct treatment interventions as our theory of the client evolves. This approach to problem solving, while it sometimes results in breakthroughs of a major order (for example, Freud's work), has many problems, not least of which is the objectivity of the observer. The inductive approach it utilizes can be highly subjective, illogical, and inaccurate (Freud's work might also be a good example).

3.2.2. *Post-Modernism*

Post-modernism, also know as relativism and post-positivism, asserts that all forms of inquiry are equally valid. In showing the subjective nature of the relativist approach to inquiry, Gellner (1992) writes, "Those who propound it or defend it against its critics, continue, whenever facing any serious issue in which their real interests are engaged, to act on the non-relativistic assumption that one particular vision is cognitively much more effective than others" (p. 70). However, as a reaction against the tightly controlled methodologies of the scientific method, Tyson (1992) believes that a significant occurrence in the applied social sciences is the "shift away from an outdated, unwarranted and overly restrictive approach to scientific social research which has long been unsatisfying to practitioners" (1992, p. 541).

Gambrill (1999), however, sees a contradiction in the way many practitioners live their lives and how the use of post-modernism affects their practices. She compares what social workers want from their personal physicians (an evidence- and knowledge-guided approach to their medical problem, which is based on best evidence from tightly controlled research studies) to what social workers want from their clients. Social workers feel comfortable using intuition, practice wisdom, folk lore, mythology, and an occasionally a badly done piece of research which validates their belief system.

Glicken (2003) describes post-modernism as a way of thinking which concerns itself with social problems that have developed in society as a result of the belief that there are rational explanations for most issues facing mankind. Post-modernism comes from a core belief that the attempt to be rational often passively accepts gender bias, discrimination, inequitable distribution of wealth, war, poverty, conflicts among peoples, and a range of problems confronting us as a people. In many ways, post-modernism is a reaction against a world that still cannot control its more primitive instincts and stems from the disillusionment of many people after the Vietnam War. Post-modernism believes that many current explanations of human behavior are incorrect and that the goal of all intellectual inquiry is to seek alternative explanations without the methodological limitations of empiricism. Those alternative explanations might include the importance of spirituality, the significance of intuition, the relevance of non-Western approaches to health, and any number of alternative views of the universe. For the post-modernist researcher, the purpose of research is to explore the world in a way that permits maximum flexibility in the use of research methodologies. In a sense, post-modernist researchers are atheoretical and value the flexibility of using a range of research methodologies to seek alternative ways of viewing the world. They believe empiricism limits more creative and intuitive approaches and discounts common experiences, observations and insights that may not be supported by objective evaluations but may, nonetheless, be true, and may add to our knowledge base.

Gambrill (1999) worries that this free-wheeling approach to research hides a more fundamental problem. Claims made by therapists that cannot be supported by hard evidence become claims supported by weak and limited research efforts that, over time, create a body of knowledge with a transparent lack of evidence. That body of knowledge is what Gambrill calls a pseudoscience, so prevalent in the human service literature because it looks like science but lacks its structure, methodology, and controls. Tanguay (2002) supports this point of view and writes:

> *No matter how reassuring, no matter how exciting the finding, no matter what hope it holds out to clients, the results of anecdotal studies, single subject trials, nonrandomized designs, and non-controlled investigations must be looked on with skepticism. Such studies may be helpful as pilot work but we are deceiving ourselves and our clients if we act on the results until they are proven. This applies to studies with negative as well as positive results. (p. 1323)*

In two opposing articles about the use of the scientific method in psychiatry, Shea (2000) and McLaren (2000) have different thoughts on how well the scientific method can be used in a discipline focusing on the human condition. Shea believes that psychiatry is badly served by the scientific method and notes that, "Any applications of that method to such essential human affairs as love, hate, religion, and the unconscious are bound to fail" (p. 227). In suggesting reasons for the lack of application of the scientific method to psychiatry, Shea argues that the scientific method assumes that everything is quantifiable and can be made rational, but that this is seldom the case in the human services. Many client behaviors defy reason and are certainly not quantifiable. People often think that science is about the use of statistics, but statistics "is for pedestrian science," (p. 228) since it does not suggest bold new theories but just breaks information into minutiae.

On the other hand, McLaren believes that Shea's arguments are spurious and that Shea has created a straw man out of issues that are meant to appeal to emotion rather than to reason. McLaren writes, "Science is mainly about bold and elegant theories which make sense of chaos, and the truly great advances in science have always vaulted far beyond the limited reach of statistics" (McLaren, 2000, p. 374). McLaren goes on to say that in Shea's attempt to vilify the scientific method in psychiatry, he makes the mistake of suggesting that there is only one scientific method when "[t]here are lots of scientific methods, some of which are applicable across a broad range of fields and which, collectively, are directed at stripping prejudice and bias from our exploratory efforts" (p. 373).

3.2.3. The Scientific Method

The scientific method, also known as critical rationalism and positivism, is a way of "thinking about and investigating the accuracy of assumptions about the world. It is a process for solving problems in which we learn from our mistakes" (Gambrill, 1999, p. 342). The scientific method requires statements, findings and conclusions to be tested so they can be accepted or rejected. In describing the scientific method, Munz (1985) says that "knowledge is not acquired by the pursuit of a 'correct' method; rather it is what is left standing when criticism has been exhausted" (p. 72). One of the key elements of the scientific approach is its willingness to critically evaluate and test knowledge and theories. By doing so, we are able to eliminate many of our mistakes and, in the process, advance knowledge.

Wuthnow (2003) writes that the scientific method "involves thinking of ways in which our cherished assumptions about the world may prove to be wrong" (p. 10). Science also involves, "candidly disclosing what we have done so others can track our mistakes" (Wuthnow, 2003, p. 10). In a statement, which not everyone will agree is representative of the scientific method but one of great importance to research on best evidence, Wuthnow goes on to say,

> *But scientific method can equally pertain to studies involving qualitative information drawn from participant observation, interviews, and archival materials. Carefully sifting through letters and diaries in an archive, or through artifacts at an archaeological dig, is ever as much science as computing regression equations or life-expectancy tables. If science is understood in this broader way, then we can identify more clearly some of the challenges in which it may usefully be employed. (p. 10)*

Tanguay (2002), however, calls for a more rigorous methodology and notes that we must be willing to maintain a "rigorous skepticism" concerning our personal beliefs regarding the effectiveness of our treatment and our cherished theories. "Professional ethics should preclude us waffling on the issues of scientific merit. A scientifically inadequate study will lead to unwarranted hope and lost incentives" (Tanguay, 2002, p. 1323). Shea (2000) goes even further and wonders if it's possible for the helping professions to use the scientific method at all. Shea writes, "No amount of wishful thinking about the scientific method is going to alter the fact that, in much of psychiatry, an indispensable element in the therapeutic process is what goes on between the therapist and the patient – the knowledge, understanding, rapport, trust and confidence that builds up over time" (p. 227). According to Shea, this subjective component of the therapeutic relationship is not open to measurement, and even if it were, the results would certainly be spurious. "Some feelings," Shay writes, "cannot be put into words that can communicate the exact nature of the experience let alone into words that can be adopted to either scientific use or logical analysis" (p. 227).

3.2.4. Justification and Falsification

In approaches that use justification, researchers gather support to prove or justify their theories or hypotheses. In approaches that use falsification, researchers try and discover errors in hypotheses or theories. The reader can readily see that falsification approaches require a much more thorough analysis than justification approaches because it takes a much more concentrated effort to disprove something than to prove it. Proving a hypothesis or theory is weighted in the direction of the methodological information the researcher is willing to share with us and is often upheld by the authority the researcher holds in having done the research. Falsification requires no authority other than the logic of the critical analysis of the research methodology.

An example of justification and falsification can be found in a famous article written by Norman Cousins in *New England Journal of Medicine* (1976). Some years ago, the well-known author was hospitalized with what was thought to be severe arthritis. In his article, Cousins contended that hospitals were bad for our health because hospital personnel were often unsupportive, that treatments tended to be uncreative, and that focusing on illness rather than wellness discouraged patients from getting better.

Failing to improve over a course of many days, Cousins convinced his doctor to release him to a hotel room where friends entertained him, many of whom were famous comedians. Cousins also watched comedies because he reasoned that laughter increased oxygen flow, which led to improved health. Gourmet meals were served on the assumption that good food improved the body's ability to heal itself. His doctor continued to see him and large doses of aspirin, the common treatment for arthritis when the article was written, were discontinued and megadoses of vitamin C were substituted. Cousins believed that vitamin C, which was thought to be a curative by such well-known advocates as Nobel Prize-winning physicist Linus Pauling, would help in his recovery.

As a result of these alternative treatments, Cousins reported that his medical condition improved significantly. The *New England Journal of Medicine* (1976, 1977) received over 3000 letters from doctors supporting Cousin's claim that hospitals were terrible places for sick people and to avoid them if possible. No one asked whether Cousins would have gone into spontaneous remission had he stayed in the hospital. Nor did anyone look at his past behavior (Cousins had a prior medical problem that made him deeply cynical about the medical establishment). Finally, no one sought to consider the validity of mega vitamin

C therapy (it has since been rejected and people now worry that large doses of vitamin C may cause kidney damage). The bias against doctors, hospitals, and the treatment of illness is so strong in American society, even among many doctors, that personal convictions caused many health care professionals to accept Cousins' findings without adequate supportive data. To be sure, some good came from the article since many people in the medical professions began to realize that hospitals needed to be more humane. Changes were made in food service, visiting hours were relaxed, consideration of the wishes of the patient regarding treatment improved, but as a piece of research, it was meant to appeal to our emotions and cannot be considered scientific. And more to the point, had Cousins used falsification and given us the many reasons his experiences were idiosyncratic to him and should not be generalized to others, the material would have been more meaningful and truthful. However, this is a good example of justification used by a figure of authority to create the illusion of good science.

3.3. MYTHOLOGIZED KNOWLEDGE

Nickerson (1986) says that knowledge serves to decrease uncertainty and that to make it useable to practitioners, it has to survive tests of its credibility which, in addition to helping us effectively treat client problems, also keeps us from making serious treatment mistakes. A serious problem in the human services is the acceptance of knowledge that is not well documented and has become mythologized through long acceptance without rigorous evaluation or debate. Gambrill (1999) points out the defining characteristics of mythologized knowledge and the ways in which champions of mythologized knowledge maintain an incorrect and even harmful belief system: (1) they discourage scientific examination of claims, arguments, and beliefs; (2) they claim to be scientific but are not; (3) they rely on anecdotal evidence; (4) they are free of skepticism or discourage opposing points of view; (5) they confuse being open with being uncritical; (6) they fail to use falsification as a way of understanding information; (7) the language they use is imprecise; (8) they rely on appeals to faith; and (9) they produce information that is not testable. In the realm of the unscientific, here are a few mythological beliefs we often see in the clinical literature without justifiable support:

1. **Belief:** Having a trained helping professional who has gone through a professional program and is licensed to practice provides more effective help than an untrained and unlicensed professional. **Reality:** As Dawes (1994) reports, there is no relationship between training, licensing, and experience. Empathic non-professionals often provide more effective help than trained professionals (Gambrill, 1999). Consequently, a study using trained and licensed professionals to prove the effectiveness of any form of treatment would be remiss if it did not compare professional help with non-professional help. Consumers of research need to know that other forms of help may be effective, and that alternative approaches, such as self-help groups or informal therapy, may work as well or better than therapy provided by trained professionals. Using

only trained people in a study limits the amount of information we can provide to consumers of research and may suggest unwarranted findings that confuse us.

2. **Belief:** The longer a client is in the therapy, the more likely important life questions will be uncovered which lead to enhanced social functioning. **Reality:** there is no relationship between length of treatment and better social functioning. In fact, Seligman (1995) found that clients with 6 months of therapy were doing as well, on self-reports, as clients with 2 years of therapy. This statement is also used to suggest that longer therapy is more in-depth, but actually, there is no evidence that this is true or that in-depth therapy is more effective than more superficial forms of therapy.
3. **Belief:** Early forms of trauma inevitably lead to problems later in life. This is one of the foundations of modern psychotherapy, and it may be true of some people, but is it true of everyone? **Reality:** research on resilience in traumatized children and adults challenges three commonly-held beliefs about human development: (1) there are universal stages of development; (2) childhood trauma inevitably leads to adult psychopathology (Benard, 1994; Garmezy, 1994); and (3) there are social and economic conditions, relationships, and institutional dysfunctions that are so problematic that they inevitably lead to problems in the social and emotional functioning of children, adults, families, and communities (Rutter, 1994).

   Perhaps the most well-known study of resilience in children as they grow into adulthood is the longitudinal research begun in 1955 by Werner and Smith (1992). In their initial report, Werner and Smith (1982) found that one out of every three children who were evaluated by several measures of early life functioning to be at significant risk for adolescent problems, actually developed into well-functioning young adults by age 18. In their follow-up study, Werner and Smith (1992) report that two out of three of the remaining two-thirds of children at risk had turned into caring and healthy adults by age 32. One of their primary theories was that people have "self-righting" capabilities. From their studies, the authors concluded that some of the factors that lead to self-correction in life can be identified. They also concluded that a significant factor leading to better emotional health for many children is a consistent and caring relationship with at least one adult. This adult (in a few cases, it was a peer) does not have to be a family member or physically present all of the time. These relationships provide the child with a sense of protection and serve to initiate and develop the child's self-righting capacities. Werner and Smith believe that it is never too late to move from a lack of achievement and a feeling of hopelessness to a sense of achievement and fulfillment.

   This finding is supported by similar findings of serious anti-social behavior in children. In summarizing the research on youth violence, the Surgeon General (Satcher, 2001) reports that "most highly aggressive children or children with behavioral disorders do not become violent offenders" (p. 9). Similarly, the Surgeon General reports that most youth violence begins in adolescence and ends with the transition to adulthood. If people did not change, then these early life behaviors would suggest that all violence in youth would certainly continue into adulthood. The report further suggests that the reasons for change in violent children relate to treatment programs, maturation, and biosocial factors (self-righting tendencies, or what has more recently been termed as resilience) that influence the lives of even the most violent youthful offenders. This and other research suggests that people do change, often on their own, and that learning from prior experience appears to be an important reason for change.

   A person's positive view of life can have a significant impact on his or her physical and emotional health, a belief supported by a longitudinal study of a Catholic order of women in the Midwest (Danner et al., 2001). Longitudinal studies of the many aspects of life span and illness among this population suggest that the personal statements written by very young women to enter the religious order correlated positively with life span. The more positive and affirming the personal statement written when applicants were in their late teens and early twenties, the longer their life span, sometimes as long as 10 years beyond the mean length of life for the religious order, as a whole, and up to 20 years or more longer than the general population. Many of the women in the sample lived well into their nineties and beyond. In a sample of 650 members of the order, six were over 100 years of age. While some members of the sample suffered serious physical problems, the numbers were much smaller than the general population and the age of onset was usually much later in life. The reasons for increased life span in this population seem to be related to good health practices (the order does not permit liquor or smoking, and foods are often fresh with a focus on vegetables) and an environment that focuses on spiritual issues and helping others. The order also has a strong emphasis on maintaining a close, supportive relationship among its members so that when illness does arise, there is a network of positive and supportive help.

4. **Belief:** The therapeutic relationship is the key to successful psychotherapy and counseling. **Reality:** noting the importance of the concept of the relationship in the professional literature, Gelso and Hayes (1998) wonder whether we have a clear understanding of what is meant by the worker–client relationship, and write:

   > *Because the therapy relationship has been given such a central place in our field for such a long period of time, one might expect that many definitions of the relationship have been put forth. In fact, there has been little definitional work. (Gelso and Hayes, 1998, p. 5)*

   In an attempt to determine the most effective approaches to treatment, not once in their work does Chambless (2001) mention the word "relationship." Interestingly, in reviewing the effectiveness of over 75 approaches to therapy, the author found little evidence that one approach worked better than another, although in arguing for a more rational approach to treatment, Chambless did find treatment protocols that seemed more effective with certain types of problems, but not with all clients and not because a therapeutic relationship was stressed.

3.4. UNDERSTANDING THE LOGICAL PROGRESSIONS IN RESEARCH IDEAS

One of my excellent students was having problems with an article on the perpetrators of family violence. The article was a post-modernist observation of men who were abusive and their relationships with their wives. The researcher sat in a court waiting room and observed couples prior to the perpetrator being called into court for a hearing involving his spousal abuse. The researcher had a protocol to guide the observations (areas of behavior to observe and evaluate) which had been developed from several articles the researcher had read, and which discussed the behavior of perpetrators with their spouses in public places. The protocol, while untested and neither valid nor reliable, was a guide the researcher used to look for certain behaviors associated with abusive men. The researcher spent an average of 20 minutes observing the couples and watched 34 couples over a 2-month period of time. Most of the couples were of color and only a few were Caucasian. The researcher concluded that the men were domineering, threatening, and exhibited potential for violence in the courthouse waiting room. Only two couples held hands or looked affectionate with one another. My student wanted to use this article as the cornerstone of her study, which was to be a similar study of men visiting their spouses in controlled circumstances while the spouse and the children lived independently in a shelter. The student's concern was how best to protect the victim and her children during these controlled setting from intimidating and potentially dangerous behavior perpetrated by the perpetrator, a very important and worthwhile issue to study. We spoke about the research article the student wanted to use.

Instructor (I): This study makes me awfully uncomfortable.
Student (S): Why?
I: Let's look at the study critically. What did you think were the parts of the study worth using?
S: It's relevant to my research.
I: That's true, but does the methodology warrant your using the findings?
S: I wonder about the lack of Caucasian subjects. About 60% of the male perpetrators in California are Caucasian. This study only had four Caucasian subjects, many fewer than the usual number I'd see in my study.
I: Good point. Why would the researcher make such an obvious mistake?
S: Maybe she doesn't like certain racial groups.
I: Maybe.
S: Maybe she didn't have time to draw a better sample. But that doesn't make sense, does it?
I: No, it doesn't. Anything else?
S: I had some problems with the protocol she used. It hardly has any positive behaviors. She's just looking for potential for violence. I think people waiting to go to a court hearing are pretty uptight. I'd guess most of us would look upset.
I: Me too. Anything else?
S: She doesn't say a word about how she selected her couples or what some of the problems might be with the research. I've noticed that most researchers have a pretty long section about the methodological problems in their study. Also, she did the analysis of the data herself. It might have been a good idea to use another person, or to have someone double check her data, or maybe even have a second person using the protocol and making independent judgments about the perpetrators' behavior.
I: A+. All very good points. Anything else?
S: Should I chuck the article and not use it for my study?
I: Ah, the eternal question. Maybe you should use it but point out the flaws and note that the subject of the article had relevance to your study but that the methodology makes the findings unreliable. That's always a wise approach in research when there are limited studies in the literature. Am I right? Are there limited studies?

S: Well, no. There are lots of them. I should go back and do a better literature review, huh?
I: Excellent idea. Better to use well-done studies than badly done studies. Basing your research on poorly-done studies just weakens your work.
S: Why did I know you'd say that?
I: It's my job to help you see the flaws in research. When you see the mistakes other people make then perhaps you won't repeat them.
S: No, I mean that I'd need to do more work.
I: Sorry, but better a little more work now than a lot more later when I read your research study.
S: There goes my weekend.

3.5. SUMMARY

This chapter on critical thinking presents several research philosophies that might help the reader understand that researchers have points of view about the meaning of research and that the approach they take in research is a result of their philosophy of research. To help the reader understand the strong and weak points of each philosophy of research, conflicting points of view ware provided. Critical thinking means that you should be able to critically evaluate all research, even the research you find appealing. Knowing about methodologies can help you do this and knowing what you should find in a study, including a discussion of weakness in the research, will help in the process of accepting best evidence from the literature review. A progression of ideas about the evaluation of a research study is also provided to show how one can approach a piece of research and, with some idea of how to evaluate a study, determine if the study is useful, well done, and a credible piece of work. Remember that the process of selecting best evidence is grounded in your desire to do what is best for the client and should not reinforce your personal belief system. If the research is compelling, it should be considered.

3.6. QUESTIONS FROM THE CHAPTER

1. Is it true that there is little well-done research on treatment effectiveness, which does not run the risk of discounting everything we read?
2. Was the study of perpetrators in the courthouse waiting room so poorly done that we would want to discount it completely?
3. How can practitioners use critical thinking when people are in life threatening crisis? Do not you do what needs to be done at the moment, and hope that it works? If you do not, you could have a suicide or homicide on your hands. What do you think?
4. Most of the research philosophies provided in this chapter seem more likely to get important information than the scientific method. At least non-empirical studies give you hope and they challenge you. Empirical studies are cold and discouraging, or are they?

5. Everybody knows that therapeutic relationships are the key to good treatment, but the author includes arguments against that belief. What is the point – that we do not have enough evidence for the belief, or that we should not accept the belief at all?

References

Astleitner, H. (2002). Teaching critical thinking online. *Journal of Instructional Psychology, 29*(2), 53–77.

Benard, B. (1994, December). *Applications of resilience*. Paper presented at a conference on the Role of Resilience in Drug Abuse, Alcohol Abuse, and Mental Illness, Washington, D.C.

Chambless, D. L. (2001). Empirically supported psychological interventions: Controversies and evidence. *Annual Review of Psychology, 52*, 685–716.

Danner, D. D., Snowdon, D. A., & Friesen, W. V. (2001). Positive emotions in early life and longevity: Findings from the nun study. *Journal of Personality and Social Psychology, 80*(5), 804–813.

Dawes, R. M. (1994). *House of cards: Psychology and psychotherapy built on myth*. New York: Free Press.

Gambrill, E. (1999, July). Evidence-based practice: An alternative to authority-based practice source: Families in society. *The Journal of Contemporary Human Services, 80*(4), 341–350.

Garmezy, N. (1994). Reflections and commentary on risk, resilience, and development. In R. J. Haggerty, L. R. Sherrod, N. Garmezy, M. & Rutter (Eds.), *Stress, risk, and resilience in children and adolescents: Processes, mechanisms, and interventions* (pp. 1–18). Cambridge, England: Cambridge University Press.

Gellner, E. (1992). *Postmodernism, reason, and religion*. London: Rutledge.

Gelso, J., & Hayes, J. A. (1998). *The psychotherapy relationship: Theory, research and practice*. New York: Wiley.

Glicken, M. D. (2005). *Improving the effectiveness of the helping professions: An evidence-based practice approach to treatment*. Thousand Oaks, Ca: Sage.

Glicken, M. D. (2003). *A simple guide to social research: First edition*. Boston: Allyn and Bacon/Longman.

McLaren, M. (2000). Psychiatry and the scientific method. *Australian Psychiatry, 8*(4), 373–375.

Munz, P. (1985). *Our knowledge of the growth of knowledge*. London: Routledge & Kegan Paul.

Nickerson, R. S. (1986). *Reflections on reasoning*. Hillside, NJ: Lawrence Erlbaum.

Rutter, M. (1994). Stress research: Accomplishments and tasks ahead. In R. J. Haggerty, L. R. Sherrod, N. Garmezy, M. & Rutter (Eds.), *Stress, risk, and resilience in children and adolescents: Processes, mechanisms, and interventions* (pp. 354–385). Cambridge, England: Cambridge University Press.

Satcher, D. (2001). Youth violence: A report of the surgeon general. U.S. Department of Health and Human Services, Office of the Surgeon General, Washington, DC.

Seligman, M. E. P. (1995). The effectiveness of psychotherapy: The consumers report study. *American Psychologist, 50*(12), 965–974.

Shea, P. (2000). Psychiatry and the scientific method. *Australian Psychiatry, 8*(3), 226–229.

Tanguay, P. E. (2002). Commentary: The primacy of the scientific method. *Journal of the American Academy of Child and Adolescent Psychiatry, 4*(11), 1322–1323.

Tyson, K. B. (1992 November). A new approach to relevant scientific research for practitioners: The heuristic paradigm. *Social Work, 37*(6), 541–556.

Werner, E., & Smith, R. S. (1982). *Vulnerable but invincible*. New York: McGraw-Hill.

Werner, E., & Smith, R. S. (1992). *Overcoming the odds: High-risk children from birth to adulthood*. Ithaca, NY: Cornell University Press.

Wuthnow, R. (2003). Is there a place for 'scientific' studies of religion?. *Chronicle of Higher Education, 49*(20), B10–B12.

Further reading

Cousins, N. (1976, December 23). Anatomy of an illness. *New England Journal of Medicine* .

4 Diagnosis and Assessment: An Evidence-Based Approach Using the Strengths Perspective with Children and Adolescents

4.1. INTRODUCTION

This chapter considers issues related to diagnosis and assessment of children and adolescents. The first part of the chapter focuses on issues related to correct diagnosis and ways of preventing bias in the diagnostic process. The second part of the chapter provides a strengths-based assessment of an adolescent young woman whose behavior suggests a variety of potential diagnoses and the process of determining the correct one for the purpose of treatment.

4.2. COMPETENCY-BASED DIAGNOSTIC TOOLS

Epidemiological studies done by the U.S. Department of Health and Human Services (1999) indicate that approximately 20% of children and adolescents younger than the age of 18 have a diagnosable mental disorder, with up to 5% of these youths experiencing profound disturbances in their functioning as a result of these emotional difficulties. Yet, according to Kataoka et al., 2002, the majority of these children and adolescents fail to receive needed services. Burns et al. (1995) found that only 25–35% of the youth who meet full criteria for a psychiatric diagnosis will be diagnosed with a problem and will receive treatment for it.

To help improve the ability of schools to recognize and treat emotional problems in youth, (Nemeroff et al., 2008) 530 students were selected by school counselors in 12 schools to be assessed with a computerized version of the National Institute of Mental Health Diagnostic Interview Schedule for Children-IV (DISCIV) (Bravo et al., 2001). The results were that 72% were confirmed to be at risk for a mental health problem while 71% had never been in treatment before. The most common problems identified by the DISCIV were symptoms related to suicide (28%), social phobia (20%), attention-deficit/hyperactivity disorder (19%), and oppositional defiant disorder (19%). Based on schools' recommendations, 82% of parents with DISCIV children agreed to make an appointment for a follow-up evaluation. Of DISCIV children whose parent agreed to seek further evaluation, 65% of them were evaluated by a health or mental health professional within 2 weeks. The National Institute of Mental Health Diagnostic Interview Schedule for Children Version IV (NIMH-DISC-IV) is a highly structured diagnostic interview, with good validity and reliability designed to assess more than 30 psychiatric disorders occurring in children and adolescents, and can be administered by non-professional interviewers after a minimal training period. The interview is available in both English and Spanish versions.

Another diagnostic tool for children and adolescents is The Scale for Assessing Emotional Disturbance (SAED) (Epstein and Cullinan, 1998), a rating scale designed to assist identifying students who may be experiencing emotional and/or behavioral problems in school. The test contains 52 items organized into seven subscales: (a) inability to (lacks self-confidence) learn; (b) relationship problems (has few friends); (c) inappropriate behavior (can be cruel to peers); (d) unhappiness or depression; (e) physical symptoms or fears (anxious, worried, tense); (f) socially maladjusted (runs away from home); and (g) school-related problems (an overall measures of school problems that affect performance). Although the validity and reliability of the SAED are good, reviewers of the measurement (Dumont and Rauch, 2000) had concerns about the selection process for determining reliability and validity of the instrument and of the usefulness of some of the scales. When the instrument was used with children who had known emotional problems, it was particularly good at identifying those problems.

Most clinicians continue to use the DSM (American Psychiatric Association, 1994) for diagnostic purposes, although there are many who believe categorizing the problems of children and young adolescents is often a mistake because of maturation and lack of complete emotional development in youth. Many clinicians have taken the position that the DSM is a guide to a diagnosis but that it should never use adult symptoms and make them comparable to those of children. The Surgeon General's report on mental health (Satcher, 1999) clearly states the problem with using adult behavior to diagnosis children, and notes:

> *Even with the aid of widely used diagnostic classification systems such as DSM-IV, diagnosis and diagnostic classification present a greater challenge with children than with adults for several reasons. Children are often unable to verbalize thoughts and feelings. Clinicians by necessity become more reliant on parents, teachers, and other professionals, who may be unable to assess these mental processes in children. Children's normal development also presents an ever-changing backdrop that complicates clinical presentation. As previously noted, some behaviors may be quite normal at one age but suggest mental illness at another age. Finally, the criteria for diagnosing most mental disorders in children are derived from those for adults, even though relatively little research attention has been paid to the validity of these criteria in children. Expression, manifestation, and course of a disorder in children might be very different from those in adults. The boundaries between normal and abnormal are less distinct and those between one diagnosis and another are fluid.*

The report goes on to note that most disorders are diagnosed by a show of symptoms and impairments but many of the symptoms and impairments of children and adolescents "such as outbursts of aggression, difficulty in paying attention, fearfulness or shyness, difficulties in understanding language, food fads, or distress of a child when habitual behaviors are interfered with, are normal in young children and may occur sporadically throughout childhood" (p. 1). The report says that effective clinicians overcome the problem by evaluating the intensity of the symptoms, the frequency, the length of time the symptoms last and whether they come at unexpected stages in the child's development. The inaccuracies of a correct diagnosis are often caused by over diagnosing normal behavior as a disorder or missing a diagnosis by failing to recognize abnormal behavior. Inaccurate diagnoses, according to the report, are more likely to occur with children who have mild forms of a disorder.

The DSM provides clinicians with easy-to-follow guidelines that permit a diagnostic category to be chosen that should, if the guidelines are followed accurately, be consistent with the diagnosis most clinicians would give for a particular emotional problem. However, the DSM has been criticized because it fails to provide an individual framework from which to fully understand many of the environmental and historical factors affecting clients. As a result, it is thought to be overly focused on pathology (Saleebey, 1996). The client's uniqueness is seldom represented by a DSM diagnosis, nor are the positive behaviors clients bring with them to treatment which often determine whether the client will improve. As most clinicians know, it's not what's wrong with the client that helps in the change process, it's what is right. As Saleebey writes (1996):

> *The DSM-IV (American Psychiatric Association, 1994), although only seven years removed from its predecessor, has twice the volume of text on disorders. Victimhood has become big business as many adults, prodded by a variety of therapists, gurus, and ministers, go on the hunt for wounded inner children and the poisonous ecology of their family background. These phenomena are not unlike a social movement or evangelism. (Saleebey, 1996, p. 296).*

Treatment paradigms, including the Strengths Perspective and Evidence-Based Practice, individualize the client by looking in a hopeful and optimistic way at the client's culture, family life, support network, coping abilities, past and current successes, and a number of otherwise ignored issues in the DSM that often contribute to good mental health and can frequently be used in the helping process. Building on the strengths of a client seems much more likely to lead to change than focusing on the negatives. Cloud (2003) has even more fundamental concerns about the DSM, and writes:

> *...[C]an even a thousand Ph.D.s gathered at a dozen conferences ever really know the significance of such vague symptoms as "fatigue," "low self-esteem" and "feelings of hopelessness"? (You need only two of those, along with a couple of friends telling the doctor you seem depressed, to be a good candidate for something called dysthymic disorder.) Though it's fashionable these days*

> *to think of psychiatry as just another arm of medicine, there is no biological test for any of these disorders. (p. 105).*

Other concerns noted by Cloud about the DSM-IV are that diagnostic categories were determined by ad hoc committee decisions that were often contentious and were only resolved by pleas for agreement and consensus, and that the DSM-IV is just a checklist of symptoms used to justify an emotional condition. To improve the DSM-IV or diagnostic manuals like it, Cloud suggests the use of four categories of disorders: "Those arising from brain disease, those arising from problems controlling one's drive, those arising from problematic personal dispositions, and those arising from life circumstances" (p. 106).

Whaley (2001) is concerned that Caucasian clinicians often see African American clients, particularly youthful clients, as having paranoid symptoms that are more fundamentally a cultural distrust of Caucasians because of historical experiences with racism. He believes that the diagnostic process with African American clients tends to discount the negative impact of racism and leads to diagnostic judgments about Black clients suggesting that they are more dysfunctional than they really are. This tendency to misdiagnose, or to diagnose a more serious condition than may be warranted, is what Whaley calls "pseudotransference," and has its origins in cultural stereotyping by clinicians who fail to understand the impact of racism. Whaley believes that cultural stereotyping ultimately leads to "more severe diagnoses and restrictive interventions" (p. 558) with African American clients. Whaley's work suggests that clinicians may incorrectly use diagnostic labels with clients they either feel uncomfortable with or whose cultural differences create some degree of hostility, casting doubt on the accuracy of diagnostic labels, with an entire range of clients who may differ educationally, racially and culturally from clinicians. These concerns reinforce the subjective nature of the diagnostic process in general and the DSM-IV in particular.

In describing incorrect diagnoses, DeGrandpre (1999) found that a diagnosis of Attention Deficit Hyperactivity Disorder (ADHD) made solely from observation of children in a physician's office routinely resulted in misdiagnosis. Sharp et al., 1999 found that boys were diagnosed with ADHD at rates three and four times higher than girls, even though ratios as low as two to one have been found in community studies. Wilke (1994) reports that young women are underdiagnosed for alcoholism because of stereotypes of drinking which apply to men but not to women. Alcoholic women are less likely to drink publicly, become violent or aggressive, or have problems with the law because of their drinking. Consequently, male behaviors that suggest alcoholism are applied to women and, having failed to note similar male patterns, a diagnosis of alcoholism is not applied to women when it should be.

Keenan et al. (2008) found high reliability and validity on the DSM-IV when diagnosing Oppositional Defiant Disorder (ODD) and Conduct Disorder (CD) in children, but noted that while there was no gender difference in the amount of ODD and CD when using the DSM-IV for diagnostic purposes, boys were still diagnosed with CD at three times the rate of girls. The researchers hypothesize that the reasons for this are that girls are not referred for treatment as often as boys and that the symptoms exhibited by boys are more severe. This is an interesting suggestion, given the fact that juvenile female crime and violence rates have been dramatically increasing over the past 20 years. It again shows that while the instrument may be reliable and valid, the use of the instrument and the willingness to use diagnostic labels that imply serious psychosocial problems with boys but not with girls may reflect social and cultural biases and inadequate diagnostic skills.

As an additional indication of misdiagnoses in the mental health field, Morey and Ochoa (1989) asked 291 psychiatrists and psychologists to complete a checklist of symptoms for a client whom they had diagnosed with a personality disorder. When the checklists were later correlated with the DSM criteria, nearly three of four clinicians had made mistakes in applying the diagnostic criteria (McLaughlin, 2002, p. 259). In a sample of 42 psychologists and 17 psychiatrists, Davis et al. (1993) had the sample read and diagnose case reports containing different symptoms of Narcissistic Personality Disorder (NPS). Ninety-four percent of the sample of the clinicians made mistakes applying the diagnostic criteria, while 25% diagnosed NPS when less than half of the DSM criteria were met.

In another example of incorrect diagnosis based upon first impressions, Robertson and Fitzgerald (1990) randomly assigned 47 counselors to watch videos of a depressed male portrayed by an actor. The only changes made in the videos were the client's type of employment (professional versus blue collar) and the client's family or origin (traditional or non-traditional). The researcher found that counselors made more negative diagnostic judgments when the actor portrayed a blue-collar worker and came from a non-traditional family. The signs and symptoms of any specific emotional disorders were secondary to the worker's bias.

In yet another example of a type of bias, self-confirmatory bias, or diagnosis based only on the information collected by the clinician that confirms his or her original diagnosis, Haverkamp (1993) had counseling and counseling psychology students watch a video of an initial counseling session and then write down the questions they wanted to ask in a follow-up session with the client. The results were that the majority of students (64%) wanted to ask questions that confirmed their original diagnostic impression of the client. A follow-up study by Pfeiffer et al. (2000) came to a similar conclusion.

While labeling for diagnostic purposes may be relevant in medicine, diagnostic labels for mental health purposes are sometimes poorly defined and pejorative. Labels often harm people, and the most vulnerable among us – the poor, minority groups, women, immigrants, and the physically, emotionally, and socially disadvantaged, are those most harmed by labels. This may be particularly true of minority clients in which harm to clients frequently occurs when labeling is used. Franklin (1992) says that African American men want to see themselves as "partners in treatment" and resent labels that suggest pathology because labels send signals to Black clients who have had to deal with labels that subtly or overtly suggest racism. Franklin strongly suggests that African American men want to be recognized for their many strengths and that clinicians should take into consideration that African American men may be doing well in many aspects of their lives. According to Franklin, African American men are particularly sensitive to male bashing and other sexist notions that berate men or negatively stereotype men in general, and Black men in particular. And while Black workers are preferable when working with Black men, Franklin urges workers to be sensitive to the Black experience and to approach Black clients with respect and awareness of the many social behaviors which create tensions in the lives of African American men, and which may also be true of other men.

Finally, we need to remember that the decision to find a child or adolescent symptomatic of an emotional problem is often ambiguous and may be tied to value judgments particular to a certain culture or society. Even within cultures, concepts of normal mental health may evolve over time if societal values or expectations change.

4.3. REDUCING ERRORS IN DIAGNOSIS

McLaughlin (2000) suggests the following ways of reducing errors in diagnosis: (1) do not make too much or too little of the evidence at hand; (2) try and note the biasing effect of your workplace which may routinely diagnose everyone in the same way; (3) use falsification to try and disprove a diagnosis; (4) consistently use all of the DSM diagnostic criteria and keep current about revisions; (5) be aware of other disorders or a dual diagnosis, and delay making a diagnosis until you have more data; (6) use symptom checklists to make certain your diagnosis adheres to DSM categories and follow a logical protocol to collect and evaluate data about the client before finalizing a diagnosis; (7) if you use psychological instruments in diagnosis, make certain they are valid and reliable with the type of client you are diagnosing (by age, gender, ethnicity, etc.); (8) make absolutely certain your expectations of clients do not reflect racial, ethnic, gender or religious bias, or self-fulfilling prophesies about certain categories of diagnosis; (9) remember the importance of social factors in diagnosis and that the DSM may have a built-in bias against certain groups; (10) consider other diagnostic possibilities and understand that the more time you take getting to know the client, the more likely you are to arrive at a correct diagnosis; (11) consider the pros and the cons of a diagnosis before formally using it with a client; (12) use multiple diagnostic instruments to determine a diagnosis and accept a diagnosis only if those instruments are in agreement with one another; (13) focus on what may be atypical about a client and follow those leads to help determine a diagnosis; (14) follow ethical standards; and (15) use training to improve your diagnostic work, particularly with diverse ethnic and cultural groups.

Grounded theory (Glaser, 1992) may be another way to help clinicians make accurate assessments of clients. In grounded theory we are not testing a predetermined belief (a hypothesis) as we normally would in most research. Instead, we are trying to come up with a theory about the client and the current problem the client is experiencing. Diagnosis develops through the following series of steps: (1) collecting sufficient information about the client, including current functioning, past functioning, and the client's theory of why he or she is experiencing difficulty now; (2) taking notes which clarify the information we have collected and referring back to the notes to see patterns or themes in the information collected. In order to help see patterns and themes in the information collected, create categories of issues, problems, and patterns; (3) summarizing the patterns and themes until an emerging theory about the client develops; (4) testing that theory against accumulating information to see if patterns and themes persist; (5) beginning to consider a diagnosis that, while theoretically accurate now, may change as more data is collected; (6) testing the diagnosis by determining if it fits the situation and whether it helps clients make sense of their experience and manage their lives more effectively; (7) having a way to double check a diagnosis (i.e., audio taping an interview and letting a colleague go through the data collection to theory process, or continually checking your notes and comparing them to emerging information); and (8) frequently asking the client to provide feedback on the information accumulated to see if your data is accurate.

Gawande (2007) reports the significant benefits of short checklists in hospital settings. Simply asking physicians to abide by several important questions posed about their practice with patients in emergency room and ICU facilities significantly reduced infections, length of stay in the facility, long-term improvement in conditions, and a number of other important areas of concern to medical practice. Gawande (2007) notes that by following simple procedures contained in a checklist, "within the first 3 months of using the checklist, the infection rate in Michigan's ICU's dropped by 66% saving hospitals 75 million dollars in costs and more than 1500 lives, a figured sustained for over 4 years because of a stupid little checklist" (p. 94). While the following checklist may not have such dramatic results, it includes the four large areas of information needed to accurately access individuals proposed by Smyer (1984): (1) biological, (2) personal/psychological, (3) physical/environmental, and (4) social/cultural. Smyer has also identified 14 different contexts in which life events occur, including family, love and marriage, parenting, health, self, friendships, social relations, finances, and work (1984, pp. 18 and 19).

4.4. A STRENGTH-BASED PSYCHOSOCIAL ASSESSMENT

Rather than using a diagnostic label with children and adolescents which may fail to accurately describe the client's unique qualities, a psychosocial assessment summarizes the relevant information we know about a client and places it into concise statements that allows other helping professionals to understand the clients and their problem(s) as well as we do. Psychosocial assessments differ from DSM-IV diagnostic statements because they provide brief historical information about the possible causation of the problem. While they are problem-focused, they also provide best evidence from the literature to support the assessment. The client's strengths are included in an assessment, as well as the problems which might interfere with the client's treatment.

For those readers unfamiliar with the strengths perspective (also called positive psychology and the wellness model), Van Wormer (1999) describes the elements of the strength approach as follows:

> *The first step in promoting the client's well-being is through assessing the client's strengths. A belief in human potential is tied to the notion that people have untapped resources – physically, emotionally, socially, and spiritually – that they can mobilize in times of need. This is where professional helping comes into play – in tapping into the possibilities, into what can be, not what is. (p. 51).*

A key idea of the strengths perspective is that skills in one area of life can be transferred to other less functional areas of life. The criticism of this capacity of people to learn from their successes is difficult to understand. Contrary to the adage that people learn from their mistakes, they generally repeat their mistakes. Success is far more instructive and motivating than failure. On the face of it, the criticism that skill in one area of life is non-transferable to other areas of life contradicts the fact that people change in life, often for the better, and that in the midst of crisis they can do amazingly wonderful things. Anderson (1997) suggests the benefits of focusing on the positive qualities of children who have been sexually abused. She believes that the focus of our work should not be on the damage done to the child but on the survival abilities of the child to cope with the abuse. This means that practitioners must look for themes of resilience in the "survival stories" of abused children and help the child recognize the active role they played in their ability to survive the abuse. Perhaps, as Anderson (1997) suggests, "[t]he psychological scars will never disappear completely; however, focusing on the child's strengths and resiliency can help limit the power of sexual abuse over the child" (p. 597).

Orsulik-Jerus et al. (2003)Orsulik-Jerus et al. (2003, p. 237) suggest a way of differentiating pathology models from wellness models such as the strengths perspective: in traditional treatment models diagnosis involves identify pathology; the focus of assessment is on illness; treatment attempts to suppress pathological symptoms while focusing is on the client's understanding of the impact of past events; the therapist is the authority, and the emphasis of treatment is on what's wrong with the client and what can be done to make things right. In the strengths-based model of treatment, the focus is on client strengths; treatment attempts to support current coping methods and strategies; the client is an active participant in treatment and the therapist is a partner in a process that considers every client be unique and possessing the necessary strength to make life enhancing changes.

4.5. A CASE STUDY: EVIDENCE-BASED PRACTICE AND THE ASSESSMENT PROCESS

This case study is used to show an evidence-based practice approach to assessing a child suffering from the aftermath of many years of abuse. The outline used in the case is for illustrative purposes only. Under each heading there is a description of the information one might include. The important thing to remember is that the assessment provides information to other professionals. It necessarily includes all of the information relevant to the case. Some of that information might pertain to ongoing difficulties or prior life problems experienced by the client. Most important, however, is that it tries to be as objective as possible to support observations, impressions, initial diagnosis, and ultimately, treatment.

4.6. A STRENGTH-BASED PSYCHOSOCIAL ASSESSMENT OUTLINE AND THE RELEVANT INFORMATION PERTAINING TO THE CASE

4.6.1. Section I: Brief Description of the Client and the Problem

In this section of the psychosocial assessment, we should include relevant socio-demographic information about the client, including the client's age, marital status, the composition of the client's family of origin and their current level of interaction, what the client is wearing, the client's verbal and non-verbal communications, his or her affect, and anything of significance that took place during the interview(s), including the defined problem(s). Interpretations are normally not made in this section. The following is an example of how this section might be written from an evidence-based practice perspective:

Patrice Alvarez is a 15-year-old young woman attending 10th grade at a local high school. She came to the interview 15 min late, was dressed in cutoffs and a blouse with holes in it, and wore no shoes. When she was asked why she was being seen she said, "My pa thinks I'm a 'ho.' He's probably right."

Patrice also said that she is failing at school after having been an honors student, and that she is the only child in a family of four children who is having problems. She said her younger brother Jack (6) and two older sisters Angel (16) and Betsy (18) are perfect and she hates them all because "they make me sick. They're such little snobs." As for her, she said, "I ain't no angel, that's for sure."

Patrice's father Lawrence (48) is the manager of a large home improvement store and makes a good living. Her mother Alfie (46) is a high school teacher in Patrice's school. Alfie asked the school social worker to see Patrice, but after four unproductive sessions, she referred Patrice for private therapy. In her referral she said that Patrice was uncooperative, angry, and dismissive. Patrice said her parents needed the help, not her. The worker also mentioned problems with depression and mood swings, which began about a year ago, confirmed by her parents and her teacher. The worker suspects, but isn't certain, that Patrice may be developing a chronic depression or perhaps bipolar disorder. Patrice was doing well until a year ago and was a loving and attentive child, but as the mood swings became more frequent with long periods of depression, her behavior became more erratic.

When asked about depression, Patrice responded, "Who wouldn't be depressed having to live with those assholes? Yeah, I feel depressed. So what? So do all my friends. It's depressing to be a teenager. Everybody knows that." When asked about other symptoms like sleep, she said she sometimes does not sleep for 3 or 4 days, but then she will sleep all day. She likes feeling high and gets a lot done. The lows are not fun but "what the hell. You take the good with the bad." When asked about self-medication, she said she took "uppers" to deal with depression and drank wine when the highs made her overly anxious.

"I know something's wrong with me," she said after about 20 min, "but I can't figure out what. I feel high and then low, and lots of time I can't think straight. I get these very big ideas when I'm high and I feel like killing myself when I'm low. I used to be a nice girl but look at me now," she said, and began crying.

4.6.2. Questions About this Initial Information

1. **Question:** Is Patrice suffering from early onset bipolar disorder?
   Answer: It's difficult to say given her age and the limited history, but the early signs are perhaps bipolar disorder 1 (DSM-IV code 296.6, DSM-IV, p. 357). We need more psychosocial history and a medical evaluation to determine if Patrice has a medical problem creating her symptoms or whether the self-medicating she's doing is greater than she says and could be responsible for her symptoms. The DSM-IV says that 10–15% of adolescents with recurrent major depressive episodes will go on to develop bipolar 1 disorder (p. 353). Whether we can give her a bipolar diagnosis now without further information is probably not recommended, but it is something to consider at this early point without making the mistake of giving her an early diagnosis and then doing everything we can to confirm it. A better approach might be to try and disprove the diagnosis and find out whether there are other reasons for her symptoms.
2. **Question:** How depressed is Patrice?
   Answer: Patrice's behavior suggests serious depression. An aspect of the DSM-IV to consider in rating her overall functioning is the global assessment functioning scale of the DSM-IV, also known as the GAF score (APA, 1994, p. 32). The GAF score ranges from 100 ("Superior functioning in a wide range of activities. Life problems never seem to get out of hand. Is sought after by others because of his or her many qualities. No symptoms") (APA, 1994, p. 32) to 10 and below ("Danger to self and to others. Inability to maintain hygiene and the possibility of suicidal acts") (APA, 1994, p. 32). In reviewing the GAF, an appropriate GAF score might be in the 50–41 range: ("Serious symptoms (e.g., suicidal ideation) or any impairment in social, occupational or school functioning") (e.g., no friends). (APA, 1994, p. 32). How serious is this score? It is serious enough to warrant treatment, and serious enough to worry about

a more extreme depression and the possibility of suicide. Let us see if we change our minds as we learn more about Patrice.

4.6.3. *Section II: Historical Issues*

This section includes any past issues of importance in understanding the client's current problems. The following might be relevant points to include in the historical section of our report:

Patrice's parents and the school confirm that Patrice was an excellent student and a positive and happy teenager until a year ago. The change in her behavior was sudden and unexpected, pointing, I thought, to a trauma. In the 2nd session with Patrice, alternating between silence and berating my work and everyone in her life, she began to discuss a painful experience she had been trying to live with. Her grandfather, a respected and much beloved member of a large extended family, had begun molesting her when she was 12. At first she thought it was harmless since it started with a lot of hugging and kissing, which she passed off as over affection by a much older person whose limit setting was perhaps blunted by age. "You know how mushy old people can get," she said. But as the affection progressed into rape with intercourse on her 14th birthday, Patrice found herself unable to tell her parents because of the impact it would have on the family. Initially she tried to repress her feelings and get on with her life but gradually she found herself becoming very depressed. To combat the depression, she began using "uppers" to create a high. Between being depressed and using "uppers" to self-medicate she has become unable to function and feels miserable. She cannot tell her parents but does not want to continue feeling as she does. She does not think her parents will believe her if she tells them about her grandfather, and she is afraid that she will become ostracized by the family even if they do believe her.

Her family is very much into placing family before the individual, and even though her sisters are doing well outwardly she thinks they are not doing as well as her parents think. Without her parent's knowledge, her older sister Betsy became pregnant by a much older man and had an abortion. Angel has been using drugs. Patrice knows that to be true since she's been getting her drugs from Angel. She thinks the family is a mess, and while everything looks good on the outside, it is a troubled family without the ability to discuss their problems. Patrice said her father has been having affairs with his employees and that her mother knows. She's heard them fighting about it. She also knows that her mother is on anti-depressives and is in therapy, although her mother has never said anything about it to anyone in the family. Patrice found the medication one afternoon with the doctor's name on the prescription. She called and found that he was a psychiatrist and, asking to check on her mother's next appointment, was told that her next "therapy" session was in a week.

Patrice has stayed away from her grandfather, but one of his employees (her grandfather has many businesses, some of which are reputed to be illegal) began walking with her after school and told her that her grandfather sent his regards, and for her to understand that what happens in the family stayed there. He smirked when he said that and Patrice knew immediately that the employee knew what had happened and that it was a veiled threat for her not to tell anyone inside or outside of the family about her grandfather's behavior.

After the second session, Patrice met with her two sisters and told them what had happened to her. They were not surprised because the same thing had happened to them, but rather than acting out, they were compliant on the outside while seething with anger and resentment on the inside. They were, they said to Patrice, as confused and disturbed as she was. They believed their mother knew about the molestations but, like them, was afraid to do anything about it. They both planned to leave home as soon as possible and they avoided their grandfather as much as possible. Betsy believed that the grandfather had also molested their mother, and that their father knew about it but was afraid to do anything.

Patrice describes her family as outwardly affectionate when other family members and close friends are present but aloof and unaffectionate when the family is by itself. She finds her father to be autocratic and controlling, and her mother to be weak and unassertive. As she has begun to open up, it seems clear that she has been unhappy far longer than the start of the molestation by her grandfather. She says that she thought about suicide when she was in elementary school, but consistent with her religious beliefs then, thought she would go to hell if she did. She no longer believes in religion or in God. "What kind of God is he to let all three of us get raped by that old man," she said at the end of the second session. "Maybe my mother too. I do not think I want to be with God, anyway."

4.6.4. Questions

1. **Question:** Is Patrice possibly suffering from PTSD as a result of the molestation?
   Answer: Possibly. According to the DSM-IV (APA, 1994), the core criteria for PTSD include distressing symptoms of (a) re-experiencing a trauma through nightmares and intrusive thoughts; (b) numbing by avoiding reminders of the trauma, or feeling aloof or unable to express loving feelings for others and; (c) persistent symptoms of arousal as indicated by two or more of the following: sleep problems, irritability and angry outbursts, difficulty concentrating, hypervigilance, and exaggerated startle response with a duration of more than a month, causing problems at work, in social interactions, and in other important areas of life (American Psychiatric Association, 1994, pp. 427–429). The DSM-IV judges the condition to be acute if it has lasted less than 3 months, and chronic if it has lasted more than 3 months. It's possible for the symptoms to be delayed. The DSM-IV notes that a diagnosis of delayed onset is given when symptoms begin to show 6 months or more after the original trauma (APA, 1994, p. 429).

   These symptoms do not exactly match Patrice's, but she is an adolescent and it's possible that PTSD shows itself with somewhat different symptoms for youth than for adults. In fact, some researchers have proposed a new category of PTSD for children called "developmental trauma disorder" or DTD, to capture what some researchers see as the central realities of life for these children: exposure to multiple, chronic traumas, usually of an interpersonal nature; a unique set of symptoms that differs from those of post-traumatic stress disorder (PTSD) and a variety of other labels often applied to such children, and the fact that these traumas affect children differently depending on their stage of development (DeAngelis, 2007). Many of the children with DTD experience depression, drug abuse, sexual acting out, and a variety of problems consistent with Patrice's symptoms, both during adolescence and later in adulthood. If one can assume that any severe trauma will result in a degree of behavioral change in most people, and if the trauma is severe and continues for a prolonged period (as in physical and sexual abuse) Ozer et al. (2003) suggest that PTSD will develop and sustain itself as a behavior when several primary reasons for developing PTSD exist. These reasons include the following: (1) a history of prior traumas; (2) existence of emotional problems prior to the traumatic event; (3) emotional problems in the victim's family of origin; (4) the extent a person believes the traumatic event will endanger his or her life; (5) the lack of a support system to help the client cope; (6) the level of emotional responsiveness of a person during and after the trauma and; (7) the existence of a dissociative state during and following the trauma. According to the authors, no single variable predicts PTSD, but a cluster of variables strengthens the probability of developing PTSD. Would the symptoms last as long as a year? Reports of lifetime rates of PTSD of between 30% and 50% have been noted in women who have been sexually assaulted or raped (Foa et al., 1995; Meadows and Foa, 1998). The Harvard Health Letter (2002) reports that PTSD is most likely to occur in those people who have experienced some form of assault. Seventy percent of the patients in the Harvard Health Letter report who had current or lifetime PTSD said that the assault was their very worst traumatic experience. So yes, the chances are good that Patrice may be suffering from PTSD.

2. **Question:** Should the grandfather be reported to child protective services and the police for child sexual abuse?
   Answer: Yes. Before this is done, however, a meeting should be held with the two sisters to confirm their molestation, and ultimately with the parents to determine their response and the degree to which they are willing to support their daughters. Without assurances that they will support their children there is a high probability that the parents will put pressure on the children to recant and that the accusation of molestation will not only divide the family but place the children in harms way from the grandfather. It is a difficult ethical issue, but our responsibility is to report the grandfather, yet to do it in such a way that the children will be protected and further harm to the family will be prevented.

4.6.5. Section III: Diagnostic Statement

The diagnostic statement is a summary of the reasons the client is experiencing problems now. The diagnostic statement combines material from the prior two sections and summarizes the most important information into a brief statement. The following diagnostic statement was written after Patrice's second session of therapy:

After two sessions of therapy, Patrice has begun sharing some very difficult information about a molestation by her grandfather that lasted 2 years, culminating with rape on her 14th birthday. She also says that her two sisters were molested by their grandfather, and believes that her parents knew but were afraid to do anything about it because of the disruptive impact it would have on the extended family and their fear of the grandfather's certain retribution because of his criminal background.

Patrice describes a long history of unhappiness and depression with suicidal thoughts that began in elementary school and started well before the molestation began. She thinks her depression is related to the dysfunctional nature of an aloof and emotionally distant family that values outward compliance and performance without providing support or emotional closeness. She describes her father as unfaithful, autocratic, and domineering, and her mother as knowledgeable of the molestation by the grandfather but too fearful, weak, and unassertive to do anything about it. She says that her older sisters appear successful and compliant outwardly but that they are both experiencing serious problems, which they blame on the dysfunctional nature of their family.

It is difficult to pinpoint a diagnosis since the molestation points to PTSD but her longer history also suggests chronic depression. My initial sense of her current functioning is that Patrice has endured a series of severe traumas that she has kept to herself until now. Her ability to openly talk about her molestation and other personal matters is a positive sign showing resilience and the desire to resolve the many problems she is experiencing at present. I have concerns about a long-standing depression, and her potential for suicide or other forms of self-destructive behavior when the family becomes involved in treatment. Her current use of drugs to self-medicate has potential for addiction leading to additional self-destructive behavior. Certainly the revelation of the molestations of all the sisters to the parents will lead to a crisis in the family. Whether Patrice or the family can weather the storm that is certain to follow is difficult to predict.

4.6.6. Question

1. **Question:** This diagnostic statement is nothing more than a recap of what we already know. Wouldn't it be helpful to give Patrice a solid diagnosis so that we know what we're dealing with?
   Answer: A diagnosis is a cluster of symptoms with indications of duration and severity. The medical model would insist that before we can treat we need a solid diagnosis, much as we would if the client had a physical problem or disease. There are symptoms of PTSD, including emotional numbing, anxiety and substance abuse, and chronic depression starting in elementary school coupled with suicidal thoughts. It's difficult to know which of these many symptoms form a complete diagnosis. Is she more prone to PTSD because of a long-standing depression, or would most adolescents suffer from PTSD as a result of being molested? These are issues we can determine, as we know more about Patrice and her development. Rather than focus on a specific diagnosis, it may be better to focus on each symptom, it's duration, frequency and severity. Self-medication and depression are a lethal mix for suicide or some other form of self-destructive behavior. Initially, the depression and the self-medication need to be

dealt with since both suggest serious problems in functioning. A suicide assessment is absolutely necessary at this point in time.

4.6.7. Section IV. The Treatment Plan

The treatment plan describes the goals of treatment during a specific period of time and comes from the agreement made between the worker and the client in the contractual phase of treatment. In this example, 12 sessions are used over a 3-month period, although in reality Patrice has the right to continue or discontinue the contact with her worker at any time. Patrice has agreed to the following treatment plan:

(1) To enlist Patrice in a cooperative effort to find the best treatment approaches for her current problems by reading the existing literature and discussing it with the worker.
(2) To discontinue the self-medication and to have Patrice seen by a psychiatrist to evaluate and prescribe, if needed, medication to treat her depression.
(3) To discuss the molestation and her feelings about it and to develop a plan to involve her sisters and her family.
(4) To discuss the cause of her early and continuing depression and to get a promise, in writing, not to commit suicide.
(5) To help her improve her school-related functioning.
(6) To meet with her sisters to discuss family functioning, their molestation by the grandfather, and whether they would support a meeting with the parents to discuss their molestations and their concerns about family life.
(7) To meet with the entire family to discuss the molestation and current family functioning.
(8) To refer Patrice to a group for adolescents having experienced molestation.
(9) To contact child protective services and the police to report the molestations of Patrice and her two sisters by their grandfather.

4.6.8. Questions

1. **Question:** Doesn't the lack of a diagnosis limit our ability to treat Patrice?
Answer: We don't know with certainty what Patrice's condition really is, other than she has experienced childhood depression, is self-medicating by using alcohol and uppers, and may have PTSD as a result of the molestation. One way to objectify the process would be to determine her level of depression by using an instrument such as the Beck Depression Inventory (BDI) (Beck et al., 1961). The BDI would help determine the level of her depression and evaluate any risk of suicide. The BDI has good reliability (.80 to .90) and good validity for measuring depression, according to Wilcox et al. (1998). Another depression inventory, the CES-D (Radloff, 1977), is also a good instrument and has a high comparative correlation (70) with the BDI when the two instruments test the same people and the test results are compared (Wilcox et al., 1998). A second professional opinion might also help. For the time being, let's consider the GAF Score of 50–41 as an indication of her current social functioning.
2. **Question:** Isn't there a good chance that using the right anti-depressant might bring about behavioral changes without the need for therapy?

Answer: We hope that treatment will lead to an improvement in functioning without medicating her with all the risks related to medication use with young adolescents, but it may not and the depression may have a physical basis. The reason for a psychiatric consultation in the treatment plan is to make certain that Patrice's depression isn't bio-chemical in nature. Given the early onset of her depression, there is a chance that the depression has a bio-chemical basis and that the correct anti-depressant might help. The issues she has identified might do well with a combination of medication and psychotherapy. The research evidence seems to suggest that anti-depressants alone are no more effective than therapy. However, we have no control over whether Patrice actually takes an anti-depressant and no way to judge her functioning unless she sees us often. That is why therapy can be highly beneficial since it keeps close tabs on the client and can help identify depression that seems to be non-responsive to medication or to therapy.

To help answer the question about the efficacy of medication for depression versus efficacy of therapy alone, several studies are provided that show the relationship between improvement in depression and the use of anti-depressants and/or therapy:

> *Study 1: It is clear that antidepressant medications produce a 60% recovery rate when prescribed within proper dosages and for adequate duration. Depression-specific time-limited psychotherapies achieve similar outcomes, even with patients experiencing moderate to severe symptomatology. Two principles emerge from this body of work: (1) major depression should not be treated with anxiolytic medications alone or with long-term psychotherapy; and (2) patient preference for a particular guideline-based treatment should be considered when it is clinically and practically feasible. (Schulberg, 1998, Internet, p. 2)*

> *Study 2: The most frequently cited results were reported by the National Institute of Mental Health Treatment of Depression Collaborative Research Program. Two hundred fifty unipolar depressed patients at three sites were randomly assigned to one of four conditions: cognitive-behavior therapy (CBT), interpersonal therapy (IPT), imipramine (a tricyclic antidepressant) plus clinical management (IMI-CM), and pill placebo with clinical management (PLA-CM). Results were generally as follows: (a) All four conditions resulted in significant improvement; (b) neither form of psychotherapy was superior to the other; (c) the only significant treatment difference for all patients occurred between IMI-CM and PLA-CM; (d) for the more severe cases, IMI-CM and IPT produced more improvement than PLA-CM whereas CBT did not; and (e) IMI-CM generally produced more rapid effects than the other conditions. (Kopta, 1999, Internet, p. 14)*

> *Study 3: Carey (2008) reports that published studies of the effectiveness of anti-depressants failed to include a third of the studies showing poor results of anti-depressant drugs. In published results, 60% of those taking ant-depressants showed positive results, as opposed to 40% of the patients on placebos. When the unpublished studies showing negative results were factored in, the drugs outperformed placebos but only by a marginal amount.*

4.6.9. Some Thoughts About Why Clients Change

Before we leave the treatment plan, a brief discussion about why clients change their behavior as a result of treatment might be helpful. McConnaughy et al. (1983) believe that client change requires both the worker and the client to be at the same state of readiness in understanding the client's problems and the emotional commitment to change them. Howard et al. (1993) suggest that clients start therapy in a state of demoralization. Through the development of trust, the therapist helps them identify their primary problems, instills hope, and helps them develop a sense of well-being. As their sense of well-being increases, problems that seemed unsolvable to the client can be discussed and remedied. Remediation suggests that clients practice new behaviors which reinforce change through stages of treatment. Howard et al. (1993) add:

> *From a psychotherapy practice point of view, the phase model suggests that different change processes will be appropriate for different phases of therapy and that certain tasks may have to be accomplished before others are undertaken. It also suggests that different therapeutic processes may characterize each phase. Therapeutic interventions are likely to be most effective when they focus on changing phase-specific problems when those problems are most accessible to change. (p. 684).*

Howard et al. (1996) caution that while these phases are distinct, they suggest different treatment goals and "thus the selection and assessment of different outcome variables to measure progress in each phase" (p. 1061). These are, of course, untested ideas from the literature, but they may help in better understanding the change process with a client like Patrice.

4.6.10. Section V. Contract

The contract is an agreement between the worker and the client that specifies the problems to be worked on in treatment, the number of sessions agreed on, and rules related to being on time, the length of each session, payment, and the cancellation policy. Many workers write up the contract and have both the client and worker sign it. A contract with Patrice might read as follows:

> *Patrice has agreed to meet with the worker for 12 consecutive one-hour weekly sessions. She agrees that more meetings might be required. The effectiveness of treatment and the progress made will be evaluated after each session and at the end of the 12 sessions using client feedback and a depression instrument. Patrice agrees to consult the research related to her current problems, share the research with her worker, and write summaries of what took place during each session. Questions to be discussed in future sessions will be sent to the worker by e-mail two days after a treatment session, or sooner. After 12 sessions, the client and worker will jointly determine whether additional sessions are*

needed. Patrice has agreed to other conditions in the contract, including the no-cancellation-of-session clause unless 24 h notice is given to the worker in writing.

4.6.11. Questions

1. **Question:** Can significant change take place in 12 sessions?
   Answer: Very often it can. Seligman (1995) found no difference in client satisfaction with treatment among clients who had been seen for an average of 6 months and those who had been seen for an average of 2 years. Kopta (1999) reports a study in which clients with severe substance abuse problems were provided 12 sessions using three different types of treatment (twelve-step-based counseling, psychodynamic therapy, and cognitive-behavioral therapy). Kopta writes, "Significant and sustained improvements in drinking outcomes were observed for all three groups" (Kopta, 1999, p. 21). Fleming and Manwell (1998) report that people with alcohol-related problems, including persistent depressions, often receive counseling from primary care physicians or nursing staff in five or fewer standard office visits with very good results. Gentilello et al. (1995) note that 25% to 40% of the trauma patients seen in emergency rooms may be alcohol dependent and depressed. The authors found that a single motivational interview at or near the time of discharge reduced drinking levels and re-admission for trauma during 6 months of follow-up. Monti et al. (1999) conducted a similar study with 18- to 19-year-olds admitted to an emergency room with alcohol-related injuries. After 6 months, all participants had decreased their alcohol consumption; however, "the group receiving brief intervention had a significantly lower incidence of drinking and driving, traffic violations, alcohol-related injuries, and alcohol-related problems" (Monti, 1999, p. 3). So yes, change might take place in as few as 12 sessions, but these are serious problems for an adolescent to handle and treatment over a longer period of time may be (probably will be) necessary. Twelve sessions is a good start.
2. **Question:** Will Patrice continue seeing the worker for 12 sessions?
   Answer: It's difficult to say, given the possibility that family pressure may result in termination from treatment once the molestation is openly discussed with her parents. Clients stop treatment when they believe it isn't helping or when the subject matter becomes too troubling. One way to help clients bridge the gap between what they think is an absence of ability to function well and a sense that change is possible is the use of bibliotherapy. Bibliotherapy uses literature to facilitate the therapeutic process. Myers (1998) defines bibliotherapy as "a dynamic process of interaction between the individual and literature, which emphasizes the reader's emotional response to what has been read" (p. 243). Pardeck (1995) gives six goals of bibliotherapy: (1) to provide information; (2) to gain insight; (3) to find solutions; (4) to stimulate discussion of problems; (5) to suggest new values and attitudes, and; (6) to show clients how others have coped with problems similar to their own. "Bibliotherapy provides metaphors for life experiences that help clients verbalize their thoughts and feelings and learn new ways to cope with problems" (Myers. 1998, p. 246). Suggesting age-appropriate books, films, and TV programs with themes that resonate with Patrice might certainly have an impact on her and could be used for discussion of their relevance to her life in treatment.

4.6.12. *Discussion of the Case*

While much of the current literature suggests that cognitive-behavioral therapy might work best with her depression, it is not entirely certain that it would work well with Patrice. The active and directive nature of cognitive therapy could remind the client of similar communication patterns used by her domineering father and her cruel grandfather. One approach that might be worth considering is the strengths perspective. Glicken (2004) defines the strengths perspective as "a way of viewing the positive behaviors of all clients by helping them see that problem areas are secondary to areas of strength and that out of what they do well can come helping solutions based upon the successful strategies they use daily in their lives to cope with a variety of issues and problems," (p.).

Understanding her parents and their behavior could also help Patrice better understand herself. The strengths approach tries to frame clients and their current problems as positively as possible, and "[w]hile clients need to understand any harm done to them by parental conduct and to understand its impact, they benefit from a more complete and potentially positive view of their parents" (Glicken, 2004, p.). The ability to understand her parents as they might have explained and defended their own behavior is an important aspect of treatment with Patrice.

By involving Patrice in a cooperative relationship where she works closely with the clinician in trying to understand herself, she may come to learn how to overcome the abuse and family dysfunction and how one moves to the next level of development: the ability to have positive feelings about herself so that she can move ahead in life and develop loving relationships with others. Her treatment calls for a positive and empathic approach, one which Saleebey believes, "obligates us to understand. .. to believe that everyone (no exceptions here) has external and internal assets, competencies and resources" (p.128), and that these resources, regardless of how dormant or untested they may be, are able to provide the wise helper with the ability to facilitate the relationship in a way that permits the client to work through relationship concerns and discomforts.

4.7. SUMMARY

In summary, the chapter discusses diagnostic issues related to developing accurate diagnoses of children and adolescents, a task made more difficult by fluctuating patterns of behavior, limited research and errors often made by clinicians which confirm incorrect observations of clients. The chapter also discusses the psychosocial assessment, which is a way of determining areas of difficulty and areas of strength in client functioning without being excessively oriented toward pathology. Used correctly, it can provide the practitioner with an understanding of the connecting elements that have created the current crisis in a client's life. The psychosocial assessment can help the clinician develop strategies that may move the client in directions that create significant changes. A key to the use of the psychosocial assessment is to focus on client behaviors, and to support assumptions about the cause of a problem and the most efficacious treatment, with recognition of best evidence available in the research literature.

4.8. QUESTIONS FROM THE CHAPTER

1. We are assuming Patrice is depressed because of the serious problems she had with her family. Are there alternative reasons for Patrice's depression?
2. We tend to assume that children of parents who have been traumatized will suffer negative consequences because parental traumas create problems in parenting. Do you believe that is necessarily true?
3. We often think of depression as an easily defined emotional state, but clearly people experience depression in unique ways. This makes one wonder if anti-depressive medications will help Patrice. What do you think?
4. The GAF score of 50–41 seems high for someone with the types of severe traumas and long term depression Patrice has endured. What might be a more accurate GAF score, in your opinion?
5. The presence of an "evil" but powerful person in an extended family has many negative ramifications for family life. What might they be?

References

American Psychiatric Association (1994). *Diagnostic and statistical manual of mental disorders* (4th edition). New York: Author.

Anderson, K. M. (1997, November). Uncovering survival abilities in children who have been sexually abused. *Families in Society: The Journal of Contemporary Human Services, 78*(6), *592–599.*

Beck, A. T., Ward, C. H., Mendelson, M., Mock, J., & Erbaugh, J. (1961). An inventory for measuring depression. *Archives of General Psychiatry, 4*, 561–571.

Bravo, M., Ribera, J., Rubio-Stipec, M., Canino, G., Shrout, P., Ramírez, R., Fábregas, L., Chavez, L., Alegría, M., Bauermeister, J. J., & Martinez, T. A. (2001, October). Test-retest reliability of the Spanish version of the Diagnostic Interview Schedule for Children (DISC-IV). *Journal of Abnormal Child Psychology, 29*(5), 433–444.

Burns, B. J., Costello, E. J., Angold, A., et al. (1995). Children's mental health service use across service sectors. *Health Affairs, 14*, 147Y159.

Carey, B. (2008, January 17). *Anti-depressant studies not published*. NYTIMES.COM at http://www.nytimes.com/2008/01/17/health/17depress.html?adxnnl=1&adxnnlx=1206810018-+aWGytkRS98+oCTtx1Usvg.

Cloud, J. (2003, January 30). How we get labeled. *Time, 161*(3), 102–106.

Davis, R. T., Blashfield, R. K., & McElroy, R. A. (1993). Weighting criteria in the diagnosis of a personality disorder: A demonstration. *Journal of Abnormal Psychology, 102*, 319–322.

DeAngelis, T. (2007, March). A new diagnosis for childhood trauma? Some push for a new DSM category for children who undergo multiple, complex traumas. *Monitor on Psychology, 38*(3). http://www.apa.org/monitor/mar07/diagnosis.html.

DeGrandpre, R. (1999). *Ritalin nation: Rapid-fire culture and the transformation of human consciousness*. New York: Norton.

Dumont, R., & Rauch, M. (2000). Test review: Scale for assessing emotional disturbance (SAED). *Communiqué, 28*(8), 24–25.

Epstein, M. H., & Cullinan, D. (1998). *The Scale for Assessing E motional Disturbance*. Austin, TX: PRO-ED.

Fleming, M., & Manwell, L. B. (1998). Brief intervention in primary care settings: A primary treatment method for at-risk, problem, and dependent drinkers. *Alcohol Research and Health, 23*(2), 128–137.

Foa, E. B., Hearst-Ikeda, D., & Perry, K. J. (1995). Evaluation of a brief cognitive-behavioral program for the prevention of chronic PTSD in recent assault victims. *Journal of Consulting & Clinical Psychology, 63*, 948–955.

Franklin, A. J. (1992). Therapy with African American men, Families in Society. *The Journal of Contemporary Human Services*, 350–355.

Gawande, A. (2007, December 30). *A Lifesaving Checklist*. Austin, TX: New York Times, *157*, 54172, Special section p.8.

Gentilello, L. M., Donovan, D. M., Dunn, C. W., & Rivara, F. P. (1995). Alcohol interventions in trauma centers: Current practice and future directions. *JAMA, 274*(13), 1043–1048.

Glaser, B. G. (1992). *Basics of grounded theory analysis: Emergence vs forcing*. Mill Valley, CA: Sociology Press.

Glicken, M. D. (2004). *Using the strengths perspective in social work practice*. Boston, MA: Pearson Education, Inc., p. 6.

Haverkamp, B. (1993). Confirmatory bias in hypothesis testing for client-identified and counselor self-generated hypotheses. *Journal of Consulting Psychology, 40*, 305–315.

Howard, K. I., Lueger, R. J., Mailing, M. S., & Martinovich, Z. (1993). A phase model of psychotherapy outcome: Causal mediation of change. *Journal of Consulting and Clinical Psychology, 61*, 678–685.

Howard, K. I., Moras, K., Brill, P. B., Martinovich, Z., & Lutz, W. (1996). Evaluation of psychotherapy: Efficacy, effectiveness, and client change. *American Psychologist, 51*, 1059–1064.

Kataoka, S. H., Zhang, L., & Wells, K. B. (2002). Unmet need for mental health care among U.S. children: Variation by ethnicity and insurance status. *The American Journal of Psychiatry, 159*, 1548–1555.

Keenan, K., Coyne, C., & Lahey, B. B. (2008, January). Should Relational Aggression Be Included in DSM-V?. *Journal of the American Academy of Child & Adolescent Psychiatry, 47*(1), 86–93.

Kopta, S. M. (1999, Annual). Individual psychotherapy outcome and process research: Challenges leading to greater turmoil or a positive transition? *Annual Review of Psychology*. http://www.findarticles.com/cf_0/m0961/1999_Annual/54442307/print.jhtml.

McConnaughy, E. A., Prochaska, J. O., & Velcer, W. F. (1983). Stages of change in psychotherapy: Measurement and sample profile. *Psychotherapy: Theory, Research and Practice, 20*, 375–388.

McLaughlin, J. E. (2000). Reducing diagnostic bias. *Journal of Mental Health Counseling, 24*(3), 256–270.

McLaughlin, J. E. (2002). Reducing diagnostic bias. *Journal of Mental Health Counseling, 24*(3), 256–270.

Meadows, E. A., & Foa, E. B. (1998). Intrusion, arousal, and avoidance: Sexual trauma survivors. In V. Follette, I. Ruzek, F. & Abueg (Eds.), *Cognitive-behavioral therapies for trauma* (pp. 100–123). New York: Guilford.

Monti, P. M., Colby, S. M., Barnett, N. P., et al. (1999). Brief intervention for harm reduction with alcohol-positive older adolescents in a hospital emergency department. *Journal of Consulting and Clinical Psychology, 67*(6), 989–994.

Morey, L. C., & Ochoa, E. S. (1989). An investigation of adherence to diagnostic criteria: Clinical diagnosis of the DSM-III personality disorders. *Journal of Personality Disorders, 3*, 180–192.

Myers, J. E. (1998). Bibliotherapy and the DCT: Co-constructing the therapeutic metaphor. *Journal of Counseling and Development, 76*, 234–251.

Nemeroff, R., Levitt, J. M., Faul, L., Wonpat-Borja, B. A., Bufferd, S., Setterberg, S., & Jensen, P. S. (2008, March). Establishing ongoing, early identification programs for mental health problems in our schools: A feasibility study. *Journal of the American Academy of Child and Adolescent Psychiatry, 47*(3), 328–338.

NIMH. (2008) Post-Traumatic Stress Disorder. http://www.nimh.nih.gov/health/publication./anxiety-disorders/post-traumatic-stress-disorder.shtml.

Orsulik-Jerus, S., Shepard, J. B., & Britton, P. J. (2003, July). Counseling older adults with HIV/AIDS: A strengths-based model of treatment. *Journal of Mental health Counseling, 25*(3), 233–244.

Ozer, E. J., Best, S. R., Lipsey, T. L., & Weiss, D. S. (2003). Predictors of posttraumatic stress disorder and symptoms in adults: A meta-analysis. *Psychological Bulletin, 129*(1), 52–73.

Pardeck, J. T. (1995). Bibliotherapy's innovative approach for helping children. *Early Childhood Development and Care, 110*, 83–88.

Pfeiffer, A. M., Whelan, J. P., & Martin, J. L. (2000). Decision-making in psychotherapy: Effects of hypothesis source and accountability. *Journal of Counseling Psychology, 47*, 429–436.

Radloff, L. S. (1977). The CES-D Scale: A self-report depression scale for research in the general population. *Journal of Applied Psychological Measures, 1*(3), 385–401.

Robertson, J., & Fitzgerald, L. F. (1990). The (mis) treatment of men: Effects of client gender role and life-style on diagnosis and attribution of pathology. *Journal of Counseling Psychology, 37*, 3–9.

Saleebey, D. (1996). The strengths perspective in social work practice: Extensions and cautions. *Social Work, 41*(3), 296–305.

Satcher, D. (1999). U.S. Department of Health and Human Services. Mental Health: A Report of the Surgeon General. Rockville, MD: U.S. Department of Health and Human Services, Substance Abuse and Mental Health Services Administration, Center for Mental Health Services, National Institutes of Health, National Institute of Mental Health.

Sharp, W. S., Walter, J. M., & Marsh, W. L. (1999). ADHD in girls: Clinical comparability of a research sample. *Journal of the American Academy of Child and Adolescent Psychiatry, 38*, 40–47.

Seligman, M. E. P. (1995). The effectiveness of psychotherapy: The consumers report study. *American Psychologist, 50*(12), 965–974.

Smyer, M. A. (1984). Life transitions and aging: Implications for counseling older adults. *The Counseling Psychologist, 12*(2), 1728.

U.S. Department of Health and Human Services. Mental Health: A Report of the Surgeon General. Rockville, MD: U.S. Department of Health and Human Services, Substance

Abuse and Mental Health Services Administration, Center for Mental Health Services, National Institutes of Health, National Institute of Mental Health; 1999.

Van Wormer, K. (1999, June). The strengths perspective: A paradigm for correctional counseling. *Federal Probation, 63*(1).

Whaley, A. L. (2001). Cultural mistrust: An important psychological construct for diagnosis and treatment of African Americans. *Psychology: Research and Practice, 32*(6), 555–562.

Wilcox, H., Prodromidis, M, and Scafidi, F. (1998, September 22). Correlations between BDI and CES-D in a sample of adolescent mothers. (Beck Depression Inventory; Center for Epidemiologic Studies Depression Scale). *Adolescence*, 7 http://www.findarticles.com/cf_0/m2248/131_33/53368535/p1/article.jhtml? term= beck+depression+inventory.

Wilke, D. (1994). Women and alcoholism: How a male-as-norm bias affects research, assessment, and treatment. *Health and Social Work, 19*, 29–35.

Further reading

Harvard Mental Health Letter (2002). What causes post-traumatic stress disorder: Two views. *Harvard Mental Health Letter, 19*(4), 8.

Schulberg, C. (2001, June 1). Treating Depression in Primary Care Practice. Applications of Research Findings. *Journal of Family Practice,* http://www.findarticles.com/cf_0/m0689/6_50/75995854/print.jhtml.

Part Three
Evidence Based Practice With Special Problems of Children and Adolescents

5 Evidence-Based Practice and the Troubled Families of America's Children and Adolescents

5.1. INTRODUCTION

Americans have many inconsistent beliefs about family life. While we treasure good family life and romanticize it in our films, novels, and on television, the fact is that many of us have had troubled experiences with our families, and as a result we have physically and emotionally distanced ourselves from them. This process of removing ourselves from our families brings about an equally American condition: loneliness and a feeling of isolation from others. As bad as family life can be, the alternative for children and adolescents can be just as bad, or worse.

As the following discussion will show, family life has been changing in America for better and for worse. Divorce rates, while declining, are still very high. Too many families lack medical insurance or suitable housing. Far too many children suffer from lack of food or abusive conditions and, more than ever, families are held to very high legal standards in terms of their ability to care for children. Yet families are the system that we believe should socialize children and teach them ethics and values. Families are supposed to house and feed children and care for them when they suffer from physical and emotional problems. And families are also supposed to promote education and teach children about citizenship and love of country and community. But when they can't or don't, we have a complex social service system to offer financial, housing and counseling services often staffed by social workers. This safety net of services is in place to help families stay together and function well. In this chapter we will explore the nature of those services and the way social work functions in the social welfare agencies and organizations most responsible for helping families in need.

5.2. THE CHANGING FAMILY IN AMERICA

Many aspects of family life in America have dramatically changed during the past 50 years. *The Journal of Pediatrics* (2003, June) reports the following data on family life in America: (1) the majority of families in America now have no children younger than 18 years of age; (2) people are marrying at an older age and the highest number of births occurs in women over the age of 30; (3) from

1970 to 2000, children in two-parent families decreased from 85% to 69%; (4) twenty-six percent of all children lived with a single parent, usually their mother; (5) the rate of births to unmarried women has gone from 5.3% in 1960 to 33.2% in 2000, and the divorce rate, while slowing, is still twice as high as it was in 1955; (6) the median income of female-headed households is only 47% of the median income of married-couple families; (7) the number of children living in poverty is now five times higher for female-headed families than for married-couple families; (8) in 2001, 36% of all U.S. households with children had one or more of the following three housing problems: physically inadequate housing, crowded housing, or housing that cost more than 30% of the household income; (9) in 2002, about 5.6 million children, or 8% of the total, lived in a household that included a grandparent. The majority of these children (3.7 million) lived in the grandparent's home; of these, two-thirds had a parent present; and (10) children living in a grandparent's home with neither parent present were more likely to be poor (30%) than children living in their parent's home with a grandparent present (12%), or children living in a grandparent's home with a parent present (15%).

While the concept of family is still well thought of in America, when social issues arise such as youth crime and lowering educational achievement, we tend to blame the family for problems experienced by children, while at the same time looking to the family for solutions. The final report of the American Assembly (2000) suggests that changing social conditions in America have not only weakened families but have over-stressed many families, resulting in increasing numbers of troubled families and with it, increasing numbers of malfunctioning children and adolescents. The idealized notion of the traditional family with one parent working and another staying at home and caring for the children has been replaced by families unable to succeed economically without both parents working; latch key children who are home alone for long periods of time after school; increasing amounts of family violence; and poorly supervised children with parents believing that so long as they clothe, feed, and provide housing for their children, anything that goes wrong with the child is the result of malfunctioning social institutions such as schools which have increasing responsibilities not only to modify poor social behavior but provide values, teach children about relationships and intimacy, and in many ways, act as surrogates for missing, chaotic, and poorly functioning families.

The social and economic pressures on American families have increased in many ways. Time, for example, which includes time to get to work and back, makes for a lengthening day for the family, complicated by the use of child care that places children in environments a distance from their homes where they respond to a number of forces that place them at risk of influences that compromise family values and result in incompatible approaches to discipline. *The Journal of Pediatrics* (2003, June) writes that, "In public opinion polls, most parents report that they believe it is more difficult to be a parent now than it used to be; people seem to feel more isolated, social and media pressures on and enticements of their children seem greater, and the world seems to be a more dangerous place" (p. 1541).

According to the National Opinion Research Center at the University of Chicago (2004), the American family has undergone a major transformation in the past generation and will likely continue to change in the future. Because of divorce, cohabitation, and single parenthood, a majority of families rearing children will probably not include the children's original two parents. Moreover, most households will not include children. Rates of marriage also are changing, and middle-class people are more likely to marry and remarry than working-class people, who are more likely to remain single or cohabit. From 1972 to 1977, 80% of working-class and middle-class adults were married. During the 1994 to 1998 period, 78% of middle-class adults were married, as opposed to 68% of working-class adults. The report goes on to say that,

> *Marriage has declined as the central institution under which households are organized and children are raised. People marry later and divorce and cohabitate more. A growing proportion of children have been born outside of marriage. Even within marriage the changes have been profound as more and more women have entered the labor force and gender roles have become more homogenous between husbands and wives. (p. 1)*

One of this generation's biggest changes is in the parental arrangements for children. In 1972, 73% of children lived with their original two parents, who were married. By 1998, 51.7% lived in such households. The number of children living with single parents went from 4.7% in 1972 to 18.2% in 1998, while the number of children living with two unmarried adults moved from 3.8% to 8.6% during this period. Cohabiting and remarried parents made up the rest of the group.

Besharov (2001) believes that the future family will include later marriage, smaller families and cohabitation and temporary relationships between people. "Overall, what I see is a situation in which people – especially children – will be much more isolated, because not only will their parents both be working, but they'll have fewer siblings, fewer cousins, fewer aunts and uncles. So over time, we're moving towards a much more individualistic society" (Besharov, 2001, p. 1)

5.3. HEALTHY FAMILIES

In developing a list of the attributes of healthy families that help develop resilient children, *The Journal of Pediatrics* (2003, June) indicates that a well-functioning family consists of two married parents who offer children secure, supportive, and nurturing environments. Children have more life success when raised by caring and cooperative parents who have adequate social and financial resources. Defining parental attributes that lead to resilient children, Spock (1985) says,

"Good-hearted parents who aren't afraid to be firm when it is necessary can get good results with either moderate strictness or moderate permissiveness.... The real issue is what spirit the parent puts into managing the child and what attitude is engendered in the child as a result" (p. 8). Baumrind (1966) believes that parents who combine warmth and affection with firm limit setting are more likely to have "children who are happy, creative, and cooperative; have high self-esteem; are achievement oriented; and do well academically and socially" (p. 887). Parents who are unresponsive, rigid, controlling, disengaged, overly permissive, and uninvolved jeopardize the emotional health of their children and these parental attributes consistently result in less emotionally strong and resilient children (Spieker et al., 1999; Simons et al., 1994). Parents who supervise their children both inside and outside of the home, who encourage growth-enhancing activities, and who then move toward shared-decision making and responsibility with children as they mature are likely to have the healthiest and most resilient children.

Chatterji and Markowitz (2000) report the negative impact of parental substance abuse, noting that it affects the social, psychological, and emotional well-being of children and their families. The researchers indicate that 10% of American adults are addicted to substances which often cause them depression and frequently lead to family life that is often disrupted, chaotic, filled with conflict, and which may ultimately result in poverty, family violence, and divorce. Children in homes where one or both parents abuse substances are themselves more at risk of abusing substances and experiencing increased amounts of behavioral problems.

5.4. FAMILIES IN POVERTY

The following data also comes from the 2003 report on the condition of America's children and families published by the Federal Interagency Forum on Child and Family Statistics in a report entitled: *America's Children: Key National Indicators of Well-Being, 2003* (Found on the Internet May 19, 2004).

(1) The proportion of children living in families with incomes below the poverty threshold was 16% in 2001. (2) In 1993, 54% of children living in female-householder families were living in poverty; by 2001, this proportion had decreased to 39%. (3) In 2001, 18% of children under age six lived in poverty, compared with 15% of older children. (4) In 2001, 8% of children in married-couple families were living in poverty, compared with 39% in female-householder families. (5) In 2001, 10% of Black children in married-couple families lived in poverty, compared with 47% of Black children in female-householder families. Twenty percent of Hispanic children in married-couple families lived in poverty, compared with 49% in female-householder families. (6) In 2001, 9% of White, non-Hispanic children lived in poverty, compared with 30% of Black children and 27% of Hispanic children. (7) Just under half a million children (0.6%) lived in households with child hunger in 2001. In 2001, 4.1% of all children

lived in households classified as food-insecure with hunger. (8) Children living in poverty are much more likely than others to experience food insecurity and hunger. In 2001, about 2.6% of the children living in poverty were in households with hunger among children, compared with 0.3% of children in households with incomes at or above the poverty line. In 2001, nearly 45.9% of children living in poverty were in food-insecure households, compared with 11.5% of children living at or above the poverty line. (9) Children in families below the poverty level are less likely than higher-income children to have a diet rated as good. In 1999–2000, for children ages two to six, 17% of those in poverty had a good diet, compared with 22% of those living at or above the poverty line.

Noting the negative effect of poverty on children, Krugman (2008, Feb. 18) reports that the poverty level is not only higher in 2006 than it was in 1969 (14% versus 17.4%) but that "many children growing up in very poor families with low social status experience unhealthy levels of stress hormones, which impair their neural development. The effect is to impair language development and memory – and hence the ability to escape poverty – for the rest of the child's life (p. 1). Krugman goes on to say that living in or near poverty is a form of exile where being poor makes one an outcast, and where American children born to parents in the bottom fourth of income distribution have a 50% chance of staying poor and a 67% chance of staying poor if the child is black. Children with high scores on standardized achievement tests who came from poor families were much less likely to go to college, according to Krugman. Poverty, he notes, trumps ability.

5.5. FAMILY HEALTH CARE DATA

The following data comes from a 2003 report on the condition of America's children and families published by the Federal Interagency Forum on Child and Family Statistics in a report entitled: *America's Children: Key National Indicators of Well-Being, 2003* (Found on the Internet May 19, 2004).

1. In 2001, 88% of children had health insurance coverage at some point during the year, maintaining the all-time high established in 2000. However, between 85% and 88% of children have had health insurance in each year since 1987, leaving 12–15% of all children consistently without health insurance.
2. The number of children who had no health insurance at any time during 2001 was 8.5 million (12% of all children), which was similar to 2000.
3. The proportion of children covered by private health insurance decreased from 74% in 1987 to 66% in 1994, then increased to 70% in 1999, but dropped down to 68% in 2001. During the same time period, the proportion of children covered by government health insurance grew from 19% in 1987 to a high of 27% in 1993. Government health insurance decreased until 1999 and then began to climb again to 26% in 2001.
4. Hispanic children are less likely to have health insurance than White, non-Hispanic or Black children. In 2001, 76% of Hispanic children were covered by health

insurance, compared with 93% of White, non-Hispanic children and 86% of Black children.

5.6. FAMILY RESILIENCE

McCubbin and McCubbin (1993, 1996) believe that family resilience consists of two important family processes: (1) *adjustment*, which includes the strength of *protective factors* in mobilizing the family's efforts to maintain its integrity, functioning, and fulfill developmental tasks in the face of risk factors; and, (2) *adaptation*, which include *recovery factors* which permit the family to effectively respond to a crisis. Family resilience is the ability of the family to deal with a crisis, to understand the potential risk factors associated with a crisis, and to develop recovery strategies that permit family members to cope and adapt to crisis situations. Family crises might include financial problems, health problems, unemployment, marital problems, abusive behavior by a caregiver, social and emotional problems of children, loss of a home, and any number of problems that affect the entire family.

In additional studies of resilience in children, Baldwin et al. (1990) note the importance of parental supervision and vigilance. Conrad and Harnmen (1993) emphasize the importance of maternal social support for children. In a study of 144 middle-class families, half of which were divorced, Hetherington (1989) indicates the importance of structured parenting. Richters and Martinez (1993) found that low-income children living in a violent neighborhood did best when living in a stable and safe home environment. Wyman et al. (1991) found that children did best when the parenting style consisted of consistent discipline and an optimistic view of the children's future. Wyman et al. (1992) found that children who were most successful in grades 4–6 had nurturing relationships with primary caregivers and stable, consistent family environments. Werner and Smith (1992) reinforce the importance of family environmental factors, including self-confident mothers who value their children, supportive alternate caregivers, and supportive spouses.

In describing the factors that assist family recovery from a crisis, Hamilton et al. (1997) believe that the critical factors are:

(1) *Family integration*: parental efforts to keep the family together and to be optimistic about the future. (2) *Family support and esteem building*: parental efforts to get community and extended family support to assist in developing the self-esteem and self-confidence of their children. (3) *Family recreation orientation, control, and organization*: a family emphasis on recreation and family entertainment. (4) *Discipline*: family life that includes organization, rules, and procedures. (5) *Family optimism and mastery:* the more families have a sense of order and optimism, the healthier the children.

In summarizing the research on family resilience, Walsh (2003) identifies the key processes in family resilience as follows: (1) making meaning of adversity by normalizing the stressful situation and understanding and managing it; (2)

having a positive outlook by being optimistic and having confidence that family crises will be resolved; (3) providing inspiration with transcendence and spirituality as new ways to resolve a crisis and often providing a bonding and supportive group that assists in resolving the crisis; (4) allowing flexibility such that families can adapt to new challenges; (5) encouraging connectedness whereby the family shows mutual support, collaboration and commitment; (6) providing social and economic resources which permit economic security and allow families to balance work with family time; (7) ensuring clarity in the way a crisis is viewed and the ability to communicate within the family to resolve difficulties; (8) allowing open emotional expression, so that family members share feelings, joke, and interact in a safe and positive way; and (9) allowing collaborative problem-solving and creative brainstorming, proactive stances, building on success and learning from failures.

In summarizing the concept of family resilience, Walsh (2003) writes,

> *Building on theory and research, on family stress, coping, and adaptation (Patterson, 2002), the concept of family resilience entails more than managing stressful conditions, shouldering a burden, or surviving an ordeal. It involves the potential for personal and relational transformation and growth that can be forged out of adversity (Boss, 2001). Tapping into key processes for resilience, families can emerge stronger and more resourceful in meeting future challenges. A crisis can be a wake-up call, heightening attention to what matters. It can become an opportunity for reappraisal of priorities, stimulating greater investment in meaningful relationships and life pursuits. Members may discover or develop new insights and abilities. Many families report that through weathering a crisis together their relationships were enriched and more loving than they might otherwise have been. (p. 3).*

5.7. FAMILY THERAPY

Although there are a number of schools of thought about how best to perform family therapy, several of the major themes in family therapy presented by Asen (2003) include the following:

1. **The Structural Approach** (Minuchin, 1974): believes that families function particularly best when certain family structures prevail, including hierarchies between the generations within a family that permit a sufficient flow of information up and down between parents and their children.
2. **Strategic Systemic Therapy** (Haley, 1963; Watzlawick et al., 1974): is based on the hypothesis that the symptom is being maintained by behaviors that seek to suppress it. Strategic therapists argue that once some changes are achieved in relation to the presenting symptom, a domino effect sets in, affecting other interactions and behaviors in the whole family and the larger system. The patient's perceived problem(s) are put into a different meaning-frame that provides new perspectives and therefore potentially makes new behaviors possible.
3. **The Milan systemic approach** (Selvini et al., 1978): focuses on questioning the various family members' beliefs and perceptions regarding relationships. Asking each

to comment and reflect on the answers given by the various family members creates feedback that changes the fabric of family interactions.

4. **The Social Constructionist Approach** (White and Epston 1990): is based on the awareness that the reality which the therapist observes is invented, with perceptions being shaped by the therapist's own cultures and his/her implicit assumptions and beliefs. This approach is influencing many systemic therapists and has led to an examination of how language shapes problem perceptions and definitions.
5. **Narrative Therapists:** narrative therapists co-construct new ways of describing the individual and related family issues so that they no longer need to be viewed or experienced as problematic.
6. **Psychoeducational Approaches** (Leff et al., 1982): in this approach family members are educated about the causes and course of a family member's emotional problems and are taught helpful ways to share experiences and solutions in family sessions.
7. **Behavioral Family and Couple Therapy** (Falloon, 1988): communication training is an example of a behavioral intervention strategy emphasizing the direct expression of positive feelings, ideas and plans. Behavioral therapists may also use structured problem-solving to formulate detailed implementation plans and to systematically review their change efforts and results.
8. **Multisystemic Treatment (MST)**: has been found to be exceptionally effective in engaging substance abusing juvenile offenders (Henggeler et al., 1996), and has produced favorable short-term (Henggeler et al., 2000) and long-term (Henggeler et al. 2002) reductions in drug use.
9. **Multidimensional Family Therapy (MDFT)**: MDFT devotes substantive resources to building an alliance with each youth (e.g., about 40% of sessions are with adolescents alone) and reestablishing emotional connections between the adolescent and his or her caregivers (Liddle, 1999). This approach focuses more on family affective processes and less on behavioral conceptualizations of problems and their solutions. Nevertheless, the roles of extra familiar systems in maintaining problems are addressed through a case management process.
10. **Contingency Management (CM)**: CM has produced promising results for substance-using adolescents (Donohue and Azrin, 2001). CM uses behavioral techniques to help youth: avoid situations associated with drug use; engage in pro-social activities incompatible with drug use; and change cognitions and feelings associated with drug use. Additionally, drug use is traced through frequent urine drug screens, and caregivers are empowered to reward abstinence and otherwise reinforce desired behavior change.
11. **Brief Strategic Family Therapy (BSFT)**: BSFT (Szapocznik and Williams, 2000) is a structural family therapy approach in which adolescent drug abuse is viewed as the result of several types of maladaptive family interventions (e.g., inappropriate alliances scapegoating the adolescent). The therapist's intervention initially aims at "joining" the family to gain an understanding of the types of repetitive family interactions that are linked with the identified problems. Later, the therapist actively restructures family relations with the goal of increasing the caregiver's authority and facilitating more effective intra-family communication. BSFT, a recent report (Santisteban et al., 2003) has demonstrated favorable short-term youth and family outcomes in comparison with group treatment (Santisteban et al., 2003).
12. **Functional Family Therapy (FFT)**: FFT integrates cognitive-behavioral therapy (CBT) strategies to teach the individual adolescent self-control and drug-refusal

skills. CBT (Carroll, 1998) is a widely used, evidence-based treatment for substance abusing adults. The results of a randomized trial, (Waldron et al., 2001), modestly supported the combined effectiveness of FFT/CBT over FFT in the reduction of adolescent drug use.

Asen (2003) conducted a meta-analysis on the effectiveness of a variety of systemic family therapy approaches. Using the following criteria for levels of evidence, he believes there is Type I evidence (at least one good systematic review, including at least one randomized controlled trial (RCT) for a number of conditions and presentations), considerable Type II evidence (at least one good RCT) and even more Type III evidence (at least one well-designed intervention study without randomization), as well as Type IV evidence (at least one well-designed observational study). Asen notes that Type V evidence (expert opinion, including the opinion of service users and careers) is increasing.

Asen's meta-analysis found that systemic family therapy has been found to be effective alone or in conjunction with other treatments in a wide range of conditions of children and adolescents, including presentations including conduct problems in children (Kazdin, 1998; Serketich and Dumas, 1996), drug and alcohol misuse in adolescents and adults (Edwards and Steinglass, 1995; Stanton and Shadish, 1997; Waldron, 1996) and marital distress (Baucom et al., 1998; Dunn and Schwebel, 1995; Jacobson and Addis, 1993). Controlled trials have shown the effectiveness of systemic therapy interventions in childhood (Gustafsson et al., 1986), enuresis and soiling (Houts et al., 1994; Silver et al., 1998), oppositional behavior problems (Serketich and Dumas, 1996) and a range of other presentations and conditions in children and their families (Carr, 2000). Systemic family and couple therapy have also been shown to be effective in the treatment of eating disorders, psychotic illnesses and mood disorders.

In determining whether family therapy systems met standards for best evidence, Dyer (2006) reports that Multidimensional Family Therapy (MDFT) (Liddle, 1999), is an approach with promising potential for work with minority youths who suffer from dual-occurring disorders. In describing MDFT, Dyer writes,

> *"MDFT is a family-based, multi-component treatment that targets the multiple systems (e.g., family, school, work, peer). At the youth level, therapists focus on building youth competencies by teaching communication and problem-solving skills. At the family level, therapists work to change negative family interaction patterns, and coach parents in ways to appropriately engage with their children." (p. 34)*

Dyer (2006) further reports that *Multisystemic Treatment* (*MST*) met Type 2 efficacy criteria for drug-abusing minority youth. Henggeler et al. (2000) studied 118 juvenile offenders with co-occurring drug abuse/dependence disorders who were randomly assigned to MST or usual community services. MST youths had lower marijuana use when outcomes were based on urine/hair samples, although there were no differences in self-reported drug use (Henggeler et al., 2002).

5.8. CASE STUDY: FAMILY THERAPY BEFORE THE IDEA OF BEST EVIDENCE

Jimmy Fox is a 10-year-old boy living with his sisters Suzanne (11) and Jane (7), and his mother Jackie (33) and father Sam (39) in suburban Chicago. Jimmy is failing at school even though he has a superior IQ. The girls are doing well in school and Jimmy is a sweet, somewhat befuddled boy who seems withdrawn but friendly and engaged in treatment. Engaged is probably not a fully descriptive term in that he comes to treatment, talks but never seems to be able to apply what we talk about. It is not resistance or lack of motivation, necessarily, but more an attempt to cope with a world he does not understand and often is not a part of.

Jimmy had to repeat first grade and is now in the 3rd grade, which he is on the verge of also having to repeat. Prior help for Jimmy by the school social worker appears to have been unsuccessful. In referring the family for treatment, the social worker wrote, "I worked with Jimmy for a full school year, and while he is a friendly boy who is never a behavioral problem in the classroom, he seems socially inept, unable to understand why he does badly academically, and frankly doesn't seem to mind failing. His teacher says that Jimmy is often so socially inept in class that the children make fun of him and call him a 'space cadet.' I have found him to be delightful, and I don't say this to suggest pathology, in a early childlike fantasy world where he always saves others from catastrophes and champions the underdog. These fantasies are sustaining to him and pleasurable."

He speaks lovingly of his family and wants badly to please his father who often, in Jimmy's rendering of events, seems unhappy with Jimmy and critical of Jimmy's many attempts to please him. He says very little about his mother but enjoys his sisters and says they're great. I've met with Jimmy's parents. His father is a jovial man who admits that Jimmy mystifies him and that he is, indeed, critical, having lost his patience with Jimmy long ago. Jimmy's mother seems detached from Jimmy and his problems. She spent a good deal of time talking about her own family, successful and prominent in her telling, and how no one failed in that family. Jimmy's problems must, she concludes, be caused by something in her husband's family, whom she characterized as socially inferior and not in the same league as her own. The husband seems to accept his wife's appraisal of the reasons for Jimmy's behavior.

The therapist who worked with Jimmy and his family said, "I'm a cognitive therapist and I try and apply cognitive-behavioral principles to my family work. After reading the referral material and speaking briefly to Jimmy's mother, I looked at the family therapy literature and thought I would apply cognitive-behavioral principles to what I could find in the literature on family therapy. From a research point of view, there wasn't much. Cognitive therapy made sense because I was having good success with individual and group patients. I saw it as an educational approach and believed that family therapy was a way of educating families into better communication patterns through problem-solving. I was pretty new to family therapy then, and when I read the literature now, what

I was doing was a kind of application of cognitive-behavioral principles adapted to family therapy or something very much like the approach used by Waldron et al. (2001) called functional family therapy."

"The first meeting was very instructive. Both parents used it to tell stories about Jimmy and his flights of fantasy. The father said that a chair at the dinner table was a bit wobbly and without telling anyone, Jimmy took the chair down to the basement, took it apart, and resembled it. Unknowingly, the father sat on it, and the chair broke, sending him sprawling to the floor and bumping his head on the table. Jimmy smiled and nodded during the telling of the story and explained that he just wanted to do something nice for his dad. As usual, his dad said, the something nice turned out to be something that made things worse."

I wondered if Jimmy could talk a bit about how he felt in the family. He looked bewildered. "I like everyone," he said.

"Do you like being made fun of," I asked.

"Sure, if I deserve it."

I looked around the room and observed that everyone was shaking their heads, and I pointed it out. "How else should we look?" his mother said, "he's just a clown."

"Are you a clown?" I asked Jimmy.

"I don't know, that's what everyone says."

"Clowns get people to laugh. I wondered if it feels like you're getting attention when others laugh at you?"

"Maybe," Jimmy said.

"And failing gets a lot of attention, too, I guess."

"Maybe," Jimmy said.

We spoke some more about the family and it soon became clear that Jimmy's role in the family was that of the scapegoat. Even the girls thought that Jimmy was strange and that they couldn't really take him seriously.

"OK, I said, your job over the next week is not to laugh, criticize or complain about Jimmy. He's a regular family person and no more putting all of your anger at the world on to Jimmy."

I can't say that Jimmy blossomed from family therapy, but when we took the burden of getting attention away for negative behavior, Jimmy's grades and his conduct improved gradually. Families that scapegoat are not happy families, and that was true of Jimmy's. There were tensions between the mother and Suzanne, who described her mother indirectly as cold, aloof and highly critical. In a meeting with each of the family members to get their feedback on how things were going at home, Suzanne said that often when she came home she would find her mother on the coach reading, and at seeing Suzanne, a look of disgust would come over the mother's face. Suzanne would hurry to her room and stay there until dinner so she wouldn't have to see her mom again and feel her mom's unmistakable, but to Suzanne, illogical hostility. "I try real hard to be good at home and school," she said, "but the more I try the more my mom seems to hate me."

The father assured me that his wife was a loving and kind mother and a good wife, but the children look skeptical when he says that in family sessions, and only Jane, the seven-year-old, occasionally says in a meek voice, "My mom's nice."

"My expectations for the family were for Jimmy to improve and for the others to form a stronger family bond. I think it happened between the father and the children, but the wife never gave me a sense that things would ever get better and she continued to look uncomfortable in therapy, ultimately telling me that she just didn't think it was doing much good and they couldn't afford more session, anyway. Jimmy, she said, was the way he was and she'd read somewhere that if you're a clown at 10 you'll be one at 40, and she guessed that was true."

"I spoke to the school social worker and suggested that she continue working with Jimmy. He seemed to respond to suggestions and homework and that working with teachers about praising his positive behavior would lower the tendency to look for negative attention. She told me a few years later that Jimmy was testing in the high 140s for IQ, but that he was still doing work just good enough to get by. "He's a sweet kid, and it makes your heart break that he isn't working at his fullest potential, but maybe when he's older. I believe," she said, "that people are resilient and once they leave troubled homes like Jimmy's, they do better."

"A mutual friend told me that after high school Jimmy joined the army and went to language school to learn Chinese. Only the brightest recruits were sent to language school and he thrived. After the army he became a computer expert. While his personal life was always touched with unhappiness and poor choices of mates, his work life flourished. I also heard the daughters did well in life and also flourished in their work life but didn't do as well in their personal lives. It's a struggle to overcome parental rejection but maybe the few months we worked together helped in the long-term ways I think therapy helps people like Jimmy and his family. I also heard that Jimmy's father died tragically at a young age and a few years after his death his wife became a recluse. I'm not surprised. She seemed like an unhappy person then, and in the three months we worked together I never felt any sense of warmth or human concern. She was, I think even then, a recluse, and believed that her children were intruders in her life."

"I wish there had been a practice literature to use when I saw the family but all I could find were descriptions of family therapy and some anecdotal evidence that it worked. I'm happy to see that there is some evidence that what I did seems to be effective but, believe me, other than going to workshops and having some supervision in family therapy, I was flying by the seat of my pants back then. I think most of us were and it made clinic wisdom take on importance it should never have had. I think the lack of dependence on research evidence continues to affect treatment to this day. It seems an odd way for the human service professions to be at a time of such criticism about what we do."

5.9. SUMMARY

This chapter discusses the changing American family and the many pressures and stressors placed on family life. Although we have made strides, too many children are still without adequate medical care, housing, finances or nutrition. A story noting problems in a family describes the impact of a child who is scapegoated by his siblings and parents.

5.10. QUESTIONS FROM THE CHAPTER

1. No society is perfect and America, for all the criticism we hear about family life, seems to be offering a great deal of help to families with a good deal of success. Do you agree or disagree with this statement?
2. We have heard the term, "two Americas," one with all the benefits of wealth (good health insurance, housing and opportunity) and the other America with limited opportunity, poor health insurance, problems in housing and insufficient income. Which America do you live in? Explain your answer.
3. It is difficult to believe that any American family goes hungry, but according to the data provided in this chapter, almost 5% of all children in America live in food scarce homes. How could this be in a country with so much excess food that a great deal of it is thrown away because of spoilage?
4. Divorce rates are declining but are still 40% of all marriages. Why do you think the divorce rate is so high and what do you think we can do to help marriages succeed?
5. Should our institutions take more responsibility for families to take some of the pressures off working parents who have limited incomes, energy, and time to do better jobs with their children? Who might those institutions be and what do you think they can do to help family life?

References

America's Children: Key National Indicators of Well-Being, 2003. The Official website of the federal interagency forum on child and family statistics. http://www.childstats.gov/. (found on Internet May 19, 2004).

American Assembly. (2000). Strengthening American Families: Reweaving the Social Tapestry. Final report of the ninety-seventh American Assembly, September 21–23, 2000. Available at: www.americanassembly.org/programs/uas_families_TOC.htm. Accessed August 9, 2001.

Asen, E. (2003). Advances in Psychiatric Treatment. *The Royal College of Psychiatrists, 8*, 230–238.

Baldwin, A. L., Baldwin, C., & Cole, R. E. (1990). Stress-resistant families and stress-resistant children. In J. Rolf, A. Masten, D. Cicchetti, K. Neuchterlein, S. & Weintraub (Eds.), *Risk and protective factors in the development of psychopathology* (pp. 257–280). Cambridge University Press.

Baucom, D., Shoham, V., Mueser, K., et al. (1998). Empirically supported couple and family interventions for marital distress and adult mental health problems. *Journal of Consulting and Clinical Psychology, 66*, 53–88.

Baumrind, D. (1966). Effects of authoritative control on child behavior. *Child Development, 37*, 887–907.

Besharov, D. (2001). *Reflections on family. A conversation with Douglas Besharov.* http://usinfo.state.gov/journals/itsv/0101/ijse/besharov.htm.

Boss, P. (2001). *Family stress management: A contextual approach.* Newbury Park, CA: Sage Publications.

Carr, A. (2000). Evidence-based practice in family therapy and systemic consultation I. *Journal of Family Therapy, 22*, 29–60.

Carroll, K. M. (1998). A cognitive-behavioral approach: Treating cocaine addiction (Publication No. NIH 98-4308). Washington, *U.S. Department of Health and Human Services, National Institute of Health* DC.

Chatterji, P. & Markowitz, S. (2000). *The impact of maternal alcohol and illicit drug use on children's behavior problems: Evidence from the children of the national longitudinal survey of youth.* Cambridge, MA: National Bureau of Economic Research Inc. (Working Paper No. 7692).

Conrad, M., & Harnmen, C. (1993). Protective and risk factors in high and low risk children: A comparison of children with unipolar, bipolar, medically ill, and normal mothers. *Development and psychopathology, 5*, 593–607.

Donohue, B., & Azrin, N. H. (2001). Family behavior therapy. In E. F. Wagner, H. B. & Saldron (Eds.), *Innovations in adolescent substance abuse* (pp. 205–227). New York: Pergamon.

Dunn, R., & Schwebel, A. (1995). Meta-analytic review of marital therapy outcome research. *Journal of Family Psychology, 9*, 58–68.

Dyer, F. (2006). Evidence Based treatment for adolescents with co-occurring disorders. *Counselor, 7*(2), 28–35.

Edwards, M., & Steinglass, P. (1995). Family therapy treatment outcomes for alcoholism. *Journal of Marital and Family Therapy, 21*, 475–509.

Falloon, I. (1988). Behavioural family therapy: Systems, structures and strategies. In E. Street, W. & Dryden (Eds.), *Family therapy in Britain.* Milton Keynes & Philadelphia: Open University Press.

Gustafsson, P., Kjellman, N., & Cederbald, M. (1986). Family therapy in the treatment of severe childhood asthma. *Journal of Psychosomatic Research, 30*, 369–374.

Haley, J. (1963). *Strategies of psychotherapy.* New York: Grune and Stratton.

Hamilton, McCubbin, McCubbin, Thompson, Sae-Young Han, and Allen (1997).

Henggeler, S. W., Pickrel, S. G., Brondino, M. J., & Crouch, J. L. (1996). Eliminating (almost) treatment dropout of substance abusing or dependent delinquents through home-based multisystemic therapy. *American Journal of Psychiatry, 153*, 427–428.

Henggeler, S. W., Pickrel, S. G., & Brondino, M. J. (2000). Multisystemic treatment of substance abusing and dependent delinquents: Outcomes, treatments, fidelity, and transportability. *Mental Health Services Research, 1*, 171–184.

Henggeler, S. W., Schoenwald, S. K., Clilngempeel, H. J., Rowland, M. D., & Cummmingham, P. B. (2002). *Serious emotional disturbance in children and adolescents: Multisystemic therapy.* New York: Guilford Press.

Hetherington, E. M. (1989). Coping with family transitions: Winners, losers and survivors. *Child Development, 60*, 1–14.

Houts, A., Berman, J., & Abramson, H. (1994). Effectiveness of psychological and pharmacological treatments for nocturnal enuresis. *Journal of Counselling and Clinical Psychology, 62*, 737–745.

Jacobson, N. S., & Addis, M. E. (1993). Research on couples and couple therapy: What do we know?. *Journal of Consulting and Clinical Psychology, 61*, 85–93.

Journal of Pediatrics. (2003). *The changing American family*. Part 2 of 3, Vol. 111 Issue 6, pp. 1541–1572. Author.

Kazdin, A. (1998). Psychosocial treatments for conduct disorder in children. In P. Nathan, J. & Gorman (Eds.), *A Guide to Treatments that Work*. New York: Oxford University Press.

Krugman, P. (2008, February 18). *Poverty is poison*. NYTimes.com http://www.nytimes.com/2008/02/18/opinion/18krugman.html?th&emc=th.

Leff, J., Kuipers, L., Berkowitz, R., et al. (1982). A controlled trial of social intervention in schizophrenic families. *British Journal of Psychiatry, 141*, 121–134.

Liddle, H. A. (1999). *Multidimensional family therapy treatment manual*. Miami, Florida: University of Miami School of Medicine.

McCubbin, M. A., & McCubbin, H. I. (1993). Family coping with health crises: The resiliency model of family stress, adjustment and adaptation. In C. Danielson, B. Hamel-Bissell, P. & Winstead-Fry (Eds.), *Families; health, and illness*. New York: Mosby.

McCubbin, M. A., & McCubbin, H. I. (1996). Resiliency in families: A conceptual model of family adjustment and adaptation in response to stress and crises. In H. I. McCubbin, A. I. Thompson, M. A. & McCubbin (Eds.), *Family assessment: Resiliency, coping and adaptation–Inventories for research and practice* (pp. 1–64). Madison, WI: University of Wisconsin System.

Minuchin, S. (1974). *Families and family therapy*. London: Tavistock.

National Opinion Research Center at the University of Chicago (2004).

Patterson, J. (2002). Integrating family resilience and family stress theory. *Journal of Marriage and the Family, 64*, 349–360.

Richters, J. E., & Martinez, P. E. (1993). Violent communities, family choices, and children's chances: An algorithm for improving the odds. *Development and Psychopathology, 5*, 609–627.

Santisteban, D. A., Coatsworth, J. D., Perez-Vidal, A., Kurtines, W. M., Schwartz, S. J., LaPerriene, A., & Szapocznik, J. (2003). Efficacy of brief strategic family therapy in modifying Hispanic adolescent behavior problems and substance use. *Journal of Family Psychology, 17*, 121–133.

Selvini. , Palazzoli, M., Boscolo, L., Cecchin, G., et al. (1978). *Paradox and counterparadox: A new model in the therapy of the family in schizophrenic transaction*. New York: Jason Aronson.

Serketich, W., & Dumas, J. E. (1996). The effectiveness of behavioural parent training to modify antisocial behaviour in children: A meta-analysis. *Behaviour Therapy, 27*, 171–186.

Silver, E., Williams, A., Worthington, F., et al. (1998). Family therapy and soiling: An audit of externalising and other approaches. *Journal of Family Therapy, 20*, 412–422.

Simons, R. L., Johnson, C., & Conger, R. D. (1994). Harsh corporal punishment versus quality of parental involvement as an explanation of adolescent maladjustment. *Journal of Marriage and Family, 56*, 591–607.

Spieker, S. J., Larson, N. C., Lewis, S. M., Keller, T. E., & Gilchrist, L. (1999). Developmental trajectories of disruptive behavior problems in preschool children of adolescent mothers. *Child Development, 70*, 443–458.

Stanton, M., & Shadish, W. (1997). Outcome, attrition and family-couples treatment for drug abuse: A meta-analysis and review of the controlled comparative studies. *Psychological Bulletin, 122*, 170–191.

Szapocznik, J., & Williams, R. A. (2000). Brief strategic family therapy: Twenty-five years of interplay among theory, research and practice in adolescent behavior problems and drug abuse. *Clinical Child and Family Psychology Review, 3*, 117–134.

Waldron, H. B. (1996). Adolescent substance abuse and family therapy outcome: A review of randomized trials. *Advances in Clinical Child Psychology, 19*, 199–234.

Waldron, H. B., Slesnick, N., Brody, J. L., Turner, C. W., & Peterson, J. R. (2001). Treatment outcomes for adolescent substance abuse at 4- and 7-month assessments. *Journal of Consulting and Clinical Psychology, 69*, 802–813.

Walsh, F. (2003). Family resilience: A framework for clinical practice – theory and practice. *Family Processes, 42*, 1–18.

Werner, E. E., & Smith, R. S. (1992). *Overcoming the odds: High risk children from birth to adulthood*. New York: Cornell University Press.

White, M., & Epston, D. (1990). *Narrative means to therapeutic ends*. New York: W.W. Norton.

Wyman, P. A., Cowen, E. L., Work, W. C., & Parker, G. R. (1991). Developmental and family milieu correlates of resilience in urban children who have experienced major life stress. *American Journal of Community Psychology, 19*(3), 405–426.

Wyman, P. A., Cowen, E. L., Work, W. C., Raoof, A., Gribble, P. A., Parker, G. R., & Wannon, M. (1992). Interviews with children who experienced major life stress: Family and child attributes that predict resilient outcomes. *Journal of the American Academy of Child and Adolescent Psychiatry, 31*(5), 904–910.

Further reading

Asen, E. (2002). Advances in Psychiatric Treatment. *The Royal College of Psychiatrists, 8*, 230–238.

US Department of Health and Human Services, Administration for Children and Families (Found on the Internet May 19, 2004). at http://www.acf.hhs.gov/programs/ofa/exsumcl.htm.

Federal Interagency Forum on Child and Family Statistics in a report entitled: *America's Children: Key National Indicators of Well-Being, 2003*. (Found on the Internet May 19, 2004).

McCubbin, H. I., McCubbin, M. A., Thompson, A. I., Han, S-Y., and Allen, C. T. (1997, June 22). *Families under stress: What makes them resilient?* 1997 American Association of Family and Consumer Sciences Commemorative Lecture on June 22, 1997, in Washington, D. C. Found on the Internet August 4, 2004 at: http://www.cyfernet.org/research/resilient.html.

Spock B., & Rothenberg, M. B. (1985). *Baby and child care*. New York NY: EP Dutton; 8.

Watzlawick, P., Jackson, D., & Beavin, J. (1967). *Pragmatics of Human Communication*. New York: W.W. Norton.

Watzlawick, P., Jackson, D., & Beavin, J. (1974). *Pragmatics of Human Communication*. New York: W.W. Norton.

6 Evidence-Based Practice with Children and Adolescents Experiencing Educational Problem

It's no secret that the U.S. educational system doesn't do a very good job. Like clockwork, studies show that America's school kids lag behind their peers in pretty much every industrialized nation. We hear shocking statistics about the percentage of high-school seniors who can't find the U.S. on an unmarked map of the world or who don't know who Abraham Lincoln was. (Gatto, 2001, p. 1)

6.1. INTRODUCTION

Schools are expected to do many things in our society. Certainly they are expected to teach children academic material that can be used to be successful in life. But additionally, schools teach children to get along, to be good citizens, to have a strong work ethic, and to help others. How well schools do is debatable because, if we know anything about schools, we know that they are not equal. The incomes of the parents whose children attend a school can make a profound difference in the quality of the education children receive and how it affects children in terms of future academic achievement and income. In 2004, only 4.5% of the children from the least affluent 25% of American families obtained a bachelor's degree, while 51% of the children from America's 25% most affluent families obtained the degree (Monteleone, 2004). Unfortunately, while public education is intended to be an equal education, as we all know, the schools in affluent American communities differ dramatically from the schools in America's poorest communities.

This difference in the quality of education places less affluent students, many of them minority students or newly immigrated students, at risk educationally. Drop out rates are much higher in less affluent schools. Rates of learning are much lower. Often, teachers in less affluent, overcrowded schools spend much of their time dealing with behavioral problems of children who act out in class and less time teaching academic subjects. No Child Left Behind, the new aphorism of education in a field full of aphorisms, has not changed the equation at all. Children in affluent schools do well while children in poor schools don't.

To show how race and income affect the educational experience, Coley (2001) reports the following: in 1998, 66% of Hispanic females and 60.5% of Hispanic males completed high school as opposed to well over 90% of Caucasian students.

In terms of completion rate of college, usually thought to be an indicator of the quality of high school preparation, while 28% of Caucasian students who completed high school completed college, 16% of African American students completed college and only 10% of the Hispanic students completing high school received college degrees.

In a Rand Corporation report on factors influencing educational achievement, Lara-Cinisomo et al. (2004) found that the most important factors associated with the educational achievement of children was not race, ethnicity, or immigrant status, but rather the level of parental education, neighborhood poverty, parental occupational status, and family income. The authors also found that parents who use less discipline but greater parental warmth have children with fewer behavior problems, regardless of ethnicity, immigrant status, or neighborhood. However, neighborhood poverty was a very strong predictor of behavior problems among young children – problems which impede school readiness. Children in poor neighborhoods, according to the researchers, are significantly more likely to exhibit both anxious and aggressive behavior, regardless of parenting behavior. The authors note that living in a poor neighborhood is very stressful for young children and increases the stress levels of parents and older siblings, which indirectly increases stress in younger children. The authors conclude that "education policies intended to benefit racial and ethnic minorities can be more successful if policymakers focus less on racial and ethnic factors and more on socioeconomic ones. Education policies alone, when not combined with socioeconomic policies, will be less successful" (p. 1).

According to O'Neill, glaring discrepancies exist among 3rd and 6th grade boys in reading, writing, and math scores, suggesting that "modern educational practices actually work against boys' best interests" (O'Neill, 2000, p. 54). To confirm the disparity between male and female performance, Allen (1993) writes, "From kindergarten to grad school girls now outperform boys in grades, admissions, student government, and extracurricular activities. Women are rapidly closing the M.D. and Ph.D. gap and make up almost half of law students," (p. 34). She then gives the following aside, "Meanwhile, boys dominate in such dubious categories as remedial education, stimulant-drug prescriptions, and suicide" (p. 34).

The US Department of Education (2004) reports that in elementary school, female fourth-graders outperformed their male peers in reading (2003) and writing (2002) assessments. At the secondary school level, the gap in the National Assessment of Educational Progress (NAEP) reading achievement grew from 10 points in 1992 to 16 points in 2002, with males performing lower than females. Additionally, the report notes that females are less likely to repeat a grade and to drop out of high school. Female high school seniors tend to have higher educational aspirations than their male peers. Females entering college baccalaureate programs were more likely than their male counterparts to graduate within 6 years. In 2001, the overall participation rate of females in adult education was higher than that of their male peers (53% versus 46%). If current trends continue, there will be 156 women per 100 men earning degrees by 2020 (Conlin, 2003).

The continuing educational disparity between the genders raises the issue of an economic imbalance which could create, "societal upheavals, altering family finances, social policies, and work–family practices" (Conlin, 2003, p. 77). As the decrease in men with comparable credentials and earning power continues, increasing numbers of women will, in all probability, never marry. Currently, 30% of all African American women 40–44 years of age have never been married (Conlin, 2003, p. 77). As women pull further ahead of men, the lack of availability of suitable men will reduce the probability of forming families.

Because boys are often considered behavioral problems in schools, many more boys than girls are diagnosed with attention-deficit hyperactivity disorder (ADHD). Conlin (2003) reports that the US uses 80% of the world's supply of Ritalin, a 500% increase over the past decade. This leads Conlin to wonder if Ritalin is the new K-12 "management tool" and quotes Paul R. Wolpe, a psychiatry professor at the University of Pennsylvania and the senior fellow at the school's Center for Bioethics as saying that in some school districts, 20–25% of the boys are taking the drug and that, "Ritalin is a response to an artificial social context that we've created for children" (Conlin, 2003, p. 81).

In describing the state of American education, Walberg (2001) says that American schools "produce the worst achievement results at the third-highest expenditures among economically advanced countries. Moreover, substantial amounts of money for special programs, more than $120 billion, have failed to reduce the achievement gap between poor and middle-class children" (p. 67). According to Walberg, American schools fail to implement new educational technologies for learning or even to do a good job of using traditional technologies.

6.2. ACADEMIC UNDERACHIEVING

Neihart (2006) argues that gifted students who underachieve are often battling cultures of class, gender, race and ethnicity that introduce contradictions that often thwart the efforts of gifted children and, in some cases, completely defeat them. She writes that Hispanic students and poor students drop out of school more frequently, are less likely to go to college, and students with the lowest abilities are more likely to have "poorly trained teachers, inappropriate curriculum and insufficient resources" (p. 196). Baldwin (1994) found that gifted students from blue-collar families may deny their abilities because to recognize them may require crossing class boundaries. Parents may tolerate the pursuit of high achievement only as long as that pursuit does not interfere with earning a paycheck or with responsibilities at home. Neihart (2006) writes that "[t]he pursuit of academic excellence has psychological costs for many minority students and for students from low socioeconomic backgrounds. These costs include feeling invisible, marginalized, isolated, or feeling powerless, being discriminated against, and even rejection from family and friends" (p. 198).

As an explanation of why so many boys underachieve, Forbes (2003) suggests that boys are experiencing a severe crisis that hampers their development and can be harmful to others. Forbes blames this crisis on restrictive male norms that:

> *... pressure male youths to prove their masculinity through stoic inexpressiveness and control, avoidance of qualities considered to be feminine, homophobia, competition, domination, and aggression. Influential and highly visible institutions, such as the government and the media, tend to favor male values such as aggression as a means to solve problems. Equally problematic is that male youths often grow up without adequate emotional and conceptual tools that enable them to distance themselves from the norm and become conscious of their own development. Recent incidents of school violence are examples of the destructive effects of boys caught up in the norm. Schools contribute to gender formation and the making of masculinities but do so in an unreflective, inchoate way. (p. 146)*

Expanding on the notion that boys underachieve in school because of male socialization, Harrison et al. (1988) indicate that while parents often believe that boys are tougher than girls, boys are far more vulnerable to illness and disease than female children. Male children are more likely to develop a variety of behavioral difficulties such as hyperactivity, stuttering, dyslexia, and learning disorders. There seems to be little evidence that these behavioral health problems experienced by boys are genetically determined. In explaining the difference in health data between men and women, Harrison et al. (1988) writes, "Male socialization into aggressive behavioral patterns seems clearly related to the higher death rate from external causes. Male anxiety about the achievement of masculine status seems to result in a variety of behaviors that can be understood as compensatory" (p. 306).

Compensatory masculinity involves copying older boys and men who represent appropriate male behavior to a young boy. Some of that behavior may result in boys doing badly in school because real men do not value education they value experience, often dangerous or destructive experience. Harrison et al. (1988) explain that "[c]ompensatory masculinity behaviors range from the innocent to the insidious. Boys naturally imitate the male models available to them and can be observed overemphasizing male gait and male verbal patterns" (p. 298). When those male models fail in school or downplay the importance of education, boys often imitate those beliefs, feeling that being a man is what defines acceptable behavior and that doing well in school is something that may feminize them to peers.

Marcus (2007) believes there are five types of underachievers. They are as follow:

1. The anxious and insecure underachievers who worry about details and experience high levels of tension which make it difficult to concentrate or to do their best work. The most effective way to help them, according to Marcus, is to lower their levels of anxiety, get them to prioritize tasks that are most important, and provide support and assurance.

2. The acting-out and manipulative underachievers who are often impulsive and lacking patience for schoolwork. Helping them achieve requires focusing on self-control, and assertively helping them see the benefits of achieving in school.
3. The unmotivated underachievers who appear to have no other significant problems – they just continue to underachieve. While they seem to be unmotivated, Marcus believes they are actually highly motivated – "not to achieve, but to maintain a kind of mediocre status quo and avoid the pains of growth, responsibility, and achievement" (p. 1). The approach Marcus has found most helpful is a careful intervention in their excuses and "working with them on the specifics of their actual, day-to-day academic preparation, linking these problems to their professed goals, and following up" (p. 1).
4. The oppositional underachievers who challenge authority, often take a defiant and angry approach towards others and view their underachievement as a rebellious act. Marcus suggests using a gentle cognitive approach but avoiding a power struggle and confrontation.
5. The introspective underachievers are students who are trying to decide who they are, where they are going, and what life means. Achievement in school is of secondary importance to resolving meaning of life issues. Marcus suggests the use of a supportive, empathetic, and reflective listening style, which focuses on helping them resolve the existential issues they face in their current lives.

The evidence for helping underachievers is scant and often based on very small samples of students. However, there are a number of important steps to take in restructuring the school experience for potential underachievers. Spielhagen (1996) found that a third of the high-potential females aged 14–16 in his study indicated that the lack of support and peer pressure were barriers to achievement and that role models and mentors were important for their achievement. Read (1991) studied 142 public school districts and gifted negative peer pressure for leaving the program in the 10th grade. Rimm et al. (1999) found that of the 1,000 talented adult women in his study, 15% deliberately did poorly on tests or failed to turn in assignments to preserve their social status. Brown and Steinberg's (1990) study of more than 8000 California and Wisconsin students indicated that they withdrew from honors classes, debate, and computer clubs to avoid being called derogatory names and other negative social consequences. Clearly there are barriers to achievement for a number of students, and therapy certainly is not the answer for schools that discriminate or permit toxic educational environments.

One way to address these barriers is for schools to develop a welcoming environment with four characteristics: they help students cope with identity issues and goals of learning; they deal with the conflicts students experience with other students and instructors; they employ skilled people who can help students and schools bridge cultural barriers; and they provide information in ways of successfully interacting with others (Hébert, 1993, 1996). Parents can also be helpful or inhibit the achievement of children with academic skills who may become underachievers. Autocratic parents have been found to inhibit the progress of gifted children, often leading to underachievement, while involved parents who support children and set standards for them are often those whose children do well academically. Obviously, the burden of work and the many pressures on economically disadvantaged students and their parents may inhibit the ideal type of parent–child interaction necessary for positive academic growth but schools, mentors and therapists are often valuable assets when parents want children to succeed but lack the time and resources to help them (Gottfried and Gottfried, 1996; Gottfried et al., 1994).

On the positive side, Datnow and Cooper (1996) found that open discussions about:

> *[I]dentity, achievement, and the psychological costs of upward mobility may help talented students grow more confident in their ability to manage affiliation/achievement conflicts, and to better control what used to "just happen" to them. Shared discourse has a liberating power that seems to grant marginalized or confused students permission to stay the course of high achievement." Neihart, 2006, p. 199)*

Many students dealing with two or more cultures may need help in learning the process of multi-cultural interaction. Code switching, the ability to change behavior to accommodate the expectations of a new environment, is something that can be taught to gifted students (Canada, 1995). Kuriloff and Reichert (2003) found that reading the work of Black writers helped Black students visualize a different future for themselves and a desire to expand their creative abilities.

6.3. BEST EVIDENCE OF THE EFFECTIVENESS OF SPECIAL EDUCATION FOR CHILDREN AND ADOLESCENTS

After evaluating the past 10 years of research on Emotional and Behavioral Problems (EBP) with children in special education classes, Kauffman (2008) concludes that special education in America is not good enough and that the life course of most youngsters with EBP is undesirable and compares unfavorably with children with other disabilities. He disagrees with the contentions that the wrong children are referred for special education, that the quality of teaching is poor because teachers are poorly prepared, or that being in special classes is stigmatizing. Rather, he believes that EBP children are very difficult to help and that much more research needs to be done to determine best practice. He writes in defense of special education that "It could be that special education simply lessens the misery of students' lives if they have EBD. If that is the case, then we would be making progress in special education if we were able to further reduce the misery or suffering that these students would otherwise experience" (p. 141).

He strongly disagrees with the following summary of what a good many people in the human services believe about special education for EBP children:

> *Special education plays a sorting role, both for those consigned to it and for those students who remain in general education. It limits expectations of the former, and gnarls the attitudes of the latter .... Thus, the system of special*

> *education, and the attitudes towards disability that undergird it, have harmful consequences for both those labeled "disabled" and those not. Among those labeled, their capacity is denied and, thus, expectations of them are limited. Those not labeled are encouraged to believe that people with disabilities are limited and, thus, they are encouraged to offer sympathy toward, but not to value the participation of, persons with disabilities. Neither view provides a basis for a society of inclusion and equity. (Lipsky and Gartner 1996, pp. 767–768)*

It is difficult not to be critical of special education classes for EBP children and adolescents when you consider the racial and gender mix of students assigned to such classes. The Elementary and Middle Schools Technical Assistance Center (2008) reports that African American children were over represented in 9 of 13 disability categories including emotional disturbance, traumatic brain injury and developmental delay, problems that would often land a child in a EBP class. American-Indian students were over represented in 9 categories of disabilities including the 3 behavioral problems cited for African American children. In K-12 education boys are more likely to be diagnosed with special education needs than girls. Among secondary students, 73% of those with learning disabilities and 76% of those who are in EBP classes for the emotionally disturbed are boys. A majority of all other disabilities (speech, mental retardation, visual impairment, etc.) are boys greater than their share of the population. It is difficult not to think that some of the reason for the lack of success of EBP classes is that certain children are dumped into special education classes less on the basis of seriousness of the problem and more on the basis of gender and racial bias.

6.4. EBP WITH AN ACADEMIC UNDERACHIEVER

Jake is a fourth grader referred by his teacher because of his acting-out behavior in class and his poor academic achievement. He has an IQ of 140 but routinely fails in all of his subjects. In my office he appears anxious and wants to know if he is seeing me because Larry, one of his classmates, accused him of hitting Larry on the playground. I assure him that this is not the reason but that his teacher *is* concerned about his work in school and his behavior in class. Jake looks glum and stares at his shoes. "Well, I try," he says, "but it's too hard for me."

I have been working with a number of boys like Jake in the school system, and while many of them have low self esteem and families that do not support their achievement in school, I have begun to think that many bright underachievers are rebellious children who compensate for poor school performance with positive activities and hobbies away from school. They learn, but use an oppositional approach to showing it by failing. It is attention seeking and not a few of them get a great deal of secondary gain from the attention they receive for being bright but doing badly in school. The contradiction drives a number of educators a little crazy since it makes little sense to them that gifted students should fail when much less gifted children do well.

Some of the children come from terrible homes and cope with assaults to their egos and to their minds one can only imagine. And yet, putting them in a position where their oppositional behavior is exposed and doing it in a fun way makes many of these children surprisingly happy to do better. Here is an example of what I used to call "wise guy" or "smart aleck" therapy, a cognitive-behavioral approach with a lot of humor and tall tale telling. Let us return to Jake's statement about how he tries in school but it is too hard for him.

Worker (W): How is it too hard?
Jake (J): I'm not very smart, you know. I'm pretty dumb and you can't expect me to get it.
W: Who says you're dumb?
J: Well, everybody.
W: Who's everybody?
J: My mom, and she used to be a teacher and she should know.
W: She says that you're dumb?
J: Well, no, but that's what she thinks.
W: I guess it's a special gift to read people's mind.
J: I don't read people's mind but every time I bring home a note from school she like says, what can you expect from someone whose dad never made it through high school.
W: Ah, so you don't read minds.
J: Nah, and my dad, he like always agrees with her. He says, "that Jake, he's just dumb like me."
W: That must be hard to listen to particularly since we both know it isn't true.
J: Yeah, it is.
W: So the computer program I saw you playing with in the library is for dumb people. I tried it and couldn't figure it out at all.
J: You're kidding. It's a snap.
W: Not for me. Not for the librarian, and not for the school technology guy who knows these things. I asked him.
J: Well, you can be dumb and still be good at computers, you know.
W: I didn't know that. I thought you had to be smart to figure out computer programs.
J: Well, you can be dumb and still know computers.
W: You don't believe that for a second, Jake.
J: Yeah I do.
W: Then why are you smiling?
J: I smile a lot.
W: I'll bet, and I'll bet you do it inside your head a lot where nobody can see you smiling.
J: I guess you're the mind reader then.
W: Yup, it comes with being a social worker.
J: What's a social worker?
W: Someone who helps smart kids like you do better in school.
J: You always help them?
W: Yup, I'm as good at helping kids as you are with computers.
J: Then why do my mom and dad think I'm so dumb?

W: I don't know, but I'll bet you've given it some thought.
J: Yeah, maybe they need to feel smarter than me because they feel dumb. It makes 'em feel better about themselves.
W: That sounds like something an adult told you.
J: Boy, you're pretty smart. A counselor told me that.
W: Sounds like baloney pies to me.
J: Yeah, me too.
W: So look, kiddo, we have some stuff to work on and we will.
J: You think it'll help?
W: For sure.
J: Boy, you're a lot better than that counselor. She wanted me to draw stuff and tell stories and I'd make these stories up.
W: I bet they were good ones, too. I'd like to hear one.
J: Yeah?
W: Yeah.
J: Well, it's like I'm a space commander and I . . .
W: Fight for justice.
J: Huh?
W: I've heard that one before. You can do better.
J: You've heard the space commander story? Were you talking to my counselor?
W: Nope, it's another of those baloney pie things kids say when they think they can pull one over on a social worker, but we have this baloney pie detector and it's impossible to pull anything over on us.
J: What's a baloney pie?
W: It's what you make out of a lot of baloney. Kids who want to keep things secret make baloney pies so they can make up stories to tell adults.
J: Well, how would you know if I was like telling the truth?
W: I'm a social worker. I'd know.
J: Well then why don't I do well in school?
W: You tell me.
J: I don't know why.
W: Sure you do.
J: Because I have low self-esteem?
W: Ha!
J: That's what the counselor said.
W: More baloney pies, señor?
J: It's boring, you know.
W: What is?
J: School. It's dumb. I know the answers to everything, and it's funny to act dumb. It makes me laugh.
W: Ah, so being a bad student is just an act. What do you get for being dumb?
J: People spend a lot of time with me. It's great.
W: Not me, señor. I only spend time with kids who want to work hard and change. Your teacher tells me you're a pain in the behind in class.
J: Oh yeah? No I'm not.
W: So if you want to work with me, señor, and I'm the best, no more baloney pies, and no more spaceship stories, and you start talking to me about why

a smart kid who fails in school because he thinks it's funny acts like a little s–t in class.

J: No I don't either.

W: I see. Telling Jean that she's fat and ugly is an example of how happy you are? Hitting Larry on the playground, a boy in a wheelchair, these are all behaviors we like to think are funny and come from a happy-go-lucky kid like you?"

J: (Puts his head down). I can be a little s–t, huh.

W: You can.

J: So are you going to help me not be a little s–t?

W: When I'm done working with you, Jake, you will not only not be a little s–t, but you'll be nice to people. It's the super social worker code. The people we work with are always nicer, happier and do better in school when we're done helping them. And you, señor, are someone social workers love because, you see, Jake, underneath all the baloney pies is a little kid who doesn't much like what he does, and when he feels that way, that's when the little s–t in him comes out.

J: So are you going to try and make me like myself better?

W: We don't try, Jake, we do. See you tomorrow, the same time.

And he *did* do better, a good deal better as did almost all of my underachievers. I was convinced a cognitive approach with humor would work with underachieving boys who desperately want to please a smart guy like me who could not be manipulated because, as a kid, I used every trick in the book to cover my own unhappiness and poor school performance. I had been attending workshops by Glaser and Ellis and Beck and I read the stoic philosophers who said that it was not what happened in life, it was how you perceived life. I could see from the behavioral literature that it made great sense to try and develop new behaviors, and that combining the cognitive with the behavioral would have good success with children. All of them? Not all, but most. I worked with kids headed for gangs, with Black and Hispanic kids, and with kids from poor or abusive families. They all loved to laugh. They all loved to imagine that this super social worker dude was actually some cartoon character sent into their lives, and that the code he shared with them was a code to become a man. I actually had a code written up, and I had them sign it and gave them a badge holding them to what the code said. Corny, but it worked. Here is the super social worker code of conduct:

1. I always try my hardest at school and at everything I do.
2. I never make excuses. If I fail I never blame anyone else and I figure out how I can do better.
3. I always tell the truth. There are no white lies. If you live your life like a super social worker, there is never a reason to lie.
4. I always treat people, well even people I don't always like. If I know them better, maybe I'll like them.
5. I respect my parents even when they aren't nice to me or when they make me do things I don't want to do. Parents are the best and I should remember that. If I say

something to my parents that hurts their feelings I will always say I'm sorry and mean it.

6. When I'm in school I always help other kids who aren't doing so well. If I don't help them then I'm cheating them and myself. I always feel better when I help other people.
7. I'm always a gentleman to girls, my teachers, older people, my friends, and my family.
8. To do your best is the highest honor of any man on earth, and to love your country and be a good citizen is what makes a man a good man.
9. Life is fun. It's good to laugh and see the funny stuff that goes on, but never laugh at other people or make fun of them. Then you're just making fun of yourself.
10. The super social worker code of conduct is for life, not just for when you're a kid. Once you take the oath, you have to follow the code even when you're a very old man.

6.5. SOME PERSONAL OBSERVATION ON UNDERACHIEVEMENT

Having worked with hundreds of underachieving children in my career, I think I can offer some of my admittedly subjective observations about why children fail to thrive in school and what we can do about it.

Families help children develop life scripts. I am afraid that all too many parents of underachievers fail to help children develop a sense of what they can do with their talents and sometimes frame school in unflattering or unhelpful ways. Some of these parents are completely disengaged from their children and from their academic experiences. One eighth-grade teacher in Tucson, Arizona told me that of 110 students, only 3–10 parents ever come for school conferences about their children. I hear similar stories from a number of teachers.

Children who get little support for their educational performance will very likely not do well without the added support of the schools and the human service personnel within the schools. Even then, without the positive involvement of parents they are not very likely to thrive. Much more needs to be done to engage parents in the education of their children. I am of the opinion that parents who neglect a child's education are neglecting their emotional development. It is a pernicious form of child neglect that has to be taken more seriously as children with real ability feel disengaged from school and either fail or drop out. It is up to the schools to be more forceful in confronting parents about their position as positive role models, and up to the community to enforce these expectations. Being a parent is not a free ride. It requires responsibilities. A society that permits parents to ignore a child's educational development is a society that will have a great number of young adults without the skills to enter the workplace.

There are parents who have such high expectations for their children that they can never meet them. Rather than trying hard but fearing that they will never meet parental expectations, they do not try at all. Many of the children I worked with fall into this category. With some help to the families to take the pressure off and some good cognitive therapy, the children often do well when the problem is noticed early. Like any reinforcing behavior, the longer it goes unchecked the more difficult it is to treat.

Most of the underachievers I have worked with are boys in elementary school. They feel bewildered by school. They are not always ready developmentally for schoolwork at five or six, and as they begin to experience failure in the early grades, they tend to give up. The educational failure of boys is tragic since so many of them have abilities and talents that could be so useful to our society. As they fail in school, so they fail elsewhere. According to Conlin (2003), men are dropping out of the workforce, abandoning children, and removing themselves from community involvement in record numbers. Since 1964, the rate of decline of men voting in presidential elections is twice that of the rate of women. More women now vote than men.

We need to take the educational failure of boys seriously and develop needed programs. As a therapist I find boys highly motivated to change when they work in a supportive environment which values rather than criticizes them. The negative view of the behavior of boys is destructive and, given the rates of ADHD and other forms of problems ascribed to boys and described in this book, the route we are taking in forming increasing categories of pathology for behavior that is historically normal for boys is very troubling. More than troubling, it is as tragic as the limits we placed on the achievement of women for so many years.

There are the boys and girls who constitute what Bly calls the sibling society, the children who feel entitled and believe that failure would not occur, and if it does, someone will take care of them. I see these children as young adults in higher education. We all do. They tell us that when we give them bad grades it affects their self-esteem. They buy essays and submit them as their own. They e-mail and text message during classes, and are detached from the serious discourse of higher education. How have they gotten so far? By a system of social passes and grade inflation that hardly makes grades meaningful anymore. That some of them go into the human services and graduate should be a message to all of us about the future of the human services in a time when everyone passes regardless of how poor their work or uninspired their effort.

The new landscape of disaffected high school students – of Goths, and invisible kids who harbor homicidal thoughts about their classmates and teachers, the school violence, and the mean girls whose destructive gossip hurts those children targeted for special abuse – presents an educational system in which it is surprising that anyone does well. The bullying, the social snubs, the putdowns, the elite who treat others like insects, none of this can be good for learning. It is a social microcosm of a troubled society and it shows how little we want to change the underlying pathologies that affect schools and our communities, large and small.

Girls in the upper grades often just tune out of education. As a school social worker I almost never saw a female client in the early grades. They did well academically or they blended in and no one noticed. By middle school many of them are your clients and the underachieving is palpable. Let us not confuse the fact that girls are doing better than boys educationally with the belief that all girls are doing well. In fact, they are not. It is gratifying to see so many women choose college and graduate school, but a good deal more can be done to bring the able but disaffected young women of middle and high school age back to serious educational effort.

Finally there are the children of color and poverty. That we help them so little is a painful reminder of our limited concern about these groups. I have given data to show how badly they fare educationally. These children have the same abilities, the same aspirations as all children but by the early grades those dreams begin to diminish. Either we commit ourselves to children succeeding, and I mean succeeding because they know the material they are expected to know and not because we give them social passes, or we can expect continued failure of our most at-risk children. When you work with these children you know they come to you with less preparation than affluent children and the children who grow up with parents dedicated to their well-being. You know you have to be more than an educator or a helping professional. You need to be the person who helps give them direction and keeps them motivated because you care about them.

6.6. REFORMING PUBLIC EDUCATION

The following discussion on reforming American education was first published in Glicken (2007, pp. 113–115). The author wishes to thank Sage Publications for permission to reprint this material.

In 1983, a presidential commission was formed to study the condition of education in America. The findings, A Nation at Risk (1983), include the following statements, many of which remain true today:

> *If an unfriendly foreign power had attempted to impose on America the mediocre educational performance that exists today, we might well have viewed it as an act of war. As it stands, we have allowed this to happen to ourselves. We have even squandered the gains in student achievement made in the wake of the Sputnik challenge. Moreover, we have dismantled essential support systems that helped make those gains possible. We have, in effect, been committing an act of unthinking, unilateral educational disarmament.*

> *The people of the United States need to know that individuals in our society who do not possess the levels of skill, literacy, and training essential to this new era will be effectively disenfranchised, not simply from the material rewards that accompany competent performance, but also from the chance to participate fully in our national life. A high level of shared education is essential to a free, democratic society and to the fostering of a common culture, especially in a country that prides itself on pluralism and individual freedom.*

Current data suggest that gains have been made in public education but that America still lags behind many industrial nations in the overall achievement of students. To improve the state of public education, Public Agenda (2005) believes that five main problems need to be rectified before public education functions well.

6.6.1. Who Controls Education?

Local control of education, while allowing creativity, often results in too many poorly-funded, underachieving schools. Should education be controlled by the federal government, who would provide uniform standards and a higher per capita child-to-teacher ratio? In countries such as France, the national government makes most of the decisions about education. "Local control means that good ideas spread more slowly and that voters may feel they can ignore problems in the community down the road" (Public Agenda, 2005, p. 1).

6.6.2. Improved Standards

For many people, "the right strategy emphasizes higher standards for students and more accountability for schools. If a school is failing to produce results, the administration should be held accountable." (Public Agenda, 2005, p. 1) Supporters say standardized tests motivate students and help improve academic performance, but critics say schools end up "teaching to the test" at the expense of other skills.

6.6.3. Improved Critical Thinking

Another set of reformers argue that children should be taught to think critically and that critical thinking, or the ability to think independently and to come up with elegant solutions to problems, is the way to make education exciting and challenging to children.

6.6.4. Make Funding Equitable

In California, a student attending the highest poverty schools from the time of kindergarten through high school will have an estimated total of $135,654 less spent on all of his or her teachers (K-12) than is spent on the K-12 teachers serving the most affluent students. A student attending the schools serving the highest numbers of Latino and African American students from the time of kindergarten through high school will have an estimated total of $172,626 less spent on all of his or her teachers (K-12) than is spent on the K-12 teachers in schools with the fewest Latino and African American students. This just covers salaries and doesn't include the significant difference in student-to-teacher ratio, the quality of school environments, availability of computers, quality of teachers, other resources or school safety (Education Trust West, 2005, p. 1).

6.6.5. *Competition*

A fifth approach suggests giving parents vouchers that could be used for students to attend either public or private schools. Parents could choose the school that's best for their child and, under a voucher system, public schools would be forced to improve in order to compete. While this approach to improving the education of American children has many supporters, The National Education Association (NEA) takes a dim view of vouchers and says:

> *Despite desperate efforts to make the voucher debate about "school choice" and improving opportunities for low-income students, vouchers remain an elitist strategy. From Milton Friedman's first proposals, through the tuition tax credit proposals of Ronald Reagan, through the voucher proposals on ballots in California, Colorado, and elsewhere, privatization strategies are about subsidizing tuition for students in private schools, not expanding opportunities for low-income children. (2005, p. 1)*

In a publication of the National Parent Teachers Association (PTA), the national organization noted that:

> *A study by the U.S. General Accounting Office (GAO) found that privately funded voucher programs do not significantly improve academic achievement for most recipients. The study examined 78 privately funded voucher programs, but focused on those in New York City, Washington, DC, and Dayton, Ohio. These findings reinforce those of an earlier study of publicly funded voucher programs in such areas as Cleveland, Milwaukee, and Florida, in which the GAO found little or no difference between the performances of voucher and public school students.*
>
> *Another cause of student attrition is dissatisfaction with the private schools themselves. Based on parents' reports, the private schools were less likely than the public schools to have a nurse's office, a cafeteria, and to provide services and programs for those students with learning disabilities, or who are English-language learners. Parent satisfaction with private schools could be traced to the characteristics of the private schools that also exist in successful public schools, such as smaller class size, individual tutoring, and better communication between parents and teachers. (Connecticut PTA, 2005, p. 1).*

However, Milwaukee has one of several court-approved voucher systems and the following suggests that the system has worked very well.

> *An analysis of the Milwaukee publicly-run voucher program by the officially appointed researcher shows the parents of "choice" kids are virtually unanimous in their opinion of the program: they love it. Parents are not only far more satisfied with their freely chosen private schools than they were with their former public schools, they participate more actively in their children's education now that they've made the move. Recently, a reanalysis of the raw data by statisticians and educational researchers from Harvard*

and the University of Houston found that choice students do indeed benefit academically from the program, showing significant gains in both reading and mathematics by their fourth year of participation. (Coulson, 2005, p. 1)

6.7. SUMMARY

This chapter provides a generally negative view of the American educational system and its failure with boys, students of color and the economically disadvantaged. A case of cognitive therapy with an underachiever was presented along with a personal discussion of why children underachieve and some thoughts on reforming the American educational system.

6.8. QUESTIONS FROM THE CHAPTER

1. Do you think it is fair to ask schools to not only teach students academic subjects, but to discipline them, fill in where their parents would not or can not, teach them good citizenship and how to get along with others, monitor their use of drugs and alcohol, and do just about everything else badly functioning families are unable or unwilling to do?
2. We blame schools for doing a bad job but is not the society we live in doing a bad job by not caring enough about kids from poor homes and troubled families?
3. The statistics about income and completion of college suggest that lower income students fail to go to or complete college because of their income levels and perhaps the quality of their academic preparation, but is not the real reason students go to college because parents want them to? Was that the case in your decision to attend college?
4. The case study about underachieving seems to suggest that children with poor self-concepts are likely to do badly in school. Do you think this is the crux of reason for underachieving and if so, what might other reasons be?
5. Do not you think that if poor children went to very high quality schools and rich children went to very low quality schools that rich kids would still do better in school and in life? Why or why not?

References

A Nation at Risk: The imperative for educational reform. (1983, April 1). *A report to the nation and the Secretary of Education, the US Department of Education by the National Committee on Excelleance in Education.* Retrieved June 26, 2006 from http://www.gov/pubs/NaAtRisk.html.

Baldwin, A. Y. (1994). The seven plus story: Developing hidden talent among students in socioeconomically disadvantaged environments. *Gifted Child Quarterly, 38*, 80–84.

Brown, B. B., & Steinberg, L. (1990). Academic achievement and social acceptance: Skirting the "brain-nerd" connection. *Education Digest, 55*, 55–60.

Canada, G. (1995). *Fist, stick, knife, gun: A personal history of violence in America.* Boston: Beacon Press.

Conlin, M. (2003, May 26). The new gender gap. *Business Week*, 74–81.
Connecticut PTA. (2005) School attrition. http://www.ctpta.org/bulletin/May-2005.pdf.
Coley, R. (2001). *Differences in the gender gap: Comparisons across racial/ethnic groups in education and work*. Princeton: Educational Testing Service, Policy Information Center, Available: http://www.ets.org/research/pic.
Coulson, A. J. (2005). *Vouchers*. Found on the Internet June 30, 2005 at http://www.schoolchoices.org/roo/vouchers.htm.
Datnow, A., & Cooper, R. (1996). Peer networks of African American students in independent schools: Affirming academic success and racial identity. *Journal of Negro Education, 65*, 56–72.
Education Trust West (2005). *Short Changing poor and minority schools*. Found on the Internet June 30, 2005 at http://www.hiddengap.org/faq/.
Elementary and Middle Schools Technical Assistance Center: (2008). *Disproportionality: The Disproportionate Representation of Racial and Ethnic Minorities in Special Education*. http://www.emstac.org/registered/topics/disproportionality/faqs.htm#overrep.
Forbes, D. (2003). Turn the wheel: Integral school counseling for male adolescents. *Journal of Counseling and Development, 81*, 142–150.
Gatto, J. T. (2001). *The underground history of American education: An intimate investigation into the problem of modern schooling*. New York: Oxford Village Press.
Glicken, M. D. (2007). *Social work in the 21st Century: An introduction to social welfare, social issues and the profession*. Thousand Oaks, CA: Sage Publications.
Gottfried, A. E., & Gottfried, A. W. (1996). A longitudinal study of academic intrinsic motivation in intellectually gifted children: Childhood through early adolescence. *Gifted Child Quarterly, 40*, 179–183.
Gottfried, A. E., Gottfried, A. W., Bathurst, K., & Guerin, D. W. (1994). *Gifted IQ early developmental aspects: The Fullerton longitudinal study*. New York: Plenum Press.
Harrison, J., Chin, J., & Ficarrotto, T. (1988). Warning: Masculinity may be dangerous to your health. In M. S. Kimmel, M. A. & Messner (Eds.), *Men's lives* (pp. 271–285). New York: Macmillan.
Hébert, T. (1993). *Ethnographic descriptions of the high school experiences of high ability males in an urban environment*. Storrs: University of Connecticut.
Hébert, T. (1996). Portraits of resilience: The urban life experiences of gifted Latino young men. *Roeper Review, 19*, 82–90.
Kauffman, J. M. (2008). Would we recognize progress if we saw it? A commentary. *Journal of Behavioral Education, 17*, 128–143.
Kuriloff, P., & Reichert, M. C. (2003). Boys of class, boys of color: Negotiating the academic and social geography of an elite independent school. *Journal of Social Issues, 59*, 751–770.
Lara-Cinisomo, S., Pebley, A. R., Vaiana, M. E., Maggio, E., Berends, M., & Lucas, S. R. (2004, Fall). *Rand corporation report: A matter of class: Educational achievement reflects family background more than ethnicity or immigration*. Report found on the Internet July 1, 2005 at: http://www.rand.org/publications/randreview/issues/fall2004/class.html.
Lipsky, D. K., & Gartner, A. (1996). Inclusion, school restructuring, and the remaking of American society. *Harvard Educational Review, 66*, 762–796.
Marcus, S. I. (2007). *Personality styles of chronic academic underachievers*. http://www.selfgrowth.com/articles/Personality_Styles_of_Chronic_Academic_Underachievers.html.

Monteleone, J. (2004, May 17). Five decades after the brown decision, the journey continues. *The Idaho Statesman,* p. 8 Local.

Neihart, M. (2006, Summer). Dimensions of underachievement, difficult contexts, and perceptions of self. *Roeper Review, 28*(4), 196–202.

O"Neill, T. (2000). Boys problems don't matter. *Newsmagazine, 27*(15), 54–56.

Public Agenda (2005). *Education at a Glance.* Found on the Internet June 30, 2005 at http://publicagenda.org/issues/overview.cfm?issue_type=education.

Read, C. R. (1991). Gender distribution in programs for the gifted. *Roeper Review, 13,* 188–193.

Rimm, S. B., Rimm-Kaufman, S., & Rimm, I. (1999). *See Jane win: The Rimm report on how 1000 girls became successful women.* New York: Crown Publishing Group.

Spielhagen, F. R. (1996). Perceptions of achievement among high-potential females between nine and 26 years of age. In K. Arnold, K. Noble, R. & Subotnik (Eds.), *Remarkable women: Perspectives on female talent development* (pp. 193–208). Cresskill, NJ: Hampton Press.

Walberg, H.J. (2001). *Achievement in American Schools.What's Gone Wrong in America's Classrooms.* Hoover Institution Press Publication. http://media.hoover.org/documents/0817999426_3.pdf.

Further reading

Allen, J. (2003, June 23). Are men obsolete. *US News and World Report,* 134(22), 33.

National Education Association (2005). Vouchers. Found on the Internet June 30, 2005 at http://www.nea.org/vouchers/index.html.

http://web.ebscohost.com.ezproxy1.lib.asu.edu/ehost/detail?vid=4&hid=22&sid=64c502a3-2336-4541-be51-4d0bfeaa9c0e%40sessionmgr8.

O'Neill, R. E., Horner, R. H., Albin, R. W., Sprague, J. R., Newton, S., & Storey, K. (1997). *Functional assessment and program development for problem behavior: A practical handbook* (Second ed.). Pacific Grove, CA: Brookes/Cole.

United States Department of Education. (1998). *National educational goals panel report.* Washington, DC: U.S. Department of Education.

Walberg, H. J., *What's Gone Wrong in America's Classrooms.* Hoover Institution Press Publication. http://media.hoover.org/documents/0817999426_3.pdf.

7 Evidence-Based Practice with Children and Adolescents Experiencing Social Isolation and Loneliness

7.1. INTRODUCTION

Estimates of loneliness among children and adolescents suggest that loneliness is a serious, often unrecognized problem. According to Asher et al. (1984), more than 10% of children in grades three through six report feelings of *loneliness* defined in part by not having anyone to play with. Moore and Schultz (1983) estimate that loneliness among high school students ranges from 8% to 16% of all students. In surveys of school counselors and social workers, Calabrese (1989) and France et al. (1984) report an increasing proportion of young people who feel alienated, isolated and alone as a result of increasing mobility, rising divorce rates, increasing numbers of single-parent families, and declining access to the extended family. Additional factors that may contribute to feelings of *loneliness* in children include: death of a parent or a significant person; divorce of parents; conflict within the home or at school; child abuse and neglect; moving to a new school or neighborhood; losing a friend, possession, or pet; immigrant status coupled with limited competence in English; poor clothing and hygiene; concerns about physical attractiveness; and routine rejection by playmates (Bullock, 1993a, 1993b). Low self-esteem, shyness, anxiety, and self-consciousness, aggressiveness, and higher sensitivity to rejection may also contribute to inadequate peer relationships and difficulty in making friends (Goswick and Jones, 1982).

Dodge (1983) studied 48 unacquainted second-graders meeting together in play groups for eight 1-h sessions. Children who were neglected approached other children frequently but ineffectively and in time decreased their contacts. Neglected children were viewed by the other children as shy, while rejected children were often aggressive, unwilling to play cooperatively, more argumentative, and more likely to engage in disruptive peer interactions. Henggeler and Borduin (1989) stress the need to differentiate children who are rejected by others from children who are neglected when we develop interventions.

7.2. UNDERSTANDING LONELINESS AND ISOLATION

Hayden et al. (1988) interviewed third through eighth grade children about the meaning of and their personal experiences with loneliness. Their descriptions of loneliness were similar to those of adults' and include such unpleasant emotions as sadness, boredom, feeling unneeded and left out – as if no one likes you, and feeling like an outsider. The researchers also noted that in describing loneliness, children used metaphorical expressions such as feeling like you are in a corner and "like you're the only one on the moon" (p. 254).

Murphy (2006)*describes loneliness* "as a condition with distressing, depressing, dehumanizing, detached feelings that a person endures when there is a gaping emptiness in his or her life due to an unfulfilled social and/or emotional life" (p. 22). Uruk and Demir (2003) define loneliness as "an unpleasant experience that occurs when a person's network of social relationships is significantly deficient in either quality or quantity (Peplau and Perlman, 1984)" (p. 179). The authors add that loneliness is "the psychological state that results from discrepancies between one's desire for and one's actual composition of relationships" (p. 179). Young (1982) defines loneliness as the "perceived absence of satisfying social relationships, accompanied by symptoms of psychological distress that are related to the perceived absence" (p. 380).

Sermat (1978) defines loneliness "as an experienced discrepancy between the kinds of interpersonal relationships the individuals perceive themselves as having and the kind of relationships they would like to have" (p. 274). A second aspect of the definition of loneliness is the distinction between issues that may serve as catalysts for loneliness, such as the loss of friends, spouses and family members, and dispositional factors such as shyness, introversion, or high expectations and demands that make individuals more vulnerable to loneliness.

Although *loneliness* can be emotionally distressing, it is also a signal that something needs to be done to increase one's social network. Uruk and Demir (2003) report a strong correlation between parents who have little time to spend with their children or fail to form attachments with their children, and the development of loneliness in adolescence that often continues into adulthood and later life. Joiner et al. (1999) believe that loneliness stems from a lack of pleasurable engagement and, as a result, a painful disconnection from trying to engage. The authors call this the "bedrock" of *loneliness*. Similarly, Jones and Carver (1991) believe that loneliness affects "one's opinion about people, life, and society in a manner suggesting that lonely people subscribe to negativistic, apathetical, and pessimistic views" (p. 400).

Weiss (1973) distinguishes *loneliness* due to emotional isolation from *loneliness* due to social isolation. Emotional isolation appears in the absence of a close emotional attachment (often related to a lack of parental attachment), while social isolation appears in the absence of an engaging social network (often related to a lack of peer support, friendships, and close social networks). Relationships with parents and peers constitute two different social contexts in which *loneliness* develops. Rubin and Mills (1991) believe that loneliness develops when a pattern made up of social anxiety, lack of dominance, and social isolation results in peer rejection and negative self-perception. Olweus (1993) reports that when children blame their own incompetence for negative social experiences with peers which result in rejection, the end effect is often social withdrawal, feelings of isolation, and depression. Rotenberg et al. (2004) found considerable evidence that loneliness correlates highly with lack of trust, particularly in young women. The author's note:

> *As we expected, the relationship between loneliness and trust is stronger for girls than it is for boys. The trust measures accounted for 57% of loneliness for girls but only 18% of loneliness for boys. These patterns are consistent with the hypothesis that if girls do not believe or rely on their same-gender peers to keep intimacies confidential and to fulfill promises then they are cut off from their preferred and prevalent form of interaction (i.e., same-gender close-peer networks) and therefore are highly prone to loneliness. Finding this pattern with girls and not with boys also is consistent with the notion that girls are more inclined to establish a network of close peers than are boys. Close peer networks may be normatively expected for girls, and thus they may be distinctly at risk for loneliness because they demonstrate both low trust beliefs in same-gender peers and low levels of reciprocal trusting behaviors with peers.*
>
> *These findings have implications for social functioning during adulthood. Women have larger intimacy networks than do men and, therefore, the observed association between loneliness and trust beliefs in same-gender peers may be stronger for women than for men during adulthood as well. (p. 235)*

Ekwall (2005) believes that it is important to differentiate social isolation from loneliness. Social isolation by choice is defined as aloneness, and can be understood as the desire to live in a way isolated from others. Social isolation without choice is defined as *loneliness, and can best be understood as a desire to have contact with others, but because of social, emotional, or geographic barriers, an inability to do so.* McWhirter (1990) suggests that loneliness can take place in both the presence and absence of social contact. Akerlind and Hornquist (1992) believe that social support research emphasizes external factors and the availability of social support while loneliness research emphasizes internal negative emotions about relationships or deficits in relationships. Regardless of the subtle differences, both loneliness and social isolation have been shown to be major negative influences on psychosocial well-being.

Ramsey (1991) found that lonely children often experience poor peer relationships and express more loneliness than peers with friends. They often feel excluded by others and frequently feel sadness, malaise, boredom, and alienation. According to Ramsey, early childhood loneliness is a predictor of loneliness in adulthood. Cassidy and Asher (1992) found that children who are minimally accepted by their peers experience the most loneliness. Bolvin et al. (1995) found that children whose loneliness increased during the school year were those children who became more rejected and more victimized over time. Bullock (1992) found links between childhood loneliness and academic failure; truancy; dropping out of school; and juvenile delinquency and mental health problems, including depression, suicide, hostility, alcoholism, poor self-concept and psychosomatic illnesses.

7.3. THE REASONS FOR LONELINESS IN CHILDREN AND ADOLESCENTS

Kochenderfer and Ladd (1996) suggest that loneliness in children may result from conflict within the home; insecure parental attachments; moving to a new school or neighborhood; losing a friend; losing an object, possession, or pet; experiencing the divorce of parents; experiencing the death of a significant person; rejection by peers; limited social skills or an understanding of how to make friends; shyness, anxiety, and low self-esteem that contribute to difficulties in making friends; victimization by peers (e.g., children who are bullied, physically or verbally attacked or taunted report high levels of loneliness, and distress). Asher et al. (1990) found that children who are aggressive report the greatest degrees of loneliness and social dissatisfaction. Rubin and Mills (1991) report that shy, inhibited and anxious children often lack social skills and confidence to interact with others and frequently report feelings of loneliness.

Sullivan (1953) believed that loneliness was a consequence of peer victimization. Lonely children communicate their withdrawn behavior to peers, who reinforce a child's feelings of loneliness by bullying, ignoring or completely leaving a child out of activities. To determine whether this construct was valid, Berguno et al. (2004) interviewed 42 children between 8 and 10 years old about their experiences of loneliness at primary school. The children were further asked to describe their experiences of being bullied, as well as to comment on their perception of the consequences of particular teacher interventions. Eighty percent of the children said they had periods of being lonely at school and that they were related to boredom, inactivity, a tendency to withdraw into fantasy, and a passive attitude towards social interactions. Children who had few friendships were more vulnerable to becoming isolated. Sixty-eight percent of the children said they had been bullied and that teacher interventions were not effective in reducing the bullying. The authors continue by noting that:

> *Teachers who intervene by punishing the bullies are similarly contributing to the child's experience of loneliness since, according to our findings punishment is not an effective long-term strategy for dealing with instances of peer aggression. It would appear that the only effective teacher interventions are those that attempt an interpersonal resolution between victim and bully. (p. 495)*

Lonely children often learn about social interactions from families who model, reinforce, and coach. Carr and Schellenbach (1993) believe that chronically lonely children may be raised in families that do not stress social learning, or the family itself may be isolated with little outside interaction with others.

In explaining a more existential reason for loneliness, Seligman and Csikszetmihalyi (2000) write that Americans "live surrounded by many more people than their ancestors did, yet they are intimate with fewer individuals and thus experience greater loneliness and alienation" (p. 9). Ostrov and Offer (1980) suggest that American culture emphasizes individual achievement, competitiveness, and impersonal social relations, and that even early loneliness may be quite pronounced in the face of such socially alienating values. Saxton (1986) argues that in contemporary American society there is a decline in the face-to-face, intimate contacts with family members, relatives, and close friends which were much more prevalent several decades ago. Mijuskovic (1992) views American society as highly mechanized with "impersonal institutions, disintegration of the family as a result of a high divorce rate, high mobility rate with its impact on family and community ties; the fast-paced living and self-centeredness of the culture interferes with people's ability to establish and maintain fulfilling relationships (RokAch, 2007, p.184).

Seligman worries that Americans have become so caught up in a personal sense of entitlement that even helping professionals have gone along with, in fact encouraged, "the belief that we can rely on shortcuts to happiness, joy, rapture, comfort, and ecstasy, rather than be entitled to these feelings by the exercise of personal strengths and virtues, which results in legions of people who, in the middle of great wealth, are starving spiritually" (ABCNews.com, 2002, online). Seligman goes on to suggest that, "[p]ositive emotion alienated from the exercise of character leads to emptiness, to inauthenticity, to depression, and, as we age, to the gnawing realization that we are fidgeting until we die" (ABCNews.com, 2002, online).

Robert Putnam (Stossel, 2000) believes that this focus on self is producing a country without a sense of social connectedness, where, "[s]upper eaten with friends or family has given way to supper gobbled in solitude, with only the glow of the television screen for companionship" (p. 1). According to Putnam:

> *... [A]mericans today have retreated into isolation. Evidence shows that fewer and fewer contemporary Americans are unionizing, voting, rallying around shared causes, participating in religious services, inviting each other over, or doing much of anything collectively. In fact, when we do occasionally gather – for twelve-step support encounters and the like – it's most often only as an excuse to focus on ourselves in the presence of an audience. (Stossel, 2000, p. 1)*

Putnam believes that the lack of social involvement negatively affects school performance, health and mental health, increases crime rates, reduces tax responsibilities and charitable work, decreases productivity and, "even simple human happiness – all are demonstrably affected by how (and whether) we connect with our family and friends and neighbors and co-workers" (Stossel, 2000, p. 1).

Commenting on the importance of understanding culture and the way cultures organize family life, belief systems, and closeness to others as factors in creating loneliness, RokAch (2007) writes,

> *Loneliness research tends to focus on individual factors, that is, either on personality factors or on lack of social contacts. However, loneliness could be expressive of an individual's relationship to the community. It is conceivable, then, that the difference between cultures and the ways in which social relations are organized within them will result in cross-cultural variations in the way people experience loneliness. The difference of the social tapestry, interpersonal interactions and the support networks which are available to individuals in various cultures are bound to affect the causes of loneliness. (p. 174)*

Although loneliness may have social and cultural antecedents, many lonely children and adolescents report feeling lonely and rejected by others from a very early age and even in the presence of others. Among lonely youth who have experienced loneliness from an early age, the absence of social contacts as they age creates a sense of despair that should not be confused with depression. The loneliness they experience is a feeling of separateness and of not fitting in that sometimes worsens with age. This type of loneliness may have its roots in failure to bond with parents or parental rejection. A case at the end of the chapter describes the treatment for this type of loneliness.

7.4. EVIDENCE BASED PRACTICE WITH LONELY AND SOCIALLY ANXIOUS CHILDREN AND ADOLESCENTS

France et al. (1984) suggest teaching youngsters to identify their feelings and understand their *loneliness* by keeping a personal journal. The journal exercise helps young clients increase their awareness of situations in which they feel lonely, particularly when and with whom they experience *loneliness*. The journal helps them find recurring themes or patterns of *loneliness*. Ponzetti (1990) suggests the use of support groups to help youthful clients cope with feelings of social anxiety, shyness, lack of self-esteem, and difficulty in making friends. Ponzetti (1990) believes that support groups help clients explore their feelings of *loneliness*, but also the "possibility that part of their problem may be their own resistance to taking control of their *loneliness*" (p. 338).

In treating lonely children, Young (1982) emphasizes the importance of cognition. Behaviors and emotions related to *loneliness* are aspects of thoughts, attributions, and assumptions that when accurately assessed help lonely children understand why they act and feel the way they do. This recognition can then be replaced by cognitive strategies to cope with feelings of loneliness and to effectively respond to situations that often increase loneliness.

Rook (1984) believes in the use of skills training to help young clients cope more effectively with social interaction, initiate social contacts, participate in groups, and enjoy themselves in social situations. Skills training teaches lonely children and adolescents to develop and maintain friendships and supportive relationships, to participate in groups, and to enjoy themselves in social situations such as dating.

Bullock (1992) believes that we can help lonely children by coaching them on ways of developing positive interactions:

> *[S]uch as telling them why each concept is important to peer interaction; asking for examples to assess children's understanding of the concept; reinforcing the examples or providing suggestions when children have trouble finding their own examples; discussing both positive and negative behavioral examples that are important to interactions; trying out some of the ideas in a play situation and assessing the situation afterwards. (Bullock, 1992, p. 94)*

It is natural to assume that depression and loneliness may be interrelated since most depressed people also experience feelings of severe loneliness and social isolation. Powell et al. (2001) studied the effectiveness of treatment with clients experiencing long-term mood disorders. They concluded that self-help groups were very important providers of positive management of mood disorders because social support forces otherwise lonely and isolated people to interact with others, often at a fairly intimate level. In considering demographic issues as a predictor of the ability to cope with mood disorders, the researchers failed to find any specific indicator other than the level of education which, the authors believe, is an important aspect of dealing with the disorder. Surprisingly, daily functioning was inversely related to the number of out-patient contacts, suggesting, according to the authors, that as people improve, they see less need for professional help. Support from families and friends also failed to predict outcomes.

Since early detection of depression is essential in learning to cope with feelings of loneliness and depression, Duffy (2000) reports several important predictors of depression:

> *A family history of major affective disorder is the strongest, most reliable risk factor for a major affective illness. Other factors associated with affective disorders include female sex (risk factor for unipolar illnesses), severe life events and disappointments, family dysfunction, poor parental care, early adversity, and personality traits.*
>
> *Based on the current state of knowledge, emphasis on identifying and treating mood disorders as early as possible in the course and particularly early-onset (child and adolescent) cases and youngsters at high risk (given a parent with*

a major mood disorder) is likely to be an effective strategy for reducing the burden of illness on both the individual and society. (p. 345)

Duffy (2000) also reports beginning evidence that brief, family-based psycho-educational interventions decrease the negative impact of parental mood disorders in children and improve family functioning in mood-disordered children. Individual treatment and family psycho-educational interventions in adult bipolar patients often decrease relapse rates and improve overall family functioning. Duffy notes that while early identification of children at risk of mood disorders is necessary, and "the most effective strategy for reducing the burden of illness on individuals and society is not clear" (p. 346). However, the serious impact of mood disorders on the individual and their families, and the high risk of suicide justify a need to develop new and more effective interventions. In the meantime, early interventions that utilize education, identification of family members at risk, and family interventions, may decrease the seriousness of the condition and reduce fears and misconceptions among family members. Harrington and Clark (1998) indicate that early intervention through the use of appropriate medications and mood disorder therapies may actually reduce the severity and reoccurrence of adolescent mood disorders.

Adams et al. (2004) studied loneliness in retirement communities and discovered that while "residence in congregate facilities affords social exposure, it does not guarantee access to close relationships, so that loneliness may be a result." (p. 475). The authors did find that when retirement communities sponsored social and leisure activities to keep older adults from being lonely and used strategies to keep them engaged with family and friends living outside the community, such activities could indirectly prevent more serious health and mental health problems. The strategies mentioned by the authors include "sending reminder notes to designated family and friends encouraging them to call or visit, holding social events where residents may invite a guest, and regularly offering informal support or informational groups at the facility for close friends or family members of residents" (p. 483). Blazer (2002b) suggests the establishment of support groups designated for those who are most likely to be lonely, including residents who have recently relocated, the bereaved, or those who are shy or lack social skills. Andrews et al. (2003) suggest the use of "befriending schemes" where volunteers meet weekly with lonely elderly persons. All of these efforts have potential to help lonely and isolated older adults, according to the literature.

Studying the importance of educational achievement, Hobfoll (1989) suggested that people who experience difficulty or failure in school early in life come to devalue education and may choose to discontinue advanced levels of training that may, as a consequence, lead to vulnerability to stressors and negative psychological outcomes. Lazarus and Folkman (1984) found that people who appraise situations as potentially threatening do so because they fail to acquire sufficient resources, often resulting in negative psychological outcomes. Consequently, education may represent an important resource contributing to positive well being in later life.

It is often assumed that loneliness is directly related to social support and that having an intimate relationship with a spouse or loved one inhibits feelings of loneliness. Bishop and Martin (2007) studied the emotional well-being of 227 older adults ages 65–94 living independently in the community who had never been married, divorced or widowed in order to determine the psychological impact of educational achievement. They found a direct relationship between educational attainment and positive well-being, including reduced feelings of loneliness that have meaning for children and adolescents as a potential way to deal with loneliness. The authors report that:

> *Three key outcomes emerged from the present study. First, past educational attainment appeared to directly reduce vulnerability to neuroticism and stress. Second, greater expression of neurotic personality traits and feelings of stress directly increases susceptibility to loneliness, whereas greater social support directly decreases loneliness. Third, past educational attainment indirectly reduces feelings of loneliness. Each of these findings provides support for educational attainment as a relevant factor of subjective well being and warrant further discussion relative to unmarried marital status. (p. 910)*

The Internet also offers a way of decreasing loneliness. White et al. (2002) believe that the Internet and, more specifically e-mail, has the potential to increase social support and the emotional well-being in youth in the following ways: they can use computers to communicate often, cheaply, and easily with family, friends, and others who have computers; they can get information about a variety of issues that are especially important to them; they can explore hobbies and find out information about their community; and they can meet new people and broaden their support system through chat rooms and bulletin boards without having to deal with the usual social anxiety felt in one-on-one contacts, small groups and other social structures that often create feelings of loneliness. The authors write "In essence, relatively isolated [people] can reconnect, strengthen and broaden their connection with the outside world by incorporating computer technology into their lives" (p. 214).

As an example applying to older adults with much less computer competence than youth in our society, in a study by White et al. (2002) to teach lonely frail older adults with a mean age of 71 to use the Internet, the authors report that 60% of the total sample and 74% of those who completed the 9-h training course were using the Internet weekly within 5 months. The authors found a decrease in feelings of loneliness and write, "Looking only at the intervention group and comparing users to non-users there were trends toward decreased loneliness and depression" (p. 219). In summary, the author's note that the Internet can enrich the lives of lonely people by providing "a source of information, social activity, and interpersonal communication, and by expanding [a persons' horizons] to provide more frequent contacts with family and friends, new opportunities to pursue interests, as well as avenues to meet new friends and to 'travel' to new places. (p. 220)

7.5. A CASE STUDY: USING EBP WITH LONELINESS AND ISOLATION

The following is a description of loneliness told to a therapist by her 17-year old client Brian (Glicken, 2006, pp. 176–177). The author wishes to thank Sage Publications for permission to reprint Brian's story. After Brian's description of his feelings of loneliness, the therapist analyzes the case, explains her treatment approach, and provides a verbatim example from several of the first few sessions with Brian.

7.6. BRIAN'S STORY

I think people who grow up in troubled families never get the hang of relationships or being with people. In my family, we were so busy surviving poverty and the illness of my mother that none of us really mastered the ability to be loved or to love someone in return. My father's favorite saying is that it's better to be home by yourself reading a good book than to be out with bad friends. Of course, he considers all my friends to be bad so I spent my childhood reading books, pretty much alone.

People sometimes think I'm stuck up when what I really am is shy and withdrawn with a few times here and there in which I can act like I'm the greatest thing since sliced bread. Pretty much I don't think people like me. Like I'm never invited to parties by the kids at school and most people just ignore me. It hurts a lot not to be liked. I do well in school because I think that's the way to get out of a troubled family and learn to live a successful life. Maybe nobody will ever like me but at least I'll have money and I'll be successful at something. The worst time when I'm lonely is after school and on weekends. I've tried going to parties with the few friends I have, but they all feel awful at parties and we make each other miserable. It's hard to explain being lonely when you're around people.

I went to see the school social worker when I was in grade school because the teacher said I looked so sad in class. She was great and I liked seeing her because she made me feel smart, but when I'd go back to class I'd feel just as lonely and weird about myself as ever.

Every once in a while I meet a girl who doesn't seem to mind my shyness, but it doesn't last long. She wants to go out where there are other people and I don't and we break up. It's not fun to break up and I guess the girls talk and the word is that I'm a psycho or something because I'm so shy. Maybe I just pick the wrong girls. Once I went out with a girl who was also very shy and lonely. After we got done telling each other how miserable we were there wasn't anything more to talk about. I guess you can choose people in your life who are exactly like you. That's what my mom says. We go to church and she points out girls she thinks would be good for me and she's probably right but the thought of asking one for a date scares me to death. I know I'd screw it up, it would get back to my mom, and then she and my dad would lecture me about not being so shy and trying harder. Like I don't know that.

I fight feeling down all the time. I force myself to get up in the morning and go to school. I try and make myself invisible so the mean kids don't say anything that hurts my feelings or the pretty girls who ignore me won't say things like "ugly or weird" under their breathes and then laugh with another girl. I don't think there's an easy answer to loneliness. It hurts all the time. You [his therapist] asked me how I cope and the best answer I can give is that I force myself to. I'm not religious but I believe God meant for me to do something special. He's given me a high IQ and lots of gifts in science and math for which I feel grateful.

I don't think there's any magical answer to loneliness. You keep on trying, you don't allow yourself to feel too sorry for yourself, and you take each day as it comes. I know those are clichés, but sometimes there's truth in a cliché, and as someone who was raised on the messages my mother got from the soap operas, I believe that sometimes the good fairy takes your lost dreams and replaces them with gold.

7.7. DISCUSSION

The therapist said, "I began my work with Brian by focusing on his many positives. He believes that he has something important to accomplish in life and that God has given him a role, as yet undefined, to do something special. Perhaps this is a spiritual aspect of Brian's search for life meaning that gives him an inner directedness that permits him to achieve even in the midst of despair. He receives satisfaction from knowing that he will succeed in life because of his determination, intelligence, and special abilities for science and math. He understands the role of his family life in contributing to feelings of loneliness but does not blame his parents or his early life experiences for his problems. He has had a good experience with a therapist, although it was difficult for him to transfer what took place in treatment into being less lonely. The therapy sounds supportive but superficial. He is able to describe, without being vindictive, the hurtful behaviors of others who treat him badly because of his shyness. He has friends, even though they all seem to be lonely and isolated like him, but at least he tries to go to social events with friends and to date.

"How best to approach his treatment?" The literature did not help much because best evidence is so limited. I wonder if researchers or clinicians think about loneliness as a serious problem. Judging by the lack of information, I doubt it. The best I could do was to assume some closeness between loneliness and depression. I actually think they are very different problems but that is what I did, focusing on any literature on social anxiety, not exactly what loneliness is, but that is what I did. I found some articles on treating loneliness using cognitive-behavioral approaches, including Young (1982), Rook (1984) and Bullock (1992). They did not give much evidence of effectiveness but their approaches were clearly described and easy enough to follow. Because of Brian's math and science skills I asked him to set up a behavioral chart that would measure his current loneliness and how it affected him socially. After several sessions of discussion, this is what he came up with, a sort of progression of where he was at present compared to where he hoped to be at the end of treatment:

Behavior	Week 1	2	3	4	5	6	7	8	9	10	11	12	13	14	15	16
1. Going to social events:	-0-															-3-
2. Dating per week:	-0-															-2-
3.Joining new people for lunch at school:	-0-															-5-
4.Going by himself To parties:	-0-															-1-
5. Joining clubs at school:	-0-															-10-

We discussed his goals and he thought clubs would be easiest for him to do since there were so many and he had been asked to join a number but felt too insecure about his social skills to join. This was an immediate goal. Using a cognitive-behavioral approach, his homework assignments all had to do with improving his social contacts and logically challenging his negative self-sentences. The following is an example from the second and third sessions of treatment.

Brian (B): I don't know, whenever I want to like join a club I start feeling like it's going to go badly. I know I'll stumble when I talk and act like a retard. I just know it because it's happened before.

Worker (W): So you're telling yourself something's going to happen before it does?

B: Yeah, well sort of. Yeah, I am.
W: It sounds like you've become a psychic and you can predict the future.
B: (Laughs). Yeah I know how it sounds, but it always happens to me.
W: Which means it *always* has to happen?
B: Well, no, I guess I can't say that.
W: And if you just heard your self-talk as self-defeating because you always predict failure, started with a clean slate, and just went into new situations hopeful that they will work out, and made a commitment not to criticize yourself if it isn't as good as you would like it to be, wouldn't that be a more hopeful way of seeing things?
B: Yeah, but it's scary.
W: I'm sure it is, Brian, but you can tell yourself good things and you can tell yourself bad things. Why not start on the assumption that with some practice, it'll work out well?
B: Yeah, that makes sense, but what if I bomb like I always do?
W: Then you bomb, tell yourself it takes a lot of practice to be good at anything, and try again. My job is to support your efforts and to always give you new ways of seeing and doing things.
B: OK, so where do we start?
W: We start tomorrow by you joining a club and staying in the club. Do you have one in mind?
B: Well, the math club, but it's for nerds like me.
W: So what's wrong with nerds? Many of our most successful people were considered nerds in high school and look at where they are now?
B: Yeah, yeah, I know. Bill Gates and guys like that.
W: Yes. Very rich, and successful, and powerful men and women like that. And who knows, maybe you'll make some friends.
B: You think?
W: I think.

Next Session

W: So how did the club joining go?
B: I joined, and not everyone was a nerd. There were even a couple of cute girls. Boy, they're all smart. Probably a lot smarter than I am.
W: Why do you say that?
B: I don't know. They seemed to know everyone and they were confident.
W: Had they belonged for a while?
B: Yeah, I was the newest one.
W: So you're psychic again, huh? You knew they were confident even when they first started?
B: (Laughs). No, I don't know that.
W: Why not ask a few how they felt when they first joined the club?
B: Yeah, maybe. I'd really like to ask that Jane Olson. She's a total babe, and smart.
W: So ask her. Start a conversation.
B: Me? With a babe? No way.
W: Yes, way. That's your homework assignment for next week.
B: She'll probably ignore me or laugh.
W: Ah, those psychic powers of yours.

B: OK, OK, I will, but then I'll feel depressed, and sick to my stomach when she laughs, and it'll be your fault.
W: I'm a big girl. I can take it. How about you, Brian?
B: I'll do it.

Next Session

W: So, how did it go with Jane?
B: I was pretty scared and I stammered and stuttered and stuff and I acted like a total jerk. And I mean total. And I was pissed at you for making me do it, and I thought I'd maybe lie and tell you I spoke to her and it went great, but then this thought came to me that it wouldn't be right, and it wouldn't help me, and that's what this was all about, helping me, and I spoke to her.
W: How did it go?
B: It went great. She's shy too. She couldn't even look at me when I started talking to her, and *she's* a babe. She told me some stuff about her family, which sounds worse than mine, and she's pretty lonely. After a while we were talking up a storm. I have a date this Friday. It's not a date exactly since we're going to a party and we'll see each other there, but she said that as soon as I came she wanted me to stand next to her, and talk, and dance with her. Man, I can't dance at all.
W: That's wonderful, Brian. Did you learn something from the experience?
B: Yeah, not to be psychotic... I mean psychic, and think I know how things will turn out before I try them. But like I'm still shy, and I feel lonely all the time.
W: No one said it would happen right away. You have a lot of practice being lonely and now you'll have to do a lot of practice not being lonely.
B: Will I ever stop feeling lonely, totally?
W: Maybe, but wouldn't it be nice to see if you can achieve the goals you've set for yourself and find out whether it makes you feel less lonely? Doesn't that possibility excite the scientist in you? We're doing a piece of research, actually, and we can evaluate the outcome in 16 weeks.
B: Yeah, it does make me feel like this is an experiment. I hope I'll stick with it and not give up.
W: I'll see to that.
B: (Gulp), I bet you will, too.

Brian's progress was good. He joined six clubs, began dating Jane and seeing her 2–3 times a week, and together they attended parties and other social events. He tries to sit with new people at lunch but finds it difficult and with some prodding from me, he can do it once or twice every 2 weeks. Has he overcome his loneliness? He says he is less lonely and has less social anxiety after 16 sessions but clearly he still has some trouble with new social situations. To provide practice for him to interact with others he is joined a group that I co-lead for adolescents with social anxiety and loneliness problems. He is quiet in the group and usually does not say anything unless asked, but he is slowly improving. He is become friendly with several of the group members who go to movies or out for a coke and says that has been a good thing. Here is how he evaluated his treatment progress:

B: You said this would be like an experiment. I think I'm busier than I used to be and having Jane in my life is great, but do I think I have the skills to deal with loneliness when I go to college? I don't know. I'm pretty uptight with people, and the thought of meeting new people still gives me knots in my stomach. I think, yeah, I'm like better, but I'm not cured. I think that will take a while, and maybe it won't happen at all. Maybe I'm one of those people who need to see someone like you all their life to keep dealing with stuff. I hope not ... not that I don't like you and all, cause I do, but what a depressing way to be ... that I'll need help the rest of my life or maybe I'll be like those lonely men at bars who drink themselves to death. Boy, I hope not. My dad says that I should just wake up one morning and be well. I wish it was that easy. Boy, do I ever. Loneliness is the pits."

7.8. SUMMARY

This chapter about loneliness provides reasons for social isolation that sometimes leads to depression over the course of the life span. Internal and external reasons for loneliness are explored and a case is presented of a lonely adolescent boy and the EBP treatment he receives for loneliness, and why it seems to be helping him.

7.9. QUESTIONS FROM THE CHAPTER

1. Do not you think that lonely people are their own worst enemy? We all have periods of loneliness but we do something about it. What stops lonely people from doing the same?
2. Why just call them depressed instead of lonely? Depressed people just do not have the energy to do anything about how lonely they feel. Do not you agree?
3. I do not believe that as many kids are lonely who say they are. All the people I know are anything but lonely. Do not you think they exaggerate their loneliness when they feel down and it throws off the data?
4. All of this stuff about women having more friends and not feeling as lonely as men sounds like nonsense to me. The women I know are always complaining about being lonely. Is not this just another example of gender political correctness?
5. Maybe kids are lonely because they are taught to be alone by their parents who may not want them to associate with other kids because of religious, racial, or ethnic difference. Do not you think that explains a lot of the reason for children feeling lonely?

References

ABCNews.com (2002). *Authentic happiness: Using our strengths to cultivate happiness.* Retrieved October 14, 2002 from the World Wide Web: http://abcnews.go.com/ sections/GMA/GoodMorningAmerica/GMA020904Happiness_feature.html.

Adams, A. K. B., Sanders, S., & Auth, E. A. (2004, November). Loneliness and depression in independent living retirement communities: Risk and resilience factors. *Aging & Mental Health, 8*(6), 475–485.

Akerlind, I., & Hornquist, J. (1992). Loneliness and alcohol abuse: A review of evidence of an interplay. *Social Science and Medicine, 34*(4), 405–414.

Andrews, G. J., Gavin, N., Begley, S., & Brodie, D. (2003). Assisting friendships, combating loneliness: Users' views on a 'befriending' scheme. *Aging & Society, 23*, 349–362.

Asher, S. R., Hymel, S., & Renshaw, P. D. (1984). *Loneliness* in children. *Child Development, 55*, 1456–1464.

Asher, S. R., Parkhurst, J. T., Hymel, S., & Williams, G. A. (1990). Peer rejection and loneliness in childhood. In S. R. Asher, & J. D. Cole (Eds.), *Peer rejection in childhood* (pp. 253–273). New York: Cambridge University Press.

Berguno, G., Leroux, P., McAinsyh, K., & Shaikh, S. (2004, September). Children's experience of loneliness at school and its relation to bullying and the quality of teacher interventions. *The Qualitative Report, 9*(3), 483, 499. http://www.nova.edu/ssss/QR/QR9-3/berguno.pdf.

Bishop, A. J., & Martin, P. (2007, October). The indirect influence of educational attainment on loneliness among unmarried older adults. *Gerontology, 33*(10), 897–917.

Blazer, D. G. (2002b). Self-efficacy and depression in late life: A primary prevention proposal. *Aging & Mental Health, 6*(4), 315–324.

Bolvin, M., Hymel, S., & Bykowski, W. M. (1995). The roles of social withdrawal, peer rejection and victimization by peers in predicting loneliness and depressed mood in childhood. *Developmental Psychopathology, 7*, 765–785.

Bullock, J. R. (1992). Children without friends: Who are they and how can teachers help? *Childhood Education, 69*, 92–96.

Bullock, J. R. (1993a). Children's *loneliness* and their relationships with family and peers. *Family Relations, 42*, 46–49.

Bullock, J. R. (1993b). Lonely children. *Young Children, 48*, 53–57.

Calabrese, R. L. (1989). The effects of mobility on adolescent alienation. *High School Journal, 73*, 41–46.

Carr, M., & Schellenbach, C. (1993). Reflective monitoring in lonely adolescents. *Adolescence, 28*, 737–748.

Cassidy, J., & Asher, S. R. (1992). Loneliness and peer relationships in young children. *Child Development, 63*, 350–365.

Dodge, K. A. (1983). Behavioral antecedents of peer social status. *Child Development, 51*, 1386–1399.

Duffy, A. (2000). Toward effective early intervention and prevention strategies for major affective disorders: A review of risk factors. *Canadian Journal of Psychiatry, 45*(4), 300–349.

Ekwall, A. (2005). Loneliness as a predictor of quality of life among older caregivers. *Journal of Advanced Nursing, 49*(1), 23–32.

France, M. H., McDowell, C., & Knowles, D. (1984, September). Understanding and coping with *loneliness. The School Counselor*, 11–17.

Glicken, M. D. (2006). *Learning from resilient people: Lessons we can apply to counseling and psychotherapy*. Thousand Oaks, CA: Sage.

Goswick, R. A., & Jones, W. H. (1982). Components *of loneliness* during adolescence. *Journal of Youth and Adolescence, 11*, 373–383.

Harrington, R., & Clark, A. (1998). Prevention and early intervention for depression in adolescence and early adult life. *European Archives of Psychiatry in Clinical Neuroscience, 248*, 32–45.

Hayden, L., Tarulli, D., & Hymel, S. (1988, May). *Children talk about loneliness.* Paper presented at the biennial meeting of the University of Waterloo Conference on Childhood Development, Waterloo, Ontario, Canada.

Henggeler, S. W., & Borduin, C. M. (1989). *Family therapy and beyond: A multisystematic approach to treating the behavioral problems of children and adolescents.* Pacific Grove, CA: Brooks/Cole.

Hobfoll, S. E. (1989). Conservation of resources: A new attempt at conceptualizing stress. *American Psychologist, 44,* 513–524.

Jr.Joiner, T. E., Catanzaro, S., Rudd, M. D., & Rajab, M. H. (1999). The case for a hierarchical, oblique, and bidimensional structure of loneliness. *Journal of Social and Clinical Psychology, 18,* 47–75.

Jones, W., & Carver, M. (1991). Adjustment and coping implications of loneliness. In C. R. Snyder (Ed.), *Handbook of social and clinical psychology.* New York: Pergamon Press.

Kochenderfer, B. J., & Ladd, G. W. (1996). Peer victimization: Manifestations and relations to school adjustment in kindergarten. *Journal of School Psychology, 34*(3), 267–283, [EJ 537 306].

Lazarus, R. S., & Folkman, S. (1984). *Stress, appraisal, and coping.* New York: Springer.

McWhirter, B. (1990). Loneliness: A review of current literature, with implications for counselling and research. *Journal of Counselling and Development, 68*(4), 417–422.

Mijuskovic, B. (1992). Organic communities, atomistic societies and loneliness. *Journal of Sociology and Social Welfare, 19*(2), 147–164.

Moore, D., & Schultz, N. R. (1983). *Loneliness* at adolescence: Correlates, attributes and coping. *Journal of Youth and Adolescence, 12,* 95–100.

Murphy, F. (2006, June). Loneliness: a challenge for nurses caring for older people. *Nursing Older People, 18*(5), 22–25.

Olweus, D. (1993). Victimization by peers: Antecedents and long-term outcomes. In K. H. Rubin, & J. B. Asendorpf (Eds.), *Social withdrawal, inhibition and shyness in childhood* (pp. 315–341). Hillsdale, NJ: Erlbaum.

Ostrov, E., & Offer, D. (1980). Loneliness and the adolescent. In J. Hartog, J. R. Audy, & Y. Cohen (Eds.), *The anatomy of loneliness* (pp. 170–185). New York: International University Press.

Peplau, L. A., & Perlman, D. (1984). Loneliness research: A survey of empirical findings. In L. A. Peplau, & S. E. Goldston (Eds.), *Preventing the harmful consequences of severe and persistent loneliness* (pp. 13–47). Rockville, MD: National Institute of Mental Health.

Ponzetti, J. J. (1990, July). Loneliness among college students. *Family Relations,* 336–340.

Powell, T. J., Yeaton, W., Hill, E. M., & Silk, K. R. (2001). Predictors of psychosocial outcomes for patients with mood disorders. *Psychiatric Rehabilitation Journal, 25*(1), 3–12.

Ramsey, P. G. (1991). *Making friends in school.* New York: Teachers College Press.

RokAch, A. (2007). The effect of age and culture on the causes of loneliness. *Social behavior and personality, 35*(2), 169–186, [Society for Personality Research (Inc.)].

Rook, K. S. (1984). Interventions for *loneliness:* A review and analysis. In L. A. Peplau, & S. E. Goldston (Eds.), *Preventing the harmful consequences of severe and persistent loneliness.* Washington, DC: U.S. Government Printing Office.

Rotenberg, K. J., MacDonald, K. J., & King, E. V. (2004, September). The relationship between loneliness and interpersonal trust during middle childhood. *Journal of Genetic Psychology, 165*(3).

Rubin, K. H., & Mills, R. S. L. (1991). Conceptualizing developmental pathways to internalizing disorders in childhood. *Canadian Journal of Behavioral Science, 23*(3), 300–317.

Saxton, L. (1986). *The individual, marriage and family*. Belmont, CA: Wadsworth Publishing.

Seligman, M. E. P., & Csikszetmihalyi, M. (2000). Positive psychology: An introduction. *American Psychologist, 55*(1), 5–14.

Sermat, V. (1978). Sources of loneliness. *Essence,* 2, 271–276.

Stossel, S. (2000, September 21). *Bowling alone*. Atlantic Unbound.

Sullivan, H. S. (1953). *The interpersonal theory of psychiatry*. New York: Norton.

Uruk, A. C., & Demir, A. (2003, March). Loneliness. *Journal of Psychology, 137*(2), 179–194.

Weiss, R. S. (1973). *Loneliness: The experience of emotional and social isolation*. Cambridge, MA: MIT Press.

White, H., McConnell, E., Clipp, E., Branch, L.G., Sloane, R., Pieper, C., & Box, T.L. (2002). *A randomized controlled trial of the psychosocial impact of providing internet training and access to older adults*.

Young, J. E. (1982). Loneliness, depression, and cognitive therapy: Theory and applications. In L. A. Peplau, & D. Perlman (Eds.), *Loneliness. A sourcebook of current theory, research and therapy* (pp. 379–405). New York: Wiley.

8 Evidence-Based Practice with Depression and Suicidal Ideation in Children and Adolescents

8.1. INTRODUCTION

This chapter on the troubling degree of depression and suicidal ideation among children and adolescents will consider depression, diagnostic factors, risk factors for depression and treatment approaches, with attention paid to prevent and recurrence after treatment. The chapter will also include a case study of a child receiving a treatment suggesting best evidence.

In a review of the research on the amount of depression in children and adolescents, Birmaher et al. (1996) found that a number of epidemiological studies reported up to 2.5% of children and up to 8.3% of adolescents in the US suffer from depression. In an NIMH-sponsored study of 9–17-year-olds, Shaffer et al. (1996) estimated that the prevalence of any severity of depression is more than 6% in a 6-month period, with 4.9% having major depression. Klerman and Weissman (1989) found that depression onset is occurring earlier in life today than in past decades. Early-onset depression often persists, recurs, and continues into adulthood, and indicates that depression in youth may also predict more severe illness in adult life. Weissman et al. (1999) found that depression in young people often co-occurs with other mental disorders, most commonly anxiety, disruptive behavior or substance abuse disorders, and with physical illnesses such as diabetes.

SAMHSA (2007, May/June) reports that in 2005, 2.2 million youth aged 12–17 experienced at least one major depressive episode. Rates of occurrence varied by age – 12-year-olds had the lowest rate (4.3%) of major depressive episodes (MDE) occurrence; 17-year-olds had the highest (11.9%) with adolescent girls having a rate of depression of 12.7% compared to the rate among adolescent boys of 4.6%. Rates were relatively similar across racial and ethnic groups. A major depressive episode is defined as a period of 2 weeks or longer during which a person has either a depressed mood or loss of interest or pleasure, and at least four other symptoms that reflect a change in functioning, such as insomnia, lack of energy or appetite, difficulty concentrating, and poor self-image.

Not surprisingly, Weissman et al. (1999) found that depression in children and adolescents is associated with an increased risk of suicidal attempts, particularly among adolescent boys, if the depression is accompanied by conduct disorder and alcohol or other substance abuse. The authors note that suicide is the third leading cause of death in 10–24-year-olds. Among adolescents who develop major depression, as many as 7% may commit suicide in their young adult years. Haines (2006, p. 1) writes:

> *Although relatively rare in youths under 12, young children do attempt suicide – and may do so impulsively when they are upset or angry. Suicide is a serious problem within the teenage population. Adolescent suicide is a leading cause of death among youth and young adults in the U.S. It is estimated that 500,000 teens attempt suicide every year with 5,000 succeeding. These are epidemic proportions. Children with a family history of violence, alcohol abuse, or physical or sexual abuse are at greater risk for suicide, as are those with depressive symptoms.*

8.2. SYMPTOMS OF DEPRESSION

Birmaher et al. (1996) believe that the diagnostic criteria and primary characteristics of major depressive disorder in youth are essentially the same as they are for adults. Ryan et al. (1987) stress the important fact that recognition of the disorder may be more difficult in youth because depressed children and young adolescents often find it difficult to describe their emotional state and may act out or show signs of irritability with others. This behavior may be misinterpreted as rebelliousness or just typical adolescent conduct, which neither the child nor the parents recognize as an underlying depressive state. The DSM-IV (APA, 1994, p. 327) notes the following symptoms of major depressive disorder in children:

> *(1) Persistent sad or irritable mood; (2) loss of interest in activities once enjoyed; (3) significant change in appetite or body weight; (4) difficulty sleeping or oversleeping; (5) psychomotor agitation or retardation; (6) loss of energy; (7) feelings of worthlessness or inappropriate guilt; (8) difficulty concentrating; (9) recurrent thoughts of death or suicide. Five or more of these symptoms must persist for 2 or more weeks before a diagnosis of major depression is indicated.*

The National Institute of Mental Health (2001, p. 1) indicates that the following are additional signs that could be associated with depression in children and adolescents: (1) frequent vague, non-specific physical complaints such as headaches, muscle aches, stomachaches or tiredness; (2) frequent absences from school or poor performance in school; (3) talk of or efforts to run away from home; (4) outbursts of shouting, complaining, unexplained irritability, or crying; (5) being bored; (6) lack of interest in playing with friends; (7) alcohol or substance abuse; (8) social isolation, poor communication; (9) fear of death; (10) extreme sensitivity to rejection or failure; (11) increased irritability, anger, or hostility; (12) reckless behavior; and (13) difficulty with relationships.

Klein et al. (2001) report that the recovery rate from a single episode of major depression in children and adolescents is quite high, but future episodes are likely to recur, particularly when brief recurring episodes of depression exist.

Depression is often associated with thoughts of suicide. Suicidal ideation refers to any self-reported thoughts of engaging in suicide-related behavior. Some investigators also consider thoughts that are less explicit in terms of wanting to take one's life (wanting to be dead, not wanting to awake) as indications of "passive" suicide ideation (Hoyert et al., 1999). While suicidal ideation may not lead to actual suicidal attempts, they are considered serious risk factors since there are an estimated 8–25 attempted suicides for every completion and suicidal ideations may move to suicidal attempts given situational conditions that may be hard for the clinician, or the family, to predict (Hoyert et al., 1999).

The rate of American male adolescent suicides has continually risen from 7.1 per 100 000 in 1986 to 11.4 per 100 000 in 1997 (CDC, 1998). From 1979 to 1992, the Native American male adolescent and young adult suicide rate in Indian Health Service Areas was the highest in the Nation, with a suicide rate of 62.0 per 100 000 (Wallace et al., 1996). It has been proposed that the rise in suicidal behavior among teenage boys results from increased availability of firearms (Brent et al., 1987, 1991) and increased substance abuse in the youth population (Birckmayer and Hemenway, 1999). However, although the rate of suicide by firearms increased more than suicide by other methods (Brent et al., 1987), suicide rates for adolescent males also increased markedly in many other countries in Europe, in Australia, and in New Zealand, where suicide by firearms is rare.

8.2.1. *Screening Tools*

Tools that are useful for screening children and adolescents for possible depression. These tools include the Children's Depression Inventory (CDI) for ages 7–17; and, for adolescents, the Beck Depression Inventory (BDI), and the Center for Epidemiologic Studies Depression (CES-D) Scale. When a youngster screens positive on any of these instruments, a comprehensive diagnostic evaluation by a mental health professional is warranted. The evaluation should include interviews with the youth, parents, and when possible, other informants such as teachers and social services personnel.

8.2.2. *Risk-Factors for Depression*

Birmaher et al. (1996) report that in childhood, boys and girls appear to be at equal risk for depressive disorders. During adolescence, however, girls are twice as likely as boys to develop depression. Harrington et al. (1997) report that children who develop major depression are more likely to have a family history of the disorder, often a parent who experienced depression at an early age, than patients with adolescent- or adult-onset depression. Adolescents who develop depression are also likely to have a family history of depression, though the correlation is not as high as it is for children. Harrington et al. indicate that other risk factors for depression include stress, divorce, abuse and neglect, chronic illness, break-up of a romantic relationship and other traumas, including natural and man-made disasters.

8.3. EVIDENCE-BASED PRACTICE WITH DEPRESSED CHILDREN AND ADOLESCENTS

In a comprehensive review of the efficacy of treatment for childhood and adolescent depression, Kaslow and Thompson (1998) found that forms of cognitive-behavioral therapy (CBT) were probably effective although none of the treatments reviewed were deemed to be well-established interventions. One form of CBT – coping skills – is based on the "Coping with Depression" course developed by Lewinsohn et al. (1996) and adapted by Clarke et al. (1992) for school-based programs to treat adolescent depression. Compared with controls on the waiting list, adolescents who received CBT had lower rates of depression, less self-reported depression, improvement in cognitions, and increased activity levels (Lewinsohn et al., 1996).

In preadolescents, two types of CBT – 12-session group interventions based on either self-control therapy or behavior-solving therapy – were compared with a control group (Stark et al., 1987). Children responded to both CBT interventions with fewer symptoms of depression and anxiety. However, the waiting list group exhibited minimal change. Self-control therapy was enhanced by doubling the number of sessions and included social skills training, assertiveness training, relaxation training and imagery, and cognitive restructuring. Monthly family meetings were also added to both the experimental and control conditions. Children receiving self-control therapy reported fewer symptoms at 7-month follow up (Stark et al., 1991).

Because depression often continues on from childhood and adolescence, with lifetime prevalence rates for major depressive disorder (MDD) of over 20% by age 18, Evans et al. (2005) believe that ages 13–14 may be a key developmental period for preventive interventions for depression. Hankin et al. (1988) report a substantial increase in diagnosed depressive disorders between ages 15 and 18 for both boys and girls. Consequently, providing effective treatments to youth prior to a period of significantly heightened risk could reduce the incidence of major depression along the life cycle.

The following is a summary of a meeting on child and adolescent depression convened by NIMH (2006) that included patient advocates and researchers in the fields of psychopharmacology, psychotherapies, clinical neuroscience, and clinical trial methodology and design. The main purpose of the meeting was to review the benefits and risks of existing treatment interventions for children and adolescents with depressive disorders and to identify gaps in current research and a future research agenda. The findings are as follows:

1. Interventions that have been proven efficacious in the treatment of major depression in youth include cognitive-behavioral therapy, interpersonal therapy, behavioral activation, cognitive restructuring, and interpersonal skill improvement. Pharmacotherapy with fluoxetine, and the combination of cognitive-behavioral therapy and fluoxetine have also been found to be effective and the risks of using these interventions are generally favorable, but careful monitoring is necessary, particularly where suicidal ideation is present.
2. Limited research is available on the treatment of depression in children under 12, particularly treatment using medication alone and medication in conjunction with therapy. Unfortunately current psychotherapeutic approaches are based largely on treatments developed for adults and may not be effective with younger children. Hopefully, new therapy approaches developed for children will be available in the near future.
3. A more precise diagnostic evaluation of depression in youth is needed, one that is sensitive to culture, gender, and age. Assessment and evaluation also needs to be individualized and gross generalizations about depression in youth should not be made based upon limited information. A thorough psychosocial history with available medical data should be available before a diagnosis is attempted.
4. Depression often co-exists with anxiety, and recovery is often hampered by untreated episodes of anxiety. More attention should be paid to understanding the impact and the effective treatment of anxiety if depression is to keep from recurring.

A major study investigated the efficacy of three types of interventions with 143 children in the 5th or 6th grade (Gillham and Reivich, 1999). The intervention group consisted of three different interventions: cognitive training skills, social problem-solving skills, and a combined treatment. All three interventions produced the same degree of improvement. The intervention group had significantly lower levels of depressive symptoms than the control group at post-intervention as well as at 6-, 18-, and 24-month follow-ups. Students in the intervention group were less likely to report moderate to severe levels of symptoms at 12-, 18-, and 24-month follow-up. However, these results were not maintained at 2.5 and 3-year follow-up assessments. Spence et al. (2005) found that treatment effects in children and adolescents generally wane over time. However, Beardslee et al. (2003) report more positive attitudes by parents and lower levels of depression in a program that offers post-treatment periodic check-ins by phone or meeting every 6–9 months during a 2.5-year follow-up.

Arnarson and Craighead (2005) studied the issue of preventing the first onset of adolescent depression. In their study of 86 students scoring between the 75th and 90th percentiles on a depression symptom measure and/or scoring above the 75th percentile on a measure of negative attributional style, just having a diagnostic interview resulted in significantly fewer cases of major depression/dysthymia during the 1-year follow-up period than did a control group receiving no intervention. Both groups scored in the same high level of potential for depression. It should be noted that the majority of the students (two-thirds of those with strong indicators of depression) refused to take part in the study.

To offset the lack of evidence that what we do in the treatment of depression is effective, Timmermans and Angell (2001) indicate that evidence-based clinical judgment should be used to make judgments based on best available evidence. Evidence-based clinical judgment has five important features: (1) it is composed of both research evidence and clinical experience; (2) there is skill involved in reading the literature that requires an ability to synthesize the information and make judgments about the quality of the available evidence; (3) the way in which information is used is a function of the practitioner's level of authority in an organization and his or her level of confidence in the effectiveness of the applied information; (4) part of the use of evidence-based practice is the ability to independently evaluate the information used and to test its validity in the context of one's own practice; and (5) evidence-based clinical judgments are grounded in the western notions of professional conduct and professional roles, and are ultimately guided by a common value system.

8.4. CASE STUDY: EVIDENCE-BASED PRACTICE WITH A DEPRESSED CHILD

Jimmy, age 10, was referred to a school social worker by his teacher because of Jimmy's depressed affect, his poor school work, and his withdrawal from the other children during the last several months. A discussion with Jimmy's mother confirmed that Jimmy was also depressed and withdrawn at home. She said that this was not unusual and that Jimmy had become increasingly sad and unhappy since the breakup of her marriage a year ago. Jimmy's father lives thousands of miles away and because the father has a low-paying job, it is difficult for him to see Jimmy as often as he would like but they stay in touch by e-mail and phone calls. A call to Jimmy's father confirmed his concern that Jimmy was showing indications of depression.

The school social worker was unable to get a psychological evaluation immediately because of the heavy caseloads and limited funding in the school system, but the psychologist met briefly with Jimmy and confirmed (without psychological testing, which would have been preferable, of course) that using the DSM-IV criteria, Jimmy certainly had a depression lasting more than 2 weeks and indicated that she thought he had a chronic depression possibly related to the divorce and urged the social worker to begin working with Jimmy immediately. A review of the literature indicated that a cognitive-behavioral approach might work best with children over 12 but there was very limited evidence of what worked well with children under 12. The school social worker had been using cognitive therapy with non-depressed children and thought she would try it with Jimmy.

She first confirmed that there was no health-related problem by asking for a physical from Jimmy's pediatrician. She then had an in-depth interview with both parents, Jimmy's father by phone, and found that Jimmy had been a happy child up the point of the divorce but that he had gradually become more and more depressed and withdrawn. He had little energy and slept 12–14 h a day. Often he complained of not feeling well and had missed 14 days of school the semester before he was seen by the social worker. Both parents confirmed that the problems they had been having in the marriage were kept from Jimmy and when the divorce took place he was taken by surprise. Jimmy is an only child and had been the "apple of their eyes" as a good athlete and student and generally popular and happy child.

The social worker began by asking Jimmy if he felt sad much of the time. Jimmy confirmed that he did. How did he know he was sad, the social worker wondered?

Jimmy (J): Because I feel tired all the time and I don't think anything good is ever going to happen to me. I feel my life won't be good.

Worker (W): Do you have a thought about why you feel that way?

J: Yeah, but there's nothing I can do about it. My dad doesn't live with us anymore, and my mother made him go away. Now I live with my mother and she's OK, but she's not like my dad. My dad spent time with me and he watched me play baseball and would teach me all kinds of things. He liked being outside and we'd do hikes together and he'd show me where animals were and the tracks they'd make. Sometimes we'd come on animals and he'd show me how you could hide from them so they wouldn't smell you and we'd watch them. He didn't believe in killing animals but we'd watch them and it was great. He calls and e-mails but it's not the same. Why can't I live with him so it can be like it was before?"

W: Have you suggested that?

J: Yeah, but my dad doesn't have any money. He lost a good job here and he's trying to find good work. My mom has a good job but I don't want to be with her. I want to be with my dad.

W: Is there anything your mom does that makes you sad?

J: No. She's a good mom but my dad and I were like very close, you know, and now we're not. He'll get married, I'll bet and he'll have kids and he'll forget about me.

W: That's one of the things you worry about?

J: All the time.

W: Have you mentioned it to your dad?

J: Oh, no. He'd be very upset. Sometimes I can tell he's crying on the phone because he misses me as much as I miss him.

W: If you lived with your father would that make you less sad?

J: Oh yeah, for sure. I wouldn't be sad at all.

The social worker contacted the parents and shared with them what Jimmy said. Could the father take Jimmy with some help from the mother? Yes, for sure he could. Would the mother mind? No, not really. Her job was demanding and she didn't have as much time to spend with Jimmy as she would like and plus, he was so depressed and he didn't seem to be any better. The parents agreed that Jimmy would live with his father and a trial arrangement was decided on for the coming semester with continued help for Jimmy.

Six months later the worker received a call from Jimmy's mother saying that he had returned home was starting school the next day and was more depressed than ever. He and his father hadn't gotten along because the father had little tolerance for Jimmy's depression. Jimmy was seen shortly thereafter.

W: Tell me what happened with your stay at your dad's.

J: It wasn't like I thought it would be. My dad just got mad at me because I was depressed so much. All the stuff we used to do together when we tried doing it again, I just didn't have, well, I was too tired to do it.

W: So you were still depressed even after you went to stay with your dad?

J: Yeah, I was. I don't know why, either. I thought I'd be pretty happy but the same stuff, the sad feelings, they just kept on going like when I was with my mom.

W: Any thoughts as to why your still feeling depressed?

J: Nope, not a one. I Just feel sad and like everything's gonna go wrong in my life, just like before.

W: One of the things I do with kids is to try and figure out why they're so sad and to help them see their lives in a better way. Can we try doing that?

J: Sure. Anything so I don't feel sad all the time.

W: OK. Let's start with some of the things you're thinking right now that tell us you're depressed. Can you tell me what those things are?

J: Yes. I feel sad all the time. I don't think I'll ever get better. I feel pretty bad about myself. I don't think I'm going to be a very happy person. My dad's mad at me and so is my mom. I feel like I did a bad job with them. Boy, when your mom and dad don't like you much, that's not a very good thing, is it.

W: OK. Let's start with how your mom and dad feel about you. You think they're mad at you and that may be so but you're going the next step and you're saying to yourself that they don't like you. You really don't know that. Being mad at a person isn't the same as not liking them. Often the people we like the most are the one's we get mad at because we care about them.

J: You mean like they still like me? Boy they don't seem to like me much. My dad hardly ever calls and my mom sort of ignores me.

W: Yes, that may be true but the idea that they don't like you is what I think we need to get at. Have you tried asking them how they feel about you?

J: No, but I have a pretty good idea.

W: Yes, that may be true but in the kind of help I give kids we try and find out if the feelings we have are actually true. Could you talk to them over the week and then let me know what they have to say?

J: Yeah I can do that but I can tell you that they don't like me much.

Jimmy came back the next week. He told the worker, "I talked to them and boy was I wrong. They think I'm mad at them for getting a divorce and that's why I'm depressed."

W: Are you mad at them for getting a divorce?

J: Well, no, but sometimes. <Pause> No, lots of time. My life was good when they were married and now it isn't. Yeah, I'm real mad at them.

W: OK, that's good that you could tell me that you're mad. It would have been much better had they stayed together because you would have been happy but they apparently weren't happy together.

J: Yeah, but they should have stayed together for me. I'm just a kid. I needed a happy family life.

W: I can understand how you feel but that just isn't what happens between grownups. It's tough to stay together when you fall out of love. Often they don't think it will affect their kids when, of course it does.

J: When you get married it's supposed to be until you die. That's what they say at church.

W: Yup, that would be nice but lots of people get divorced. Do you know any kids at school or church where their parents got divorced?

J: Lots of them.

W: Are the kids all unhappy?"

Jimmy thinks for a while.

J: Well, no. Lots of them are like they were before.

W: So it's possible for a kid to go through a divorce and not be unhappy. Why do you think you're so unhappy then?

J: Well, they just should have stayed married.

W: Do you think that maybe your thinking is wrong about your parents? Maybe you're thinking that people haven't the right to do things that make you unhappy?

J: Yeah, well, doesn't everybody think like that?

W: Many people do but when you think about it, we can't control what other people do. We can only control how we think about it.

J: We can? You mean I don't have to be sad about the divorce?

W: Yes, that's exactly what I mean. You can feel badly about the fact that two people who once loved each other fell out of love but they still love you.

J: Yeah, they do but shouldn't you feel sad when bad things happen?

W: Yes, but not for a long time. You should be able to get over it just like your friends at school. Could you ask them how they were able to deal with their sad feelings when their parents got divorced?

J: I already know. They just said that they were able to be happy even when their parents weren't. A lot of them knew their parents weren't happy way before they got divorced and they just started practicing being happy.

W: How did they do that?

J: They got good friends and did stuff at school and they knew they're parents loved them and they'd be OK.

W: That sounds like wonderful advice. Would you like to try thinking that way?

J: Yeah, but sometimes the sad feelings won't let me.

W: I understand but when that happens maybe you can start thinking about the happy things. Maybe you can just tell your mind to forget what's sad and think about happy things. Or maybe you can watch a happy movie or read a happy book or go back to playing sports. Anything that makes you happy.

J: You think that will help?

W: Yes, I do. And in the coming weeks you'll find out that you'll kinda feel the same way.

8.5. DISCUSSION

According to the worker, Jimmy's improvement has been slow but steady. It took several months for him to stop blaming his parents for his unhappiness and to recognize that they had been unhappy together long before the divorce. He wishes they had been more upfront about their problems because he might have been able to help. He also thought that he had something to do with their divorce but was able to resolve that belief after a few sessions. Jimmy has begun to deal with his thoughts and to return to many of the activities he was involved with before he became depressed. He still has intrusive thoughts that cause sadness but it is usually over in a day or two. He has stopped missing school.

The worker said that her use of cognitive therapy has been largely positive. Children, she said, take to it well and learn to use it quickly. She wishes there had been more research to help her select an approach to use with childhood depression and admits that using something with best evidence for adolescents and adults created some concerns on her part. "A full-blown depression isn't your ordinary school problem. What works with rebellious or low achieving kids may or may not work with childhood depression. I have to admit that what I did wasn't classical cognitive therapy because I used other approaches and I was very supportive. We did a lot of homework assignments, which Jimmy liked and largely completed. I spoke to some colleagues who were doing treatment with depressed children and some were using play therapy and others were just doing straight analytic therapy. Neither appealed to me, which I know isn't a good attitude, but until we have better research I guess I choose the approach that works best for me and hopefully the research will start taking childhood depression seriously."

8.6. SUMMARY

This chapter on childhood depression discusses the amount of depression in youth, the cause of so much depression in America's children and adolescents, and the best evidence of treatment efficacy from the research literature. Unfortunately, research providing best evidence of treatment effectiveness is still in process but further research efforts offers hope that treatment approaches with strong efficacy will be found to offer effective psycho-social interventions. A case study shows the use of cognitive therapy with a depressed 10-year old boy.

8.7. QUESTIONS FROM THE CHAPTER

1. Do not you think it is pretty natural for kids to feel down once in a while, and do not you think what we call depression in children is really more a part of the natural developmental cycle of kid's emotions trying to catch up with the changes in their bodies?

2. There is tremendous pressure on America's youth in school to be popular, wear great clothes, and act cool. Do not you think the depression many adolescents experience could be eliminated by making schools more user friendly, less prone to bullying, and less socially competitive?
3. Cognitive therapy seems like a pretty assertive way of treating children. Would not it be better just to give the child in this case study a lot of positive and unconditional support and feedback to bolster his low self-esteem?
4. It seems likely that depression is a learned behavior taught to children by depressed parents. Would not we get a lot more mileage from treatment if parents were treated for their depression along with their children?
5. Medicating young children for depression with drugs that have little proven efficacy seems cruel and ineffective. Do not you think that once children begin to use medications for their depression that they will be hooked on ever more potent anti-depressives for life?

References

American Psychiatric Association. (1994). *Diagnostic and statistical manual of mental disorders (DSM-IV)* (4th ed.). Washington, DC: American Psychiatric Press.

Arnarson, E. Ö., & Craighead, W. E. (2005). *Prevention of depression: A preliminary study*. Unpublished manuscript, University of Colorado at Boulder.

Beardslee, W. R., Gladstone, T. R. G., Wright, E. J., & Cooper, A. B. (2003). A family-based approach to the prevention of depressive symptoms in children at risk: Evidence of parental and child change. *Pediatrics, 112*, 119–131.

Birckmayer, J., & Hemenway, D. (1999). Minimum-age drinking laws and youth suicide, 1970–1990. *American Journal of Public Health, 89*, 1365–1368.

Birmaher, B., Ryan, N. D., & Williamson, D. E., et al. (1996). Childhood and adolescent depression: A review of the past 10 years. Part I. *Journal of the American Academy of Child and Adolescent Psychiatry, 35*(11), 1427–1439.

Brent, D. A., Perper, J. A., & Allman, C. J. (1987). Alcohol, firearms, and suicide among youth. Temporal trends in Allegheny County, Pennsylvania, 1960 to 1983. *Journal of the American Medical Association, 257*, 3369–3372.

Brent, D. A., Perper, J. A., Allman, C. J., Moritz, G. M., Wartella, M. E., & Zelenak, J. P. (1991). The presence and accessibility of firearms in the homes of adolescent suicides. A case-control study. *Journal of the American Medical Association, 266*, 2989–2995.

Centers for Disease Control and Prevention. (1998). *Youth risk behavior surveillance—United States, 1997*. CDC Surveillance Summaries, August 14, 1998. MMWR, 47 (no. SS-3).

Clarke, G. N., Hops, H., Lewinsohn, P. M., Andrews, J., Seeley, J. R., & Williams, J. (1992). Cognitive-behavioral group treatment of adolescent depression: Prediction of outcome. *Behavior Therapy, 23*, 341–354.

Evans, et al. (2005). In D. L. Evans, E. B. Foa, R. E. Gur, H. Hendin, C. P. O'Brien, & M. E. P. Seligman (Eds.). *Treating and preventing adolescent mental health disorders: What we know and what we don't know*. New York: Oxford University Press.

Gillham, J. E., & Reivich, J. E. (1999). Prevention of depressive symptoms in school children. *Psychological Science, 10*, 461–462.

Haines, C. (2006, November, 24). *Depression in children*. WEBMD. http://www.webmd.com/content/article/118/112886.htm?printing=true

Hankin, B. L., Abramson, L. Y., Moffitt, T. E., Silva, P. A., McGee, R., & Angell, K. E. (1988). Development of depression from preadolescence to young adulthood: Emerging gender differences in a 10-year longitudinal study. *Journal of Abnormal Psychology, 107*, 128–140.

Harrington, R., Rutter, M., & Weissman, M. M., et al. (1997). Psychiatric disorders in the relatives of depressed probands. I. Comparison of prepubertal, adolescent and early adult onset cases. *Journal of Affective Disorders, 42*(1), 9–22.

Hoyert D. L., Kochanek K. D. & Murphy S. L. (1999). Deaths: Final data for 1997. *National Vital Statistics Report, 47*(19). Hyattsville, MD: National Center for Health Statistics. DHHS Publication No. (PHS) 99-1120.

Kaslow, N. J., & Thompson, M. P. (1998). Applying the criteria for empirically supported treatments to studies of psychosocial interventions for child and adolescent depression. *Journal of Clinical Child Psychology, 27*, 146–155.

Klein, D. N., Schwartz, J. E., & Rose, S., et al. (2001). Five-year course and outcome of dysthymic disorder: A prospective, naturalistic follow-up study. *American Journal of Psychiatry, 157*(6), 931–939.

Klerman, G. L., & Weissman, M. M. (1989). Increasing rates of depression. *Journal of the American Medical Association, 261*, 2229–2235.

Lewinsohn, P. M., Clarke, G. N., Rhode, P., Hops, H., & Seely, J. (1996). A course in coping: A cognitive-behavioral approach to the treatment of adolescent depression. In D. Hibbs, & P. S. Jensen (Eds.), *Psychosocial treatments for child and adolescent disorders: Empirically based strategies for clinical practice* (pp. 109–135). Washington, DC: American Psychological Association.

National Institute of Mental Health. (2001). *Working toward better understanding and treatment of mental illness*.

National Institute of Mental Health Meeting Summary. (2006, February). *Benefits, limitations, and emerging research needs in treating youth with depression*.

Ryan, N. D., Puig-Antich, J., & Ambrosini, P., et al. (1987). The clinical picture of major depression in children and adolescents. *Archives of General Psychiatry, 44*, 854–861.

Substance Abuse and Mental Health Services Administration (SAMHSA) News. (2007, May/June). *Depression: reports offer statistics, 15*(1).

Shaffer, D., Fisher, P., & Dulkan, M. K., et al. (1996). The NIMH diagnostic interview schedule for children version 2.3 (DISC-2.3): description, acceptability, prevalence rates and performance in the MECA study. *Journal of the American Academy of Child and Adolescent Psychiatry, 35*(7), 865–877.

Spence, S. H., Sheffield, J. K., & Donovan, C. L. (2005). Long-term outcome of a school-based, universal approach to prevention of depression in adolescents. *Journal of Consulting and Clinical Psychology, 73*, 160–167.

Stark, K. D., Reynolds, W. M., & Kaslow, N. J. (1987). A comparison of the relative efficacy of self-control therapy and a behavioral problem-solving therapy for depression in children. *Journal of Abnormal Child Psychology, 15*, 91–113.

Stark, K. D., Rouse, L., & Livingston, R. (1991). Treatment of depression during childhood and adolescence: Cognitive-behavioral procedures for the individual and family. In & P. Kenall (Ed.), *Child and adolescent therapy* (pp. 165–206). New York: Guilford Press.

Timmermans, S., & Angell, A. (2001). Evidence-based medicine, clinical uncertainty, and learning to doctor. *Journal of Health & Social Behavior, 42*(4), 342.

Wallace, J. D., Calhoun, A. D., Powell, K. E., O'Neil, J., & James, S. P. (1996). *Homicide and suicide among Native Americans, 1979–1992* (Violence Surveillance Series, No. 2). Atlanta: Centers for Disease Control and Prevention, National Center for Injury Prevention and Control.

Weissman, M. M., Wolk, S., & Goldstein, R. B., et al. (1999). Depressed adolescents grown up. *Journal of the American Medical Association, 281*, 1701–1713.

Further reading

Lewinsohn, P. M., Clarke, G. N., Hops, H., & Andrews, J. (1990). Cognitive-behavioral treatment for depressed adolescents. *Behavior Therapy, 21*, 385–401.

Wallace, L.D., Calhoun, A.D., Powell, K.E., O'Neil, J., & James, S.P. (1996). *Homicide and suicide among Native Americans, 1979–1992*. Violence Surveillance Series, No. 2. Atlanta: Centers for Disease Control and Prevention, National Center for Injury Prevention and Control.

Weissman, M.M., Wolk, S., & Goldstein, R.B., et al. (1999). Depressed adolescents grown up. *Journal of the American Medical Association, 281*, 1707–1713.

Further reading

Lewinsohn, P.M., Clarke, G.N., Hops, H., & Andrews, J. (1990). Cognitive-behavioral treatment for depressed adolescents. *Behavior Therapy, 21*, 385–401.

9 Evidence-Based Practice with Children and Adolescents Experiencing Anxiety

9.1. INTRODUCTION

Anxiety is a substantial problem for children and adolescents. The combined prevalence of anxiety disorders is higher than that of virtually all other mental disorders of childhood and adolescence (Costello et al., 1996). The 1-year prevalence of anxiety disorders in children ages 9–17 is 13%. Kashani and Orvaschel (1988) found an 8.7% rate of one or more anxiety disorder among adolescents, making it one of the most prevalent emotional disorders among children and adolescents (Albano et al., 2003). Kendall et al. (2000) believe that anxiety may continue into adulthood, causing significant impairment if left untreated. The Brown University Psychopharmacology Update (2007, January) reports that anxiety affects physical health and that a clear relationship exists between anxiety in children and adolescents and at least one and often multiple somatic complaints, usually restlessness, stomachaches and palpitations.

Complicating the assessment and treatment of childhood anxiety is research suggesting that parents and children often disagree on the existence of the problem and its severity. Safford et al. (2005) write "A growing body of research on parent–child agreement for reporting psychological problems suggests that the agreement, even when using structured or semistructured interviews, is quite low, especially when assessing internalizing disorders such as anxiety" (p. 747). According to the researchers, the assessment process to determine the existence and severity of an anxiety disorder must consider the child's ability to report the symptoms of anxiety and whether the self-report is affected by the child's desire to please the clinician or the parent's tendency to over emphasize, underemphasize, or deny the existence of anxiety as a result of the parent's own emotional states at the time. The congruence between the child's perception and the parent's is therefore frequently at odds, often because the child is more aware of his or her inner life and how the anxiety affects it.

The Eating Disorder Review (March/April 2003) reports that 60% of the clients seeking help for eating disorders suffered from childhood anxiety problems. Obsessive compulsive disorder (OCD) was reported by 40% of 650 clients seeking help for eating disorders. When clients were asked which anxiety disorder affected them before the onset of the eating disorder, most reported OCD, phobias and social phobias. Following the recognition of the eating disorder, many suffered from panic attacks and PTSD.

This chapter discusses common child and adolescent anxiety problems, including separation anxiety disorder, generalized anxiety disorder, social phobia, and OCD, as well as the more effective treatment approaches from the research literature.

9.2. TYPES OF ANXIETY PROBLEMS

9.2.1. Separation Anxiety Disorder

Separation anxieties are common among infants and toddlers. When they affect older children or adolescents, the behavior may represent separation anxiety disorder. In order for a person to be diagnosed with separation anxiety disorder, the anxiety must cause emotional distress or affect social and educational functioning for at least one month (DSM-IV). Children who experience separation anxiety may find it difficult to leave parents and often have difficulty falling asleep because of fear of being abandoned. Often children with separation anxiety obsessively worry that their parents have been involved in an accident, have become too ill to care for them, or are in "lost" to the child forever. The need to stay close to their parents often makes going to school or to a friend's home stressful. Young children with separation anxiety often experience nightmares or fears at bedtime. Other symptoms include depression, withdrawal, apathy, or difficulty in concentrating. Young children experience nightmares or fears at bedtime. Separation Anxiety should not be diagnosed when children or adolescents are living in dangerous situations where they could be hurt when they are away from home.

About four percent of children and young adolescents suffer from separation anxiety disorder (DSM-IV). The disorder is more common in girls (DSM-IV). The problem often disappears as children mature but there are a number of instances in which the disorder lasts for a number of years and transitions to serious adult problems, most specifically panic disorder with agoraphobia, worry about separation from their own children and partners, and other obsessions which cause emotional pain in adulthood. Goenjian et al. (1995) suggest that separation anxiety is often associated with physical and sexual trauma, death or illness in the family, and because the disorder often runs in families, genetic and environmental factors that have not been established but may relate to overprotective parenting brought about because of parental traumas.

The Harvard Mental Health Letter (2007, Jan.) reports "Children who are insecurely attached – lacking this confidence in their parents – are more likely to develop anxiety disorders, especially separation anxiety" (p. 1). Furthermore, parents with intrusive emotional problems may promote insecure attachment through over-protectiveness and reluctance to allow age-appropriate independence. Similarly, parents who are abusive, neglectful, or alternate between affection and rejection may not only promote anxiety but may fail to respond to a child's signals of distress. Other parents may just lack competence in dealing with the extra encouragement and special coaching a timid child might need to deal with separation anxiety when it occurs, and the lack of an adequate response may trigger longer and more severe episodes.

9.2.2. *Generalized Anxiety Disorder*

Children with generalized anxiety disorder excessively worry and obsess about a variety of events in their lives, including their school performance, being on time, terrorism and numerous natural and manmade disasters that inhibit their social functioning. Physical symptoms can include tremors, sweating, multiple somatic complaints, and exhaustion. Generalized anxiety sometimes leads to perfectionism, conformity, the need for continual reassurance, and low self-esteem (DSM-IV). The one-year prevalence rate for all generalized anxiety disorder sufferers of all ages is approximately three percent. The lifetime prevalence rate is about five percent (DSM-IV). About half of all adults seeking treatment for this disorder report that it began in childhood or adolescence, but whether childhood anxiety continues into adulthood is not known. However, the remission rate for children suffering from generalized anxiety is not as high as it is for separation anxiety disorder.

9.2.3. *Social Anxiety Disorder*

Children with social anxiety disorder persistently worry about being embarrassed in social situations. The worry often relates to fear of being judged by others, or public behavior that might cause embarrassment or lead to ridicule. Social anxiety may produce such physical reactions as palpitations, tremors, sweating, diarrhea, blushing, muscle tension, and even full-blown panic attacks. Young children are often unable to discuss their fears and instead may cry, appear timid in new social settings, and stay close to familiar adults. Black and Noyes, 1997 report that children with social anxiety may do badly in school, avoid going to school, or avoid social interactions with other children. The avoidance of social situations often interferes with a many aspects of a child's life. Black and Noyes (1997) report a lifetime prevalence rate of 3–13%, with females in the majority of those with social anxiety. For many people with social anxiety the problem may last a lifetime, although many people report remission or a lessening of the disorder as they achieve in life.

9.2.4. *Obsessive-compulsive Disorder*

OCD is characterized by repetitive and time-consuming obsessive or compulsive behaviors that cause heightened anxiety when not completed. The obsessions are intrusive images, thoughts, or impulses. The compulsive behaviors (i.e., hand-washing or cleaning rituals) are an attempt to displace the obsessive thoughts (DSM-IV). Flament et al. (1988) estimate the prevalence of OCD as being from 0.2% to 0.8% in children, and up to two percent of adolescents. Lenane et al.

(1990) found a strong familial component to OCD from twin studies of both genetic susceptibility and environmental influences. Lenane et al. (1990) found that if one twin has OCD, the other twin is more likely to have OCD if the children are identical twins rather than fraternal twins. There is an increased occurrence of among first-degree relatives of children with OCD, particularly among fathers (Lenane et al., 1990). Leonard et al. (1997) report that the incidence of OCD in families does not appear to be just a matter of the child imitating relatives since OCD patterns are often different from those of relatives with the disorder. Rauch and Savage (1997) and Grachev et al. (1998) report that many adults with either childhood or adolescent onset of OCD show evidence of abnormalities in a neural network known as the orbitofrontalstriatal area.

9.2.5. Panic Disorder and Agoraphobia

Panic disorder is present when a child has recurrent, frequent (at least once a week) panic attacks. Panic attacks are discrete spells lasting about 20 min, during which the child experiences somatic or cognitive symptoms. Panic disorder can occur with or without agoraphobia. Agoraphobia is a persistent fear of being trapped in situations or places without a way to escape easily and without help. Panic disorder is rare in prepubertal children compared to adolescents. Because many panic symptoms are somatic in nature, many children undergo medical assessments before a panic disorder is suspected. This diagnosis is further complicated in children who have a concurrent medical illness, especially asthma; a panic attack can trigger an asthma attack and vice versa. Panic attacks also can occur in the context of other anxiety disorders such as OCD or separation anxiety.

Panic attacks usually develop spontaneously, but over time, children begin to attribute them to certain situations and environments. Affected children then attempt to avoid those situations, which can lead to agoraphobia. Agoraphobia is diagnosed when the child's avoidance behaviors are of such a degree that they greatly impair normal functioning, such as going to school, visiting the mall, or doing other typical activities. In adult panic disorder, concerns about future attacks, the implications of the attacks, and changes in behavior are important features of the diagnostic criteria. Children and younger adolescents usually lack the sufficient insight and forethought necessary to evolve these additional manifestations. Behavioral changes, when they occur, typically involve avoiding circumstances or situations related (in the child's belief) to the panic attack.

9.2.6. Phobias

Children and adolescents with phobias have unrealistic and excessive fears of certain situations or objects. Many phobias have specific names, and the disorder usually centers on animals, storms, water, heights, or situations such as being in an enclosed space. Young people with phobias will try to avoid the objects and situations they fear, so the disorder can greatly restrict their lives. Severe fears are present in about 10–15% of children and specific phobias are found in about five percent of children (Bourne, 2005). Children with specific phobias experience an intense fear of an object or situation that does not go away easily and continues for an extended period of time. Children often have specific phobias of the dark, spiders, bees, heights, water, choking, snakes, dogs, birds, and other animals. For many children, these fears and phobias interfere with their participation in and enjoyment of various activities. It may also interfere with their education, family life, or their social life.

Rainey (1997) notes that a variety of cognitive-behavioral treatments have been used for phobias with some success. Marks (1987) found that simple or specific phobias have been quite effectively treated with cognitive-behavioral therapy. Foa and Kozak (1986) found exposure treatment (discussed in more detail under the treatment of PTSD later in the chapter) to be effective with phobias. Some patients cannot handle the process of flooding the client with thoughts of the phobia used in exposure therapy, and an alternative conditioning technique can be used called counter-conditioning (Watson, 1924). In this form, the client is trained to substitute a relaxation response for the fear response in the presence of the phobic stimulus, an incompatible response to feeling fearful or having anxiety. Wolpe (1958) developed a systematic way to gradually introduce the fear-producing stimulus in a step-by-step fashion known as systematic desensitization. Systematic desensitization involves three steps: (1) training the client to physically relax; (2) establishing an anxiety hierarchy of the stimuli involved; and (3) employing counter-conditioning relaxation as a response to each feared stimulus beginning with the least anxiety-provoking stimulus and moving to the next least anxiety-provoking stimulus, until all of the items listed in the anxiety hierarchy have been dealt with successfully. Systematic desensitization in a variety of forms has been commonly used to treat specific phobias and, in some cases, can be achieved in a single therapeutic session (Ost, 1989; Zinbarg et al., 1992).

9.2.7. Post-Traumatic Stress Disorder (PTSD)

PTSD is thought to be linked to a highly traumatic experience or life-threatening event that produces intrusive thoughts related to a very disturbing aspect of the original traumatic event. These thoughts are difficult to dislodge once they reach conscious awareness. In many cases of PTSD, the child or adolescent physically and emotionally re-experiences the original traumatic event and is frequently in a highly agitated state of arousal as a result. Symptoms of PTSD usually begin within three months of the original trauma. In half the cases, complete recovery occurs within three months of the onset of symptoms, but many cases last more than 12 months (APA, 1994, p. 426).

According to the DSM-IV (APA, 1994), the core criteria for PTSD include distressing symptoms of, (1) re-experiencing a trauma through nightmares and intrusive thoughts; (2) numbing by avoiding reminders of the trauma, or feeling aloof or unable to express loving feelings for others and; (3) persistent symptoms of arousal as indicated by two or more of the following: Sleep problems, irritability and angry outbursts, difficulty concentrating, hyper-vigilance, and an exaggerated startle response with a duration of more than a month, which causes problems at work, in social interactions, and in other important areas of life (American Psychiatric Association, 1994, pp. 427–429). The DSM-IV judges the condition to be acute if it has lasted less than three months, and chronic if it has lasted more than three months. It is possible for the symptoms to be delayed. The DSM-IV notes that a diagnosis of delayed onset is given when symptoms begin to appear six months or more after the original trauma (APA, 1994, p. 429). Symptoms of PTSD in children and adolescents are as follows (Mental Health Association of Westchester, 2008):

1. *Children 5 years and younger*: Fear of being away from parents; crying, shaking or bedwetting; fear of darkness; trouble sleeping and nightmares.
2. *Children 6–11 years old*: Not wanting to be around other children; irritability and fighting; distractibility and trouble concentrating; nightmares and difficulty sleeping; refusing to go to school; stomachaches or headaches; flashbacks; memories of the frightening event that seem real; bed wetting.
3. *Adolescents 12–17 years old*: Nightmares and trouble sleeping; flashbacks or frightening memories that feel as if the trauma is happening again; refusing to go places or do things that remind the adolescent of the trauma; not getting along with friends; difficulty concentrating; trouble with school work; feeling sad and not wanting to be with friends.

Cohen (1998) believes that certain PTSD symptoms, such as dissociation, self-injurious behaviors, substance abuse, and/or conduct problems, may obscure the original trauma and clinicians may miss the existence of PTSD. Children going through abrupt changes in development may demonstrate some of the signs of PTSD. To meet the criteria for a diagnosis of PTSD, the child must first have been exposed to an extremely traumatic event that results in re-experiencing the event, avoidance and numbing, and increased arousal when memories of the event are triggered. Cohen (1998) suggests that re-experiencing the trauma may show itself in repetitive play with traumatic themes, recurrent upsetting dreams about the trauma, and intense anxiety when conscious and unconscious cues remind the child of the trauma. Avoidance and numbing may be observed in the child who is withdrawing from his or her usual activities and who uses techniques to avoid thinking about the trauma, which may become obsessive. This may also be true of children who have a complete loss of memory about the event or seem detached and lack future thinking. Persistent symptoms of increased arousal, if they are to be considered part of the response to PTSD, must be newly observed symptoms that may include sleep problems, irritability or angry outbursts, difficulty concentrating, hyper-vigilance, and exaggerated startle response. Symptoms must be present for at least one month and cause clinically significant distress or impairment in normal functioning to be diagnosed as PTSD.

Cohen (1998) believes that clinicians often fail to ask children about a traumatic life event because it may trigger severe anxiety. The children are not likely to tell clinicians about traumatic events because they may feel shamed by the event, as in the case of sexual molestation by a family member. In situations that involve litigation, a discussion of the precipitating event that may confuse the child's memory could result in liability concerns about the clinician's role in the child's confusion about the event. Because of this, Cohen believes that we often miss important evidence of the presence of PTSD. Cohen believes that several semi-structured interviews are necessary to find out about traumatic events in a child's life. Cohen suggests that clinicians pay close attention to the criteria for PTSD when they collect information from the interviews.

Gist and Devilly (2002) worry that PTSD is being predicted on such a wide basis for every tragedy that occurs that we have watered down its usefulness and write,

> *Progressive dilution of both stressor and duration criteria has so broadened application that it can now prove difficult to diagnostically differentiate those who have personally endured stark and prolonged threat from those who have merely heard upsetting reports of calamities striking others (p. 741).*

The authors go on to say that many early signs of PTSD are normal responses to stress that are often overcome with time and distance from the event. Interference by professionals in the treatment of PTSD could make the problem more severe and prolonged. In determining whether PTSD will actually develop, children need time to cope with the trauma on their own. Gist and Devilly (2002) note that the predictions of PTSD in victims of the World Trade Center bombings turned out to be almost 70% lower than what actually occurred, four months after the event. Susser et al. (2002, August) report that 2001 New Yorkers were interviewed by telephone between January 15 and February 21, 2002. The interview indicated a significant decrease in the stress-related symptoms subjects experienced during and after the World Trade Center bombings only several months earlier, and write, "Many affected New Yorkers are clearly recovering naturally, a tribute to the resilience of the human psyche" (p. 76). Of course, symptoms of PTSD may develop much later than four months after a trauma. Still, the point is well taken. Children often heal on their own and a premature diagnosis of PTSD may be counterproductive.

There may be other factors that determine whether PTSD develops following a trauma. McGaugh & Cahill (1997) found that memory formation during a traumatic event can be blocked, reducing the likelihood of PTSD. If this is the case, the authors wonder if we can predict who will be most likely to experience PTSD as a result of the variables related to its formation. In a review of studies determining the impact of traumatic experiences, *The Harvard Health Letter* (2002, October) reports that "[t]he people most likely to have symptoms of PTSD were those who suffered job loss, broken personal relationships, the death or illness of a family member or close friend, or financial loss as a result of the disaster itself" (p. 8). However, several studies reported in the Harvard Health Letter also note that a person's current emotional state may influence the way they cope with the trauma. Environmental concerns (living in high crime areas, for example) and health risks (disabilities which make people vulnerable, as another example) raise the likelihood of repeated traumatization that may increase the probability of developing PTSD. Stein (2002, December) suggests that one significant event that influences the development of PTSD is that of being exposed to assaultive traumatic events such as serious fights, domestic violence, child abuse, muggings, sexual trauma, and other forms of traumatic violence. Stein believes that vulnerability to repetitive acts of violence significantly increases the probability of developing PTSD. Ozer et al. (2003, p. 69) conclude:

> *There is a common thread between exposure to prior traumatic stressors, family history of psychopathology, and the exposed person's own psychological difficulties as predictors of PTSD symptoms. This thread is that psychological difficulties, perhaps also manifested in or as a consequence of poorer social support, play some role in conferring risk of developing PTSD symptoms after exposure to a traumatic stressor. It is tempting to make an analogy to the flu or infectious disease: Those whose immune systems are compromised are at greater risk of contracting a subsequent illness. Similarly, this cluster of variables may all be pointing to a single source of vulnerability for the development of PTSD or enduring symptoms of PTSD-a lack of psychological resilience.*

9.3. EVIDENCE-BASED PRACTICE WITH PROBLEMS ANXIETY OF IN CHILDREN AND ADOLESCENTS

The author wishes to thank Sage Publication for permission to reprint the following discussion of exposure therapy, which first appeared in Glicken (2005, pp. 153–156).

In 1995, the Task Force on Promotion and Dissemination of Psychological Procedure identified empirically supported treatments for children (Chambless and Ollendick, 2001). Although Chambless and Ollendick (2001) concluded that "well-established treatments" did not exist for anxiety disorders in children and adolescents (separation anxiety, avoidant disorder, overanxious disorder), CBT and CBT plus family anxiety management training were classified as "probably efficacious treatments." Similarly, in the category of phobias, CBT was classified as "probably efficacious treatment." In a meta-analysis of over 20 studies believed to meet high research standards, Ishikawa et al. (2007) came to the same conclusion. In a review of the existing research on the treatment of childhood and adolescent anxiety, Compton et al. (2002) reported substantial evidence of the effectiveness of cognitive-behavioral interventions. Cartwright-Hatton et al. (2004), in their systematic review of the effectiveness of CBT with anxiety disorders in children and adolescents, found that the odds were good that CBT would lead to recovery and that it was an effective intervention for anxiety disorders in children and adolescents.

In treating PTSD, Rothbaum et al. (2002, Winter) describe a type of treatment based on an emotional-processing theory which believes that PTSD develops as a result of memories eliciting fear that trigger escape and avoidance behaviors. This treatment has been used with adults and whether it would be useful for children and adolescence is difficult to say, given the lack of research. However, it is included here for the reader to understand the approach and determine through further evaluation whether it would help (or potentially hurt) children and adolescents experiencing symptoms of PTSD as a result of a trauma.

Since the development of a "fear network" functions as a type of obsessive condition, the child continues to increase the number of stimuli that serve to increase fear. To reduce the number of stimuli that elicit fear, the child must have his or her "fear network" activated so that new information can be provided that rationally contradicts the obsessive network of emotions reinforcing the PTSD symptoms. The authors believe that the following serve to reduce the client's fear network: (1) Repeated reliving of the original trauma helps to reduce anxiety and correct a belief that anxiety will necessarily continue unless avoidance and escape mechanisms are activated; (2) discussing the traumatic event reduces negative reinforcement of the event and helps the client see it in a logical way which corrects misperceptions of the event; (3) speaking about the trauma helps the client realize that it's not dangerous to remember the trauma; and (4) the ability of the client to speak about the trauma provides the client with a sense of mastery over his or her PTSD symptoms. The authors call this type of treatment, "exposure therapy."

Several types of exposure therapies show promise in the treatment of PTSD. Stress inoculation therapy (SIT) is an approach that includes relaxation, cognitive restructuring, preparing for a stressor, thought-stopping, covert modeling, and role-playing. Cognitive-processing therapy (CPT) provides traditional cognitive therapy and exposure in the form of writing and reading about the traumatic event (Resick, 1992; Resick and Schnicke, 1992). In CPT, ideas and perceptions about the traumatic event are challenged and more accurate and logical perceptions are encouraged. Additionally, clients are encouraged to write about their traumas and read them aloud to the therapist. The repetition of writing and reading about the trauma tends to reduce its emotional impact on the client and hopefully leads to a lessening of symptoms through an understanding of "sticking" points that may serve to reinforce anxiety. Hensley (2002, p. 338) provides an explanation of exposure therapy as it might be given to a client who has been raped:

1. Memories, people, places, and activities now associated with the rape make you highly anxious, so you avoid them.
2. Each time you avoid them you do not finish the process of digesting the painful

experience, and so it returns in the form of nightmares, flashbacks, and intrusive thoughts.
3. You can begin to digest the experience by gradually exposing yourself to the rape in your imagination and by holding the memory without pushing it away.
4. You will also practice facing those activities, places, and situations that currently evoke fear.
5. Eventually, you will be able to think about the rape and resume your normal activities without experiencing intense fear. (Hensley, 2002, p. 338).

In describing a typical application of exposure therapy in a number of the studies reviewed with positive results, Rothbaum et al. (2002, p. 63) write:

> *Prolonged exposure treatment consisted of nine biweekly individual sessions. The first two sessions were devoted to information gathering, explaining the treatment rationale, and treatment planning, including the construction of a hierarchy of feared situations for in vivo exposure. During the remaining sessions, survivors were instructed to relive, in their imagination, the traumatic experiences, describing it aloud "as if it were happening now." Exposure continued for about 60 min and was tape-recorded so that survivors could practice imaginal exposure as homework by listening to the tape. The survivors were also given homework assignments, instructing them to approach feared situations or objects that were realistically safe. Detailed instructions for conducting exposure therapy with PTSD patients can be found in Foa and Rothbaum (1998).*

Reviews of the current literature using exposure therapy for PTSD have been quite positive. In the annual review of important findings in psychology, 12 studies found positive results using exposure therapy with PTSD. Eight of these studies received special recognition for the quality of the methodology and for the positive nature of the outcomes (Foa and Meadows, 1997). Several of the studies were done with Viet Nam veterans and showed a significant reduction in the symptoms of PTSD following exposure therapy (Keane et al., 1989). The same positive results were found in studies with rape victims in which exposure therapy was used (Foa et al., 1991, 1999). Exposure therapy has been used with a variety of PTSD victims, including victims of combat traumas, sexual assaults, child abuse, and other forms of violence. Exposure therapy has the most consistently positive results in reducing symptoms of PTSD when compared to other forms of treatment (Rothbaum et al., 2000).

Exposure therapy was compared to cognitive restructuring (Deblinger et al., 1990; Foa et al., 1995). Both types of treatment were considered highly effective, but exposure therapy alone was more effective than cognitive restructuring. Better than 50% of the clients receiving exposure therapy achieved over a 70% improvement of PTSD symptoms after nine sessions, while clients receiving cognitive restructuring alone needed an additional three sessions to achieve the same results. Rothbaum et al. (2000) report that in the past 15–20 years, exposure therapy has been used with a variety of patients experiencing a number of traumatic events leading to symptoms of PTSD. Rothbaum et al.

(2002) write that "[e]xposure therapy has more empirical evidence for its efficacy than any other treatment developed for the treatment of trauma-related symptoms" (p. 65).

9.3.1. Debriefing

One form of treatment with potential for use in work with PTSD victims following a tragedy such as 9–11 is single session treatment, or what has also been called debriefing. In this approach, clients who have experienced a trauma are seen in a group lasting one to three hours, and within a week to a month of the original traumatic event. Risk factors are evaluated and a combination of information and opportunity to discuss their experiences during and after the trauma are provided (Bisson et al., 2000). Most debriefing groups use crisis intervention techniques in a very abbreviated way and may provide educational information to group members about typical reactions to traumas, what to look for if group members experience any of these symptoms, and who to see if additional help is needed. They may also attempt to identify group members at risk of developing PTSD (Van Emmerik et al., 2002).

Despite the considerable appeal of this approach, there is almost no evidence that debriefing works to reduce the number of people who experience PTSD following debriefing sessions, and some evidence that it may increase PTSD over other forms of treatment (Van Emmerik et al., 2002). In fact, debriefing is less effective than no treatment at all following a trauma and may actually lead to an increase in PTSD (Van Emmerik et al., 2002). Gist and Devilly (2002) support these findings and write, "immediate debriefing has yielded null or paradoxical outcomes" (p. 742) because the approaches used in debriefing are often those "kinds of practical help learned better from grandmothers than from graduate training" (p. 742). The authors report that while still high, the estimates of PTSD after the 9–11 bombing dropped by almost two-thirds within four months of the tragedy and conclude that:

> *These findings underscore the counterproductive nature of offering a prophylaxis with no demonstrable effect, but demonstrated a potential to complicate natural resolution, in a population in which limited case-conversion can be anticipated, strong natural supports exist, and spontaneous resolution is prevalent (p. 742).*

There are several primary reasons for the lack of effectiveness of debriefing: (1) Debriefing interferes with natural healing processes and sometimes results in bypassing usual support systems such as family, friends, and religious groups (Horowitz, 1976); (2) upon hearing that PTSD symptoms are normal reactions to trauma, some victims of trauma actually develop the symptoms as a result of the suggestions provided in the debriefing session, particularly when the victim has not had time to process the various feelings he or she may have about the trauma (Kramer and Rosenthal, 1998); and (3) clients seen in debriefing include both those at risk and those not at risk. Better results may be obtained by screening clients at risk through a review of past exposure to traumas that may have served as catalysts for the current development of PTSD (Brewin et al., 2000).

9.3.2. Combinations of Therapy

Resick et al. (2002) tested two forms of cognitive therapy with women who had been raped. They used a waiting list of women as a control group who were told that they would need to wait at least six weeks for treatment, but were contacted every 2 weeks to make certain they did not need emergency help. Women on the waiting list were encouraged to call if they needed help and a therapist, using a non-directive approach, would provide telephone counseling. If frequent calls indicated an inability to cope with stress or suicidal thoughts, the person was terminated from the study and offered immediate help, although the authors reported that this never happened in the study.

The authors found that cognitive therapy using exposure techniques was very successful in treating PTSD in this sample, and that the success of this approach would bode well for PTSD caused by traumas other than sexual assault and rape. Many of the women in the study who showed marked improvement had histories of other traumas and were considered to be chronically distressed. Therapy was equally effective for recent traumas (three months earlier) and prior traumas (thirty years earlier). In contrast, the women on the waiting list did not improve at all.

Lee et al. (2002) tested the effectiveness of stress inoculation training with prolonged exposure (SITPE) as compared to eye movement desensitization and reprocessing (EMDR). The authors report that 24 participants with PTSD were randomly assigned to one of the treatment approaches. Outcome measures included self-reports by subjects, ratings by observers, and self-reported measures of depression. There was no significant difference in the improvement rate for the two therapies at the end of treatment. However, on the degree of intrusive symptoms, EMDR did much better than SITPE, and at follow-up, EMDR produced greater gain in lessening all symptoms of PTSD (Lee et al., 2002, p. 1071).

In the treatment of PTSD with children and adolescents, Cohen (1998) reports only limited evidence of the effectiveness of psychotherapy, although she refers to three recent studies that provide empirical support for the use of cognitive-behavioral therapy in treating children with PTSD. Even though there is little data to guide clinicians in their work with children and adolescents with PTSD, Cohen (1998) notes that experts in the field suggest that the major treatment components that work with children are, "direct exploration of the trauma, use of specific stress management techniques, exploration and correction of inaccurate attributions regarding the trauma, and inclusion of parents in treatment" (Cohen, 1998, p. 755). Parents can benefit from education regarding the child's PTSD symptoms and learning how they might help in managing them.

9.3.3. *Final Thoughts on Treatment*

Dadds and Barrett (2001) emphasize that clinicians treating anxiety problems in children and adolescents recognize that the following treatment issues can affect outcomes regardless of the approach used: Because children may be in denial about the problem or feel threatened by discussing it, a certain amount of resistance may be noted in treatment. Because many anxious children feel threatened by the lack of structure in treatment sessions in which they are expected to discuss the problem with limited help from the clinician, the authors suggest that treatment increases in effectiveness by talking about positive issues or topics that do not produce anxiety and improve rapport. By explaining treatment as skill-building rather than an attempt to reduce pathology, the child will more likely embrace the process. The authors also note that high levels of anxiety in parents can impede treatment. Involving parents in concurrent work on their own anxiety problems can be a very positive experience that leads to more durable change. The clinician's ability "to engage the parents at the level of their own coping, without conveying blame and incompetence, will be a critical factor in the use of adjunctive family interventions" (Dadds and Barrett, 2001, p. 108).

9.4. CASE STUDY: EBP WITH AN ANXIOUS CHILD

I was a school social worker in suburban Chicago for two years in the mid-1960s. The year prior I'd become very interested in cognitive therapy and attended workshops by Ellis and by Glasser and read everything I could read about cognitive therapy. It frankly made a lot more sense than the psychodynamic approach I had resisted learning in graduate school, and the play therapy approaches my supervisor wanted me to learn in my clinical work with children. Growing up in North Dakota is a grounding experience, I suppose. I did what I thought would work with the children and their families I'd grown up with. Dolls with removable parts and concerns about the Oedipal complex were pretty far removed from the poor kids I grew up with who could talk, and think, and who were fiercely committed to doing better regardless of their often abusive or alcoholic home lives.

When I began to get hundreds of children referred for counseling largely for what struck me as normal problems of low self-esteem related to over-worked families with too little income, I immediately decided to use what I thought was a practical approach, or the hundreds of needy children in my care would never receive help. I settled on cognitive therapy and humor since they were all I had to go on.

One of my children, a second-grade boy (we'll call him Robert), was pulling the hair out of his scalp and was partly bald. His mother asked me to work with him and informed me that he had a heart defect, and that I had to be very careful not to exert him physically. She gave me the name of his doctor, who confirmed he'd had a congenital heart defect at birth but that it was repaired and there was no reason other than his mother's overprotective behavior to let him do what other kids did. His doctor ended the conversation by saying that his mother's over-protectiveness was "screwing the child up badly" and if she didn't stop filling him full of stories of how he'd die if he did what the other kids did, that Robert would be a non-functioning adult overwhelmed with anxiety. He'd seen it before, and she was doing everything possible to give Robert death anxiety.

Robert was a small child, anxious, serious, worried about his looks, and afraid, he continually told me, of dying if he played too hard, so he did not play at all.

I was just learning cognitive therapy, so I made a few stabs at explaining the theory and helping him spot irrational behavior in what his mother was telling him. It seemed to have no impact. Because of the huge numbers of children I was working with as the only male worker in a large school district with no mental heath or family service agencies close by, I performed a type of triage in which I placed children in groups with similar children and did a type of recreational/cognitive/silliness therapy in which the whole idea was to have fun. I suppose I was in some ways influenced by my own silly behavior and just enjoyed having fun with such serious and hurting children. And it worked. We told jokes, had secret handshakes, played games, had burping contests, and interspersed with the fun was an attempt to give some cognitive direction and support.

Robert could hardly wait to come to group. Having fun was an antidote to his mother's morbid predictions of his early demise. His hair grew back, he started doing well in class, and best of all, he thought, he could burp better than anyone in a group of exceptional burpers. I also worked with his severe and serious mother who complained that I was turning Robert against her. Instead of being the compliant boy he used to be, he was acting – well – he was acting like a boy, for heaven sakes. "Do you know that he could die anytime and that you, Mr. Glicken, will be to blame?" She told me her husband had left her because he could not stand the way she overprotected Robert, and if she could put up with him leaving then she could also put up with my leaving.

By hook and by crook I was able to see Robert for almost an entire school year, and he thrived, even though his mother wrote letters to the school superintendent about the evilness of my work, and how I was taking the child away from her. His teachers and the superintendent were astonished at his improvement and supported my work. I wish I'd had better skills at working with his mother, and I wish she'd embraced the improvement Robert made, but in the seven months I worked with Robert I began to develop a therapy style that has stayed with me, for better or worse, to this day. The style uses logic and humor. I still tell jokes. A laughing client is much more open to change than a crying client, in my view. Humor places us in a child ego state where we can be very open to change. I saw that personally in my own therapy with Robert and Mary Goulding, whose training program opened many of us to new recognitions about ourselves through laughing, dancing, and just having a helluva good time for a few weeks.

I'm happy to see that cognitive-behaviroal therapy is one of the major treatments for a variety of child and adolescent problems. When I began doing it in the mid-1960s, many people told me it wouldn't work with children because they were too unformed to think rationally about problems. I found just the opposite–that they were much more open than adults were to examining self-defeating thoughts and seeing the illogic of certain life perceptions.

I look back on the two years I spent working with Robert, who would now be diagnosed with a severe anxiety disorder, or worse, and I revel in the thought of how easy therapy seemed when it was just about a new worker trying to apply what he thought children would respond to without the need to focus on pathology, but rather to recognize the elegance of children doing the best they could, and when someone praised them for it, being able to leap tall buildings in a single bound.

Before summer break Robert came by and gave me a card he'd made himself. On the outside of the card he'd drawn a man surrounded by boys. On the inside of the card he'd written: "Little boys like to laugh and have hair and feel good. Big boys like to laugh and help them."

9.5. SUMMARY

This chapter on anxiety examines the types of anxiety disorders, their possible origins, and best evidence for treatment effectiveness. The importance of working closely with children and their parents in stress and the severity of anxiety is noted in both its prevalence and the associated mental health problems that develop if anxiety is not dealt with early in life. A case study using EBP is also included in the chapter.

9.6. QUESTIONS FROM THE CHAPTER

1. It is hard to believe that so many of America's youth have problems with anxiety. Is not it possible, that like depression, anxiety is just a function of emotions catching up with quickly developing bodies and that once development is complete that anxiety will go away in most people?
2. Flooding people with thoughts of the trauma that originally caused anxiety (exposure therapy) sounds pretty cruel. Do not you think that in many people it could increase and not decrease anxiety?
3. Phobias, PTSD, panic disorders: It all sounds like baloney to me. Why do we have to create so many categories of anxiety when just saying you are anxious would be as effective? Do not you agree that we are diagnosing emotional problems to death?
4. I can hardly believe that debriefing does not work. What is wrong with helping kids who have has a traumatic experience by giving them some suggestions for handling anxiety they have from the experience?
5. Do not you think that most anxiety problems would go away on their own if we did not keep reminding kids that they should feel anxious because of something that

happened to them? Natural healing takes place when we let people heal in their own ways after a trauma. The best treatment is no treatment in my view. Do not you agree?

References

Albano, A. M., Chorpita, B. F., & Barlow, D. H. (2003). Childhood anxiety disorders. In E. J. Mash, R. A. & Barkley (Eds.), *Childhood psychopathology*(2nd ed.) (pp. 279–329). New York: Guilford Press.

American Psychiatric Association. (1994). *Diagnostic and statistical manual of mental manual* (4th ed.). Washington, DC: American Psychiatric Press.

Author. (2003, March/April). Anxiety disorder in children may foretell eating disorders. *Eating Disorder Review*, *14*(2), 1.

Bisson, J. I., McFarlane, A. C., & Rose, S. (2000). Psychological debriefing. In E. B. Foa, T. M. Keane, M. J. & Friedman (Eds.). *Effective treatments for PTSD* (pp. 39–59). New York: The Guilford Press, *2000*.

Black, D. W., & Noyes, R. (1997). Obsessive-compulsive disorder and axis II. *International Review of Psychiatry, 9*, 111–118.

Bourne, E. J. (2005). *The anxiety & phobia workbook* (4th ed.). New York: New Harbinger Publications.

Brewin, C. R., Andrews, B., & Valentine, J. D. (2000). Meta-analysis of risk factors for posttraumatic stress disorder in trauma-exposed adults. *Journal of Consulting Clinical Psychology, 68*, 748–766.

Brown University Psychopharamcology Update, (2007), January. pp. 4–5 http://web.ebscohost.com.ezproxy1.lib.asu.edu/ehost/pdf?vid=4&hid=102&sid=d6a260ce-7aa8-4670-b215-542875783977%40sessionmgr102.

Cartwright-Hatton, S., Roberts, C., Chitsabesan, P., Fothergill, C., & Harrington, R. (2004). Systematic review of the efficacy of cognitive behaviour therapies for childhood and adolescent anxiety disorders. *British Journal of Clinical Psychology, 43*, 421–436.

Chambless, D. L., & Ollendick, T. H. (2001). Empirically supported psychological interventions: Controversies and evidence. *Annual Review of Psychology, 52*, 685–716.

Cohen, J. A. (1998, September). Summary of the practice parameters for the assessment and treatment of children and adolescents with posttraumatic stress disorder. *Journal of the American Academy of Child and Adolescent Psychiatry, 37*(9), 747–752.

Compton, S. N., Burns, B. J., & Robertson, E. (2002). Review of evidence base for treatment of childhood psychopathology: Internalizing disorders. *Journal of Consulting and Clinical Psychology, 70*, 1240–1266.

Costello, E. J., Angold, A., Burns, B. J., Stangl, D. K., Tweed, D. L., Erkanli, A., & Worthman, C. M. (1996). The Great Smoky Mountains Study of Youth. Goals, design, methods, and the prevalence of DSM-III-R disorders. *Archives of General Psychiatry, 53*, 1129–1136.

Dadds, M. R., & Barrett, P. M. (2001). Psychological management of anxiety disorders in childhood. *Association for child psychology and psychiatry* (pp. 999–1011). New York: Cambridge University Press, *Vol. 42*, (x).

Deblinger, E., McLeer, S. V., & Henry, D. (1990). Cognitive behavioral treatment for sexually abused children suffering from post-traumatic stress: Preliminary findings. *Journal of the American Academy of Child & Adolescent Psychiatry, 29*, 747–752.

Flament, M. F., Whitaker, A., Rapoport, J. L., Davies, M., Berg, C. Z., Kalikow, K., Sceery, W., & Shaffer, D. (1988). Obsessive compulsive disorder in adolescence: An epidemiological study. *Journal of the American Academy of Child and Adolescent Psychiatry, 27*, 764–771.

Foa, E. B., Dancu, C. V., Hembree, E. A., Jaycox, L. H., Meadows, E. A., & Street, G. P. (1999). A comparison of exposure therapy, stress inoculation training, and their combination in reducing posttraumatic stress disorder in female assault victims. *Journal of Consulting and Clinical Psychology, 67*, 194–200.

Foa, E. B., Hearst-Ikeda, D., & Perry, K. J. (1995). Evaluation of a brief cognitive-behavioral program for the prevention of chronic PTSD in recent assault victims. *Journal of Consulting & Clinical Psychology, 63*, 948–955.

Foa, E. B., & Kozak, M. J. (1986). Emotional processing of fear; Exposure to corrective information. *Psychological Bulletin, 99*, 20–35.

Foa, E. B., & Meadows, E. A. (1997). Psychosocial treatment for post-traumatic stress disorder: A critical review. In J. Spence, J. M. Darley, D. J. & Foss (Eds.). *Annual Review of Psychology* (pp. 449–480). Palo Alto, CA: Annula Reviews, *48*.

Foa, E. B., & Rothbaum, B. O. (1998). *Treating the trauma of rape: A cognitive behavioral therapy for PTSD*. New York: Guilford.

Foa, E. B., Rothbaum, B. O., Riggs, D., & Murdock, T. (1991). Treatment of post-traumatic stress disorder in rape victims: A comparison between cognitive-behavioral procedures and counseling. *Journal of Consulting and Clinical Psychology, 59*, 715–723.

Gist, R., & Devilly, G. J. (2002). Post-trauma debriefing: the road too frequently traveled. *Lancet, 360*(9335), 741–743.

Glicken, M. D. (2005). *Improving the effectiveness of the helping professions: An evidence-based approach to practice*. Thousand Oaks, CA: Sage Publications.

Goenjian, A. K., Pynoos, R. S., Steinberg, A. M., Najarian, L. M., Asarnow, J. R., Karayan, I., Ghurabi, M., & Fairbanks, L. A. (1995). Psychiatric comorbidity in children after the 1988 earthquake in Armenia. *Journal of American Academy of Child and Adolescent Psychiatry, 34*, 1174–1184.

Grachev, I. D., Breiter, H. C., Rauch, S. L., Savage, C. R., Baer, L., Shera, D. M., Kennedy, D. N., Makris, N., Caviness, V. S., & Jenike, M. A. (1998). Structural abnormalities of frontal neocortex in obsessive-compulsive disorder [Letter]. *Archives of General Psychiatry, 55*, 181–182.

Harvard Mental Health Letter. (2007, January), 23(7), 1–2. http://web.ebscohost.com.ezproxy1.lib.asu.edu/ehost/pdf?vid=4&hid=102&sid=d6a260ce-7aa8-4670-b215-542875783977%40sessionmgr102.

Hensley, L. G. (2002). Treatment for Survivors of Rape: Issues and Interventions. *Journal of Mental Health Counseling, 24*(4), 331–348.

Horowitz, M. J. (1976). *Stress response syndromes*. New York: Aronson.

Ishikawa, S., Okajima, I., Matsuoka, H., & Sakano, Y. (2007). Cognitive behavioural therapy for anxiety disorders in children and adolescents: A meta-analysis. *Child and Adolescent Mental Health, 12*(4), 164–172.

Kashani, J. H., & Orvaschel, H. (1988). Anxiety disorders in mid-adolescence: A community sample. *American Journal of Psychiatry, 145*, 960–964.

Keane, T. M., Fairbank, J. A., Caddell, J. M., & Zimering, R. T. (1989). Implosive (flooding) therapy reduces symptoms of PTSD in Vietnam combat veterans. *Behavior Therapy, 20*, 245–260.

Kendall, P. C., Chu, B., Pimentel, S. S., & Choudhury, M. (2000). Treating anxiety disorders in youth. In P. C. Kendall (Ed.), *Child and adolescent therapy: Cognitive-behavioral procedures* (2nd ed., pp. 235–287). New York: Guilford Press.

Kramer, S.H., Rosenthal, R. (1998). Meta-analytic research synthesis. In Bellack, A.S., Hersen, M., series eds, Schooler, N.R., volume ed. *Comprehensive clinical psychology: vol 3–research and methods*, 1st edn. Oxford: Pergamon, 1998: 351–368.

Lee, C., Gavriel, H., Drummond, P., Richards, J., & Greenwald, R. (2002). Treatment of PTSD: Stress inoculation training with prolonged exposure compared to EMDR. *Journal of Clinical Psychology, 58*(9), 1071–1089.

Lenane, M. C., Swedo, S. E., Leonard, H., Pauls, D. L., Sceery, W., & Rapoport, J. L. (1990). Psychiatric disorders in first degree relatives of children and adolescents with obsessive-compulsive disorder. *Journal of the American Academy of Child and Adolescent Psychiatry, 29*, 407–412.

Leonard, H. L., Rapoport, J. L., & Swedo, S. E. (1997). Obsessive-compulsive disorder. In J. M. & Weiner (Ed.), *Textbook of child and adolescent psychiatry* (2nd ed.) (pp. 481–490). Washington, DC: American Academy of Child and Adolescent Psychiatry, American Psychiatric Press.

Marks, I. M. (1987). *Fears, phobias, and rituals: Panic, anxiety, and their disorders*. New York: Oxford University Press.

McGaugh, J. L., & Cahill, L. (1997). Interaction of neuromodulatory systems in modulating memory storage. *Behavioral Brain Research, 83*, 31–38.

Mental Health Association of Westchester (2008). *Anxiety disorders – children and adolescents*. http://mhawestchester.org/diagnosechild/canxiety.asp.

Ost, L. G. (1989). One-session treatment for specific phobias. *Behavioral Research and Therapy, 27*, 1–7. In Gray, P. (1994). *Psychology* (2nd. ed.). New York: Worth.

Ozer, E. J., Best, S. R., Lipsey, T. L., & Weiss, D. S. (2003). Predictors of posttraumatic stress disorder and symptoms in adults: A meta-analysis. *Psychological Bulletin, 129*(1), 52–73.

Rainey, R. (1997). *Treatment for phobias*. http://www.phobialist.com/treat.html.

Rauch, S. L., & Savage, C. R. (1997). Neuroimaging and neuropsychology of the striatum. Bridging basic science and clinical practice. *Psychiatric Clinics of North America, 20*, 741–768.

Resick, P. A. (1992). Cognitive treatment of a crime-related PTSD. In R. D. Peters, R. J. McMahon, V. L. & Quinsey (Eds.), *Aggression and violence throughout the life span* (pp. 171–191). Newbury Park, CA: Sage.

Resick, P. A., Nisith, P., Weaver, T. L., Astin, M. C., & Feuer, C. A. (2002). A comparison of cognitive-processing therapy with prolonged exposure and a waiting condition for the treatment of chronic posttraumatic stress disorder in female rape victims. *Journal of Consulting and Clinical Psychology, 70*(4), 867–879.

Resick, P. A., & Schnicke, M. K. (1992). Cognitive processing therapy for sexual assault victims. *Journal of Consulting and Clinical Psychology, 60*, 748–756.

Rothbaum, B. O., Meadows, E. A., Resick, P., & Foy, D. W. (2000). Cognitive-behavioral therapy. In E. B. Foa, M. Friedman, T. & Keane (Eds.), *Effective treatments for posttraumatic stress disorder: Practice Guidelines from the International Society for Traumatic Stress Studies* (pp. 60–83). New York, NY: Guilford.

Rothbaum, B., Olasov, C., & Schwartz, A. C. (2002). *American Journal of Psychotherapy, 56*(1), 59–75.

Safford, S. M., Kendall, P. C., Flannery-Schroeder, E., Webb, A., & Sommer, H. (2005). A longitudinal look at parent-child diagnostic agreement in youth treated for anxiety disorders. *Journal of Clinical Child and Adolescent Psychology, 34*(4), 747–757.

Stein, M. B. (2002). Taking aim at posttraumatic stress disorder: Understanding Its nature and shooting down myths. *Canadian Journal of Psychiatry, 47*(10), 921–923.

Susser, E. S., Herman, D. B., & Aaron, B. (2002). Combating the terror of terrorism. *Scientific American, 287*(2), 70–78.

Van Emmerik, A. P., Kamphuis, J. H., Hulsbosch, A. M., & Emmelkamp, P. M. (2002). Single session debriefing after psychological trauma: A meta-analysis. *Lancet, 360*(9335), 766–772.

Watson, J. B. (1924). *Behaviorism*. Chicago: University of Chicago Press.

Wolpe, J. (1958). *Psychotherapy by reciprocal inhibition*. Stanford: Stanford University Press.

Zinbarg, R. E., Barlow, D. H., Brown, T. A., & Hertz, R. M. (1992). Cognitive-behavioral approaches to the nature and treatment of anxiety disorders. *Annual Review of Psychology*, *43*, 235–267. In Gray, P. (1994). *Psychology* (2nd ed.). New York: Worth.

Further reading

Harvard Mental Health Letter. (2002). What causes post-traumatic stress disorder: two views. *Harvard Mental Health Letter*, *19*(4), 8.

10 EBP with Child and Adolescent Eating Disorders

10.1. INTRODUCTION

Eating disorders are a serious problem for America's children and adolescents. As many as a third of them are overweight and many more suffer the serious consequences of bulimia, anorexia and binge eating. This chapter will discuss the diagnoses, causation and best evidence for treatment efficacy. At the end of the chapter is a case study on binge eating, a new category of eating disorder with its origins in childhood and which affects millions of Americans, often leading to obesity.

10.2. BULIMIA NERVOSA

Bulimia nervosa, also called bulimia, is an emotionally based eating disorder characterized by periodic episodes of binge eating, during which a child or adolescent consumes large quantities of food followed by purging as a weight loss mechanism. Purging may include vomiting, fasting, the use of enemas, excessive use of laxatives and diuretics, or compulsive exercising. Bulimia usually develops in adolescent girls whose binge and purge behavior is done in secret and is associated with disgust at binging and relief at purging. Sanders (1996) reports that bulimia in 1–3% of adolescent young women in the United States, and bulimic behaviors in 10–20% of adolescent young women in the United States. Children and adolescents with bulimia usually have normal weight but are often very unhappy with their bodies.

The symptoms of bulimia may include: (1) eating uncontrollably followed by purging; (2) vomiting or abuse of laxatives or diuretics in an attempt to lose weight; (3) using the bathroom frequently after meals; (4) excessive exercising; (5) abnormal pre-occupation with body weight; (6) dental problems; (7) sore throat; (8) depression or mood swings; (9) swollen glands in the neck and face; (10) heartburn, indigestion and bloating; (11) irregular periods; and (12) weakness, exhaustion and bloodshot eyes (Haines, 2005, p. 1).

Serious complications of bulimia may include: (1) erosion of tooth enamel because of repeated exposure to acidic gastric contents; (2) dental cavities; (3) swelling and soreness in the salivary glands (from repeated vomiting); (4) stomach ulcers; (5) ruptures of the stomach and esophagus; (6) disruption in the normal bowel release function; (7) dehydration; (8) irregular heartbeat; (9) heart attack (in severe cases); (10) lower libido (sex drive); and (11) higher risk for suicidal behavior (Haines, 2005, p. 1).

10.3. EVIDENCE-BASED PRACTICE WITH BULIMIC YOUTH

Stunkard and Stellar (1984) found that almost 90% of bulimia clients suffer from moderate to severe depression and that bingeing and purging is a way to reduce depression. Huebner (1993) used the therapeutic triad to reduce symptoms of bulimia. In part one of the triad the bulimic patient is asked to keep a daily log which displays (1) the amount of food and fluid intake, (2) the number of binge–purge episodes, (3) states of mind, and (4) exercising. Using this method, the clinician can associate bulimic activity and the emotional states that may have triggered the activity. While the approach seems to work, Huebner (1993, p. 146) reports that many bulimics find it very difficult to keep logs.

In part two of the triad, the bulimic experiments with her binge–purge behavior and observes the reinforcing and addictive nature of the disease. At this point, hopefully, the client begins to develop cognitive control over the bulimia. Part of the process includes a strict diet of 1200–1400 calories and an educational process helping the client see the difference between food as a healthy and necessary part of life and food as addictive. If the bulimic feels the need to binge, she is instructed to wait at least 1 h after her healthy meal. Once the client is able to control his or her binge eating, the frequency of binge–purge episodes declines. Part three of the triad involves the treatment of the individual and her family to identify the possible life issues that caused the bulimia and to offer support and encouragement.

Wilson and Fairburn (1993) report that cognitive-behavioral therapy (CBT) has consistently been shown to be applicable and effective in treating bulimia nervosa. Treasure et al. (1994) note that cognitive-behavioral treatment has been found to produce significant reductions in the frequency of binge eating, vomiting, and other compensatory behaviors used by bulimics to control their weight. Waller et al. (1996) found that not only does CBT result in rapid improvement in eating patterns of bulimics, but also improvement maintains itself over time. Thackwray et al. (1993), randomly assigned 47 women to a cognitive-behavioral or a behavioral treatment group. At the end of treatment, 92% of the women who received CBT had ended their binge/eating/purging behavior, compared to 100% of those who received behavioral therapy. However, at follow-up, 69% receiving CBT maintained their abstinence compared to 38% in the behavioral group.

Cooper and Steere (1995) conducted a similar study comparing cognitive-behavior therapy with an exposure plus response prevention behavioral treatment. Both treatments worked in the short run, but 1 year later only the CBT group had not relapsed. Interestingly, neither therapy approaches changed the treatment group's attitudes toward body shape and ideal weight, nor could the researchers use changes in attitude to predict relapse. Fairburn et al. (1993) compared the effects of CBT with IPT, a psychodynamically oriented therapy, and CBT with BT (behavioral therapy). Half the clients assigned to the BT group discontinued their treatment. For those who remained, few had good outcomes. Clients assigned to CBT and IPT made equivalent, substantial, and lasting changes, although IPT took longer to produce results. The researchers concluded that bulimia can be effectively treated without focusing on the individual's eating habits and attitudes regarding body shape and weight.

10.4. ANOREXIA NERVOSA

Carey (2006) reports that 1%, or about 3 million mostly young women will at some point suffer from self-starvation that characterizes anorexia, a life-threatening eating disorder characterized by self-starvation and excessive weight loss. The disorder is diagnosed when a person weighs at least 15% less than his or her normal body weight, and typically begins around the onset of puberty. Extreme weight loss in people with anorexia nervosa can lead to dangerous health problems and even death. Anorexia literally means "loss of appetite," a misleading term since those with anorexia nervosa are often hungry but refuse food anyway. People with anorexia nervosa have intense fears of becoming fat and see themselves as fat even when they are very slender. These individuals may try to correct this perceived "flaw" by strictly limiting food intake and exercising excessively in order to lose weight.

Anorexia is commonly seen as a disorder of white, affluent teenaged girls and young women, and in fact up to 90% of anorexics are female, with the onset of symptoms typically occurring between ages 11 and 20. But male anorexics do exist, and anorexia has been diagnosed in children as young as seven, and in middle-aged and even elderly women. It affects people of all races, ethnic groups, and social classes. People with anorexia nervosa are often very high achievers, performing very well in school, sports, work and other activities (Siegfried et al., 2003).

To be diagnosed as having anorexia nervosa, according to the DSM-IV-TR, a person must display:

1. A refusal to maintain appropriate body weight, leading to a body weight less than 85% of that expected.
2. An intense fear of gaining weight or becoming obese.
3. A disturbance in the way in a person views his or her body weight or shape, coupled with denial of the seriousness of current low body weight.
4. In women who have had their first menstrual period but are not yet menopausal, the absence of at least three consecutive menstrual cycles.

The DSM-IV-TR specifies two subtypes of anorexia:

1. Restricting type: during a current episode of anorexia nervosa, the person has not regularly engaged in binge eating or self-induced vomiting, over-exercise or the misuse of laxatives, diuretics or enemas.
2. Binge-eating type or purging type: during the current episode, the person regularly binge eats or engages in self-induced vomiting, over-exercise or the misuse of laxatives, diuretics, or enemas.

Although it is thought that anorexia is caused by feelings of unattractiveness and overweight that are maintained by various cognitive biases (Rosen et al., 1995), a review of research by Skrzypek et al. (2001) suggests that the problem is not perceptual but relates to the way perceptual information is evaluated. This could lead to what Jansen et al. (2006) refer to as a lack of overconfidence bias in which most of us see ourselves as more attractive than others see us, a bias that it also referred to as illusory glow. Anorexics judge their own attractiveness more in keeping with the way others would judge them, and are therefore thought to lack an overconfidence bias that boosts self-esteem. Wonderlich et al. (2005) found that the following describes people who suffer from anorexia: intrusive thoughts about food and weight-related issues, the ability to fight off the temptation to eat, and pathological levels of the need to pursue high standards and maintain control. O'Brien and Vincent (2003) found common emotional problems exist in tandem with anorexia, including clinical depression, obsessive-compulsive disorder, high levels of anxiety, substance abuse, and one or more personality disorders.

Some ways of determining whether a child or adolescent is suffering from anorexia include the following (Hoek, 2006): (1) rapid weight loss over several weeks or months; (2) continuing to diet even when thin or when weight is very low; (3) intense fear of gaining weight; (4) strange eating habits or routines, such as eating in secret; (5) feeling fat, even if underweight; (6) striving for perfection and being very self-critical; (7) undue influence of body weight or shape on self-esteem; (8) laxative, diuretic or diet pill use; (9) irregular menstrual cycles; (10) wearing loose clothing to hide weight loss; (11) compulsive exercising; and (12) physical symptoms including intolerance to cold weather, brittle hair and nails, dry or yellowing skin, anemia, constipation, swollen joints, and a new growth of thin hair over the body.

The dangerous side effects of starving oneself are described by Katzman (2005), who reports that anorexia can put a serious strain on the structure and function of the heart and cardiovascular system, with slow heart rate (bracycardia) and elongation of the QT interval seen early on. People with anorexia often have electrolyte imbalance, which has been linked to heart failure, muscle weakness, immune dysfunction, and ultimately death. Anorexia in adolescents may result in stunted growth, low levels of essential hormones (including sex hormones), and chronically increased cortisol levels. Osteoporosis develops as a result of anorexia in 38–50% of cases, and poor nutrition leads to the lowering of essential bone structure bone mineral density. Changes in brain structure and function are early signs of the condition. Untreated anorexia may result in damage to the heart and kidneys, irregular heart beat, low blood pressure, and, ultimately, death from starvation or suicide.

10.5. EVIDENCE-BASED PRACTICE WITH ANOREXIC YOUTH

Carey (2006) reports that fewer than a third of anorexics treated with antidepressants like Prozac and ongoing therapy remain healthy for a year or more.

These discouraging results are reinforced by reports of high dropout rates for anorexics receiving therapy. Halmi et al. (2005) characterize dropout rates for anorexics in treatment as "astronomical." Wilson et al. (2007) reinforce the difficulty of helping clients suffering from anorexia by noting that although cognitive therapy and a specific form of family therapy have been used with some success with anorexic adolescents, even the most effective interventions "fail to help a substantial number of patients" (p. 199). To add to the lack of best evidence to help clients suffering from anorexia, the authors indicate that only 15 comparative studies on the treatment of anorexia have been completed and published in the past 20 years. The researchers go on to say

> *The persistent deficit of controlled treatment research in anorexia nervosa is attributable to distinctive features of the disorder, including its rarity, the presence of medical complications that sometimes require inpatient management, and the extended period of treatment necessary for full symptom remission in established cases. Patients' ambivalent attitudes about recovery compound these challenges at every phase of research, making it more difficult to recruit samples, prevent attrition, and secure participation in follow-up assessments (Agras et al., 2004; Wilson et al., 2007, p. 199)*

Several representative studies are summarized here, including the following: Eisler et al. (2000) found that the longer a client had evidence of anorexia, the more negative the treatment results. In his study, clients with anorexia for 8 months or less were likely to improve, while patients with evidence of anorexia of longer than 16 months had intermediate to poor treatment results. Dare et al. (2001) found that treatment effects 6 years after initiation of treatment were poor. Pike et al. (2003) found that cognitive-behavioral therapy was superior to nutritional counseling for preventing relapse after inpatient treatment. Compared with patients assigned to nutritional counseling, patients receiving cognitive-behavioral therapy were less likely to drop out or be withdrawn (22% versus 73%), slower to relapse, and more likely to achieve a good outcome (44% versus 7%).

An approach to the treatment of anorexia in adolescents with promise is a type of family therapy known as the Maudsley model (Dare and Eisler, 1997; Lock and le Grange, 2005). Lock et al. (2001) published a detailed manual that outlines treatment procedures. The intervention involves 10–20 family sessions spread over 6–12 months. In phase one of treatment, parents are told to take complete control over their child's eating and weight and are helped to find effective approaches. When the child begins to comply with parental control over weight and eating, parental control fades and the adolescent's ability practice to age-appropriate autonomy is linked to resolving the eating disorder. In reviewing the evidence that the Maudsley model works, Wilson et al. (2007) point out that methodological problems including small sample size limit our ability to say that the model is a form of best evidence of treatment effectiveness. Still, initial findings are cause for optimism in an otherwise troubling lack of good effectiveness data.

10.6. BINGE EATING

Children and adolescents who binge or compulsively overeat is a serious eating disorder characterized by frequently eating large amounts of food (beyond the point of feeling full) while feeling a loss of control over their eating. Needless to say, one of the serious side effects of binge eating is obesity. Haines (2005) notes that many people with binge-eating disorder are also depressed or have high levels of anxiety. It is thought binge overeating is a way to cope with both problems. Additional symptoms of binge eating in children and adolescents are as follows: (1) frequently eating what others would consider an abnormally large amount of food; (2) frequently feeling unable to control what or how much is being eaten; (3) eating much more rapidly than usual; (4) eating until uncomfortably full; (5) eating large amounts of food, even when not physically hungry; (6) eating alone out of embarrassment at the quantity of food being eaten; (7) feelings of disgust, depression or guilt after overeating; (8) fluctuations in weight; and (9) frequent dieting.

Haines (2005) reports that estimates of binge overeating are as high as 2% of all adults, but 10–15% among the overweight attending self-help groups for weight loss. The exact number of children and adolescents is unknown, but the disorder very likely begins in early life and data similar to that of adults would not be unrealistic. Many people report that anger, sadness, boredom, anxiety or other negative emotions can trigger an episode of binge eating. Impulsive behavior and certain other psychological problems also seem to be more common in people with binge-eating disorder. From emerging research, Grilo et al. (2005) believe that binge eating begins in childhood and adolescence and contributes to obesity. Individuals with binge-eating disorder, they report, often have multiple co-occurring problems, including low self-esteem and impulsivity.

10.7. EVIDENCE-BASED PRACTICE WITH BINGE EATING

Few well-controlled studies on the treatment of binge-eating disorder have been performed to date. However, cognitive-behavioral therapy seems to be the best-supported approach for treating binge eating. Cognitive-behavioral therapy is generally thought to result in high treatment completion rates (roughly 80% across different methods), remission from binge eating in over 50% of patients, and broad improvements in associated depression and psychosocial functioning (Agras et al., 1997; Wilfley et al., 1993, 2002). Evidence exists that clients who suffer from binge-eating disorder are very emotionally complex and suffer from multiple emotional problems. For example, Grilo et al. (2005) reported that 73% of their research participants had at least one additional lifetime psychiatric disorder (e.g., 46% had major depressive disorder, 32% had an anxiety disorder, and 24% had an alcohol use disorder), and 32% had at least one personality disorder.

Several other treatments have been found to be effective in treating binge eating. Wilfley et al. (1993, 2002) found that the use of interpersonal psychotherapy has shown strong short-term and longer term outcomes identical to those for cognitive-behavioral therapy of over 70% remission through 12 months of follow up. Telch et al. (2001) also found dialectical behavior therapy useful in treating binge eating, with remission rates of 56% remission within 6 months after treatment completion. Dialectical behavior therapy places strong emphasis on training clients in self-awareness and emotional constraint. There is no evidence to support the effectiveness of other psychological approaches to treatment. Interestingly, programs that focused primarily on weight loss and not the underlying problems related to binge eating do not fare as well (Devlin et al., 2005) when dealing with binge eating. A case study on the treatment of binge eating in a child is reported at the end of this chapter.

10.8. OBESITY

In just two decades, the prevalence of overweight American children aged 6–11 doubled, and that for American teenagers tripled. One-third of all US children are overweight or at risk of becoming overweight. In total, about 25 million US children and adolescents are overweight or nearly overweight (Mayo Clinic, 2006). Although there are some genetic and hormonal causes of childhood obesity, most excess weight is caused by kids eating too much and exercising too little. If children consume more calories than they expend through exercise and normal physical development, they gain weight. Far less common than lifestyle issues are genetic diseases that can predispose a child to obesity. These diseases, such as Prader-Willi syndrome and Bardet-Biedl syndrome, affect a very small proportion of children. In the general population, eating and exercise habits play a much larger role.

Concern for weight problems is considered when a child or adolescent is above the 85th percentile for weight and the term obesity is applied when a child or adolescent is above the 95th percentile. Thirty-two percent of all American youth were either at risk of being overweight or are actually overweight (Journal of Adolescent Health, 2006). The impact of childhood obesity is well known by now, and includes diabetes, cardio-vascular problems, and generalized health problems related to lack of exercise and poor nutrition.

Research into the reasons for obesity suggests a number of responsible factors. Akerman et al. (2007) found that parents often have difficulty recognizing weight problems in children. The researchers concluded that parents with overweight children, underestimated weight and parents with thin children overestimated weight. Parents of children with normal BMI scores had the strongest relationship between perceived and actual BMI scores. Mikhailovich and Morrison (2007) found that parents from a higher socio-economic status were more likely to regulate and restrict certain types of foods while parents with lower socio-economic status were more concerned with the socialization of meal times and the quantity of food, rather than the quality of food. In a randomly selected study of 50 000 children ages 6–17, Barlow and Chang (2007) found that a high level of parental aggravation contributed to a higher risk of child obesity. Children were ignored or told to watch television during these periods, which may have contributed to overeating and a sedentary lifestyle. The most aggravated parents (about 9% of the sample) had children with BMI in the 95th percentile.

Jordan (2008) found that a positive parenting style defined as high displays of sensitivity, emotional warmth, and involvement coupled with high expectations of achievement, maturity and self-control were associated with a lower risk of overweight children by the first grade. Laessle et al. (2001, p. 447) found that "eating behavior of obese children differed significantly from normal weight children only when the mother was present." The researchers found that "Overweight children ate faster with larger bites and showed an acceleration of their eating rate toward the end of the meal" (Laessle et al., 2001, p. 447). Rhee (2008) indicates that 17% of US children aged 2–19 are currently overweight and that another 17% are at risk of becoming overweight. Rhee found that the ages during which weight becomes a noticeable problem are 2–11 or the very times parents have the most influence on their children. The researchers found three specific reasons for obesity in children: permissive behavior toward the amount of food intake by the child, modeling overeating as a positive approach to food, and family difficulties which use food and overeating to reduce family tension.

10.9. EVIDENCE-BASED PRACTICE WITH OBESE YOUTH

Summerbell et al. (2003) reviewed selected randomized controlled trials of lifestyle interventions for treating obesity in children with a minimum of 6 months duration. Examples of lifestyle interventions include dietary, physical activity and/or behavioral therapy interventions, with or without the support of associated family members. Interventions from any setting and delivered by any professional were considered. The authors reviewed 18 randomized controlled trials with 975 participants. Five studies ($N = 245$ participants) investigated changes in physical activity and sedentary behavior. Two studies ($N = 107$ participants) compared problem-solving with usual care or behavioral therapy. Nine studies ($N = 399$ participants) compared behavioral therapy at varying degrees of family involvement with no treatment or usual care or mastery criteria and contingent reinforcement. Two studies ($N = 224$ participants) compared cognitive-behavioral therapy with relaxation. According to the authors, most of the studies were too small to actually determine the effects of the treatment. A meta-analysis was not done since so few of the trials included the same comparisons and outcomes. Although 18 research studies were found, most of these were small studies, and therefore evidence is limited and no conclusions can be drawn with confidence.

Coates and Thoresen (1978) report on the effects of cognitive-behavioral approaches to the treatment of obesity in youth. These procedures, they note, are designed to alter eating and to increase activity. "Persons are instructed in methods for changing specific features of their personal, social, and physical environment as a means of altering their eating and exercise behaviors" (p. 146). Although there are few studies applicable to youth, and most are quite small, several did find promising results. Rivinus et al. (1973) treated 10 black lower socio-economic children in ten 2-h weekly group meetings which included a weigh-in, a group meeting with parents and children, group suppers in which appropriate eating habits were modeled and discussed, and material reinforcement for habit change. Subjects self-monitored the application of these procedures in their homes and were rewarded for meeting pre-selected goals. Although the magnitude of the weight changes was small (only two subjects lost more than 10 pounds), nine subjects did report weight loss, a significant finding given the racial and socio-economic characteristics of the sample employed. Aragona et al. (1975) reported promising short-term results with 5–10-year-old females. Parents were trained in nutrition, exercise, and ways to alter the physical and social environment. A money deposit was refunded for attending weekly group meetings, completing homework assignments, and when their children met weight loss goals. One group of parents was also trained to reinforce habit changes in their children, while a third group served as a no-contact control. Both experimental procedures produced clinically significant short-term losses over the 12 weeks of treatment (average losses of 11.3 and 9.5 pounds in the two treatment groups as compared to an average gain of 0.9 pounds in the control group). At the 46-week follow-up evaluation, most subjects returned to or exceeded baseline weights and this could not be attributed to normal growth patterns.

Wheeler and Hess (1976) designed an individually tailored behaviorally oriented program with 2–10-year-old children. Three factors are notable: (1) mothers and children were treated in pairs; (2) programs were tailored to the needs of the individual child based on a careful behavior analysis; and (3) the program emphasized gradual changes and long-term involvement. After 7 months of treatment, treatment subjects ($N = 14$) averaged a 4.1% reduction in percentage overweight, while dropouts ($N = 12$) gained an average of 3% and no-treatment controls ($N = 14$) gained an average 6.3% above normal weight.

Gross et al., 1976 treated 10 obese adolescent girls in 10 weekly sessions, which included self-monitoring, rearranging the physical and social environment, nutritional information, and individual problem solving. At the end of 10 weeks, four subjects had gained or maintained, three subjects had lost from 2 to 8 pounds, and three lost more than 15 pounds. At a 27-week follow-up: (1) of those maintaining or gaining immediately following treatment, three continued to gain, while one lost ten pounds; (2) the losses of those losing two to eight pounds ranged from 6 to $14\frac{1}{4}$ pounds; and (3) of those losing 15 or more pounds, the losses now ranged from 21 to 40 pounds. In general, continued success could be predicted from weight losses during the program. Average percent overweight at the beginning of treatment was 39.2; at the end of treatment it was 34.5; and at follow-up it was 31.5. The authors conclude that while behavioral therapy shows hopeful signs, "maintenance of changes or continued losses may still be the rare exception rather than the rule" (p. 147).

Recognizing the limited evidence that our treatment approaches work for obese youth, Coates and Thoresen (1978) summarize the problems facing treatment professionals, which include the following: (1) limited research evidence on what actually works; (2) the difficulty of treating food addictions due to the many outside pressure on children to eat. These outside pressures include TV advertising and the availability of an overabundance of food with poor nutritional benefits which are highly addictive; (3) the need to change family eating habits. This change in eating habits intrudes on the habits of other members of the family, who may believe the problem is just a matter of the child's self-control to stop eating when he or she is full; (4) poor research designs that confuse the issue of best evidence and stop us from developing truly effective approaches to treating obesity in youth; and (5) a recognition that some foods are addicting and that they should be labeled in a way which provides enough information so that families and schools can keep them out of kitchens and menus.

10.10. CONCLUSIONS

Wilson et al. (2007) believe that although significant gain has been made in the use of EBP with eating disorders over the past 25 years, particularly with bulimia nervosa and binge-eating disorder in adults, there still remains a great deal of work to do in order to determine best treatment approaches for work with children and adolescents. Since most eating disorders have their beginning in early life, the lack of best evidence for work with children and adolescents, particularly those suffering from anorexia and obesity, should form a research agenda for the coming years. Wilson et al. (2007) conclude that despite the progress made to date,

> *[F]ormal opportunities for professional training in evidence-based psychological treatment of eating disorders remain very limited. Few doctoral programs in psychology [or the remaining human services] in the United States offer a systematic focus on eating disorders despite the widespread interest among some of the most talented undergraduate students aspiring to careers in clinical psychology." (p. 212)*

10.11. CASE STUDY: EVIDENCE-BASED PRACTICE AND BINGE EATING IN AN 8-YEAR-OLD CHILD

Michael is an 8-year-old child referred by his parents for treatment because of binge eating. Michael came for his first session with his father but spoke to me alone. The following is a summary of our work together.

Michael is a pleasant child with normal weight and height who is articulate and clearly concerned about his binge-eating problem. He readily admits that he compulsively eats to the point of vomiting when he attends parties and functions where there is a great deal of food. He thinks it is wrong to leave food because of all the starving people in the world and believes he is doing his part not to be wasteful. He also told me later in the interview that the idea of eating all the food he can possibly eat overwhelms him when he is at parties and cannot resist the temptation. Still, it upsets him that he eats far more than he normally does at home to the point of becoming sick. His mother is hospitalized often because of severe asthma and the house, while it has enough food, never has the type of "fancy" food, as he calls it, that he finds at parties. Once he starts eating, he stuffs himself with food and is unable to stop. He eats normally at home because the food, "Well, it just isn't very good when my mom's gone and there's not much to eat at home."

I wondered why he thought it was necessary to eat everything just to not be wasteful, and I reminded him that most of us save leftovers for another meal. He looked stymied and shook his head. Finally, he said, "I don't know why. I guess when I'm eating it makes me feel good – until I get sick." I asked him to explain how food made him feel good. "I like the way it tastes, and there's so much to eat, and I worry I won't get enough to eat, and maybe I'll be full before I eat everything I want to eat." But there usually is enough food, I suggested. "Yeah, but when I'm at a party I always worry that the food will run out so I eat as much of it and as fast as I can."

I asked him if he had like to learn how to not eat so much and he nodded. "Yes. The kids aren't inviting me to parties any more because I get sick all the time. My dad gets mad at me, too, and won't let me go to parties if I keep getting sick." I wondered if anything was making him sad or worry a lot. He thought for a while and then haltingly said, "Well, my dad is mad a lot. He makes fun of me sometimes, and my mom isn't home very much, and when she is, she can't come outside or go to stuff with me like she used to. We all have to work hard and sometimes the kids make fun of us because we don't have a car and we have to shop using my old wagon. And like, because we're Jewish, you know, kids say awful stuff, like do we bury our dead standing up and drink the blood of dead babies. I thought we were pretty nice people, but I guess some of the kids don't think so."

"That must be tough to listen to knowing that Jews are pretty special people." He nodded his head. "Is it hard to sleep at night," I asked.

"Yeah, a lot of times I worry that someone will come into the house and kill us like they did to my mom's family when they lived in Poland, and I guess I feel scared and I can't sleep."

"Do you feel sad, much?"

"I cry a lot like when the rabbi makes us stay late at Hebrew School and we can't go home in time to see cartoons on TV. It always goes away when I eat something delicious. I guess I like to eat and sometimes we have really good food at home like the Chinese noodles my dad brings home or that herring in white stuff. Boy, I could eat a ton of that, but my dad gets mad at me when I eat too much at home so I do it at parties and stuff like that."

It seemed clear to me that Michael was feeling a great deal of pressure at home. One way to go in dealing with his problem was to pursue best evidence on the treatment of child anxiety and depression. The concept of binge eating was new to me so before the second session I went to the limited literature on binge eating. I found an article by Agras (1997) that discussed binge eating as a new diagnostic category and noted that many binge eaters were able to abstain from binge eating after treatment. Agras suggested that binge eating is often caused by underlying pathology and that the therapist needs to determine the pathology before starting the treatment. The author noted that binge eating was difficult to control because food was a reinforcer, and many of us use food to calm our anxiety or to reward ourselves when rewards were used to reinforce self-esteem and achievement. I also found an excellent article by Horowitz and Garber (2006) on the treatment of depression in children, and one by DeAngelis (2002) that noted the two different directions clinicians were taking in treating binge eating:

> *Because binge eating disorder involves both weight and eating disorder concerns, researchers in both the obesity and eating disorders fields perceive treatment goals through the lens of their own training. On one side of the debate, eating disorder experts believe binge eating is best treated by traditional eating disorder approaches, such as helping patients reduce or eliminate bingeing, improving their self esteem and body acceptance, and treating underlying psychological problems such as depression and anxiety. On the other side, obesity experts maintain, it's better to treat the obesity first. They believe that tackling psychological problems without addressing excess weight puts the cart before the horse. (p. 1)*

The approach I used was a combination of work on the binge eating and work on Michael's underlying feelings of depression and anxiety using a cognitive-behavioral approach. We discussed the need for restraint in eating and the consequences of becoming too fat. He knew a few very fat kids at school, and everyone made fun of them, so becoming fat was not something he wanted. I asked him to keep track of how much he ate, and when, and to bring his record with him each week to therapy. He readily complied.

The treatment for his depression and anxious feelings were made much more difficult by the presence of serious family problems. Because his mother was ill and expenses had far outstripped his father's ability to pay, the real possibility existed that Michael and a younger brother might be placed in foster care. The thought frightened him. He had heard terrible stories about the mistreatment of children in foster care and had decided that the only way for that not to happen was to do as much to help out around the house as possible. He wondered continually if his mom would ever come home from the hospital and if he made her sick. To cope with his worries Michael read books well beyond his grade level and loved Sherlock Holmes stories because solving mysteries excited him. We approached his binge eating, consequently, as a way of solving a mystery.

"Can you understand the reasons for your compulsive eating from the things you've told me about your life?" I asked.

"Well, food tastes good so I guess eating makes me feel better? Maybe when I eat and feel full I feel happy? Lots of kids go to bed without enough food. That must make them feel sad. My mom's sick, and she isn't ever at home, and my dad isn't very nice lots of time and makes fun of me so I guess maybe that doesn't make me very happy, huh?"

"I guess that's so, Michael. You've done a very good job of understanding some things about yourself. I do wonder why you're so scared at night when you go to bed."

"Well, the Cossacks could come like they did at my mom's house, and they hate Jews, and it would be pretty bad, so I stay up and I have my play knife with me in case they come."

Using a cognitive approach I began to show how some of his ideas were probably not entirely true while others, unfortunately were. The best way to deal with untrue problems was to think them through like Sherlock Holmes. He liked the idea. "So," I said, "you're afraid of the Cossacks but there aren't any Cossacks in Iowa. I've never seen a single one, have you?" He admitted he had not. "So it's not Cossacks you're afraid of, I guess. Can you remember what you say to yourself when you go to bed and you can't sleep?"

He thought for a while. "I say to myself that they'll come take me to a foster home at night when I'm sleeping so I won't put up a fuss. That's what I say."

I wondered if there was a chance he had be placed in a foster home. "Yeah, one of the kids in my class, his mom's a social worker and she came to the house last week and talked to my dad about a foster home for me and Harold."

"That was something that could make a little kid worry a lot," I said, "so let's get your dad in and talk to him about it."

"The father told us quite frankly that he wasn't doing well and that his wife's illness had put a terrible strain on him, but that after talking to the social worker he would never ever put his kids in foster care, no matter what happened and for Michael to not think about it."

When his father left Michael nodded and said, "I guess I don't have to worry about the Cossacks anymore, huh?" I agreed and wondered about the other things he had mentioned. "I guess I have to think about them like Sherlock Holmes would and figure it out for myself."

I can help," I told him.

"Yup, I know."

We treated the binge eating in a cognitive-behavioral manner by having him keep a record of how much he had overeaten, the way he felt at the time, and how he felt after he had over eaten. He confessed he felt awful. "My tummy hurts, and I feel like the other kids and their moms think I'm a freak 'cause I eat so much and get sick." I suggested that it would be wise to remember how he felt after he had eaten too much before he started to overeat. We worked on what would be a normal amount to eat and he was clearly pleased that he had been able to attend five functions without binge eating, but it is a difficult problem. After 6 months he said he had not overeaten once, but that he always wanted to. The urge to overeat was very strong, and in many ways I began to see it as an addiction.

I did periodic follow-ups with my child patients and Michael admitted that he had binge eaten several times when things were really tough at home. A chat with his father confirmed that the father was unwilling to reduce his pressure on Michael or his negative comments. "I grew up in a house where there was plenty of criticism and it didn't hurt me," he said. "American kids can learn about life by being a part of the problems the family is having, not by us protecting them. It'll make him stronger – a survivor like the rest of his family. That's what we Jews are – survivors – and the sooner he learns to defend himself from the 'Goyim' (non-Jews), the better."

By all measures, Michael is doing better. His weight is still within the normal range, and he reports not being scared as much, or as sad. His mother has been home for almost a year because of a new medication, and things at home are better. "My mom kind of makes up for my dad when he's mean. That really helps." The binge eating has decreased about 90%, and hopefully, unlike all too many binge eaters, it would not move into a seriously addictive stage in which obesity is the end result.

10.12. SUMMARY

This chapter discusses the wide-spread problem of eating disorders among America's children and adolescence. In addition to eating disorders in which weight is kept from accumulating including purging practices and starvation, the chapter discusses the more prevalent problems of binge eating and obesity, problems that constitute very real long term health problems as today's youth ages. Best evidence of treatment effectiveness is provided for four types of eating disorders and a case study shows the use of cognitive therapy with an 8 year old child who is binge eating.

10.13. QUESTIONS FROM THE CHAPTER

1. We seem to be obsessed with anorexia and bulimia because, in many ways they are more compelling disorders than obesity. Do not you agree, however, that because of its long-term health implications, obesity is the more serious problem?
2. You can blame anorexia and bulimia with our national obsession with being skinny. Do not you agree that young women need better models of how to look than anorexic professional models and movie actresses?
3. You can blame obesity on our constant advertising of junk food on TV. Do not you agree that if it were not for TV advertising, few children would overeat or become obese.

4. Is not it true that the reason so many children are obese is that parents feed them too much, do not oversee their eating, and probably set bad role models by overeating themselves.
5. People with anorexia are probably mentally ill and have distorted views of reality that make it impossible for them to see how dangerously thin they have become. Do not you think that is the reason treatment is so ineffective: Anorexics are being treated for an eating disorder when, in fact, they have a mental illness?

References

Agras, S. (1997). Treating binge eating (1997). *Journal of Consulting and Clinical Psychology, 65*, 343–347.

Agras, W. S., Telch, C. F., Arnow, B., Eldredge, K., & Marnell, M. (1997). One-year follow-up of cognitive-behavioral therapy for obese individuals with binge eating disorder. *Journal of Consulting and Clinical Psychology, 65*, 343–347.

Agras, W. S., Brandt, H. A., Bulik, C. M., Dolan-Sewell, R., Fairburn, C. G., & Halmi, K. A., et al. (2004). Report of the National Institutes of Health Workshop on overcoming barriers to treatment research in anorexia nervosa. *International Journal of Eating Disorders, 35*, 509–521.

Akerman, A., Williams, M. E., & Meunier, J. (2007). Perception versus reality: An exploration of children's measured body mass in relation to caregivers' estimates. *Journal of Health Psychology, 12*(6), 871–882.

Aragona, J., Cassady, J., & Drabman, R. S. (1975). Treating overweight children through parental training and contingency contracting. *Journal of Applied Behavior Analysis, 8*, 269.

Barlow, S. E., & Chang, J. (2007). Is parental aggravation associated with childhood overweight? An analysis of the national survey of children's health 2003. *Acta Paediatrica, 96*(9), 1360–1364.

Carey, B. (2006, June 14). Study sees no gain in using antidepressant to treat anorexia. *N. Y. Times.com.* http://www.nytimes.com/2006/06/14/health/14prozac.html?_r=1&adxnnl=1&oref=slogin&adxnnlx=1210093297-d3mSf1xoSb10rg2NNK15RA

Coates, T. J., & Thoresen, C. E. (1978). Treating obesity in children and adolescents: A review. *American Journal of Public Health, 68*, 143–151.

Cooper, P., & Steere, J. (1995). A comparison of two psychological treatments for bulimia nervosa: implications for models of maintenance. *Behaviour Research Therapy, 33*(8), 875–885.

Dare, C., & Eisler, I. (1997). Family therapy for anorexia nervosa. In D. Garner, & P. E. Garfinkel (Eds.), *Handbook of treatment for eating disorders* (2nd ed.) (pp. 333–349). Chichester, England: Wiley.

Dare, C., Eisler, I., Russell, G., Treasure, J., & Dodge, L. (2001). Psychological therapies for adults with anorexia nervosa: Randomised controlled trial of out-patient treatments. *British Journal of Psychiatry, 178*, 216–221.

DeAngelis, T. (2002, March). Binge-eating disorder: What's the best treatment? *Monitor on Psychology, 33*(3). http://www.apa.org/monitor/mar02/binge.html.

Devlin, M. J., Goldfein, J. A., Petkova, E., Jiang, H., Raizman, P. S., & Wolk, S., et al. (2005). Cognitive behavioral therapy and fluoxetine as adjuncts to group behavioral therapy for binge eating disorder. *Obesity Research, 13*, 1077–1088.

Eisler, I., Dare, C., Hodes, M., Russell, G., Dodge, E., & le Grange, D. (2000). Family therapy for adolescent anorexia nervosa: The results of a controlled comparison of two family interventions. *Journal of Child Psychology and Psychiatry and Allied Disciplines, 41*, 727–736.

Fairburn, C., Jones, R., Peveler, R., Hope, R., & O'Connor, M. (1993). Psychotherapy and bulimia nervosa: Longer-term effects of interpersonal psychotherapy, behavior therapy, and cognitive behavior therapy. *Archives of General Psychiatry, 50*, 419–428.

Grilo, C. M., Masheb, R. M., & Wilson, G. T. (2005). Efficacy of cognitive behavioral therapy and fluoxetine for the treatment of binge eating disorder: A randomized double-blind placebo-controlled comparison. *Biological Psychiatry, 57*, 301–309.

Gross, M. A., Wheeler, M., & Hess, K. (1976). The treatment of obesity in adolescents using behavioral self-control. *Clinical Pediatrics, 15*, 920.

Haines, C. (2005, July). *Eating disorders.* Web M.D. http://www.webmd.com/content/article/118/112906.htm?printing=true 11-24-06

Halmi, K. A., Agras, W. S., Crow, S., Mitchell, J., Wilson, G. T., Bryson, S. W., & Kraemer, H. C. (2005). Predictors of treatment acceptance and completion in anorexia nervosa: Implications for future study designs. *Archives of General Psychiatry*, 62, 776–781.

Hoek, H. W. (2006). Incidence, prevalence and mortality of anorexia nervosa and other eating disorders. *Current Opinion in Psychiatry, 19*(4), 389–394.

Horowitz, J. L., & Garber, J. (2006). The prevention of depressive symptoms in children and adolescents: A meta-analytic. *Vanderbilt University Journal of Consulting and Clinical Psychology, 74*(3), 401–415.

Huebner, H. F. (1993). *Endorphins, eating disorders, and other addictive behaviors.* New York: W.W. Norton & Co..

Jansen, A., Smeets, T., Martijn, C., & Nederkoorn, C. (2006). I see what you see: The lack of a self-serving body-image bias in eating disorders. *The British Journal of Clinical Psychology, 45*(1), 123–135.

Jordan, A. B. (Ed.) (2008). Overweight and obesity in America's children: Causes, consequences, solutions. *The Annals of the American Academy of Political and Social Science, 615*, 6–243.

Journal of Adolescent Health (2006). Position Paper: Treating and preventing adolescent obesity: A position paper of the Society for Adolescent Medicine, *38*, 784–787.

Katzman, D. K. (2005). Medical complications in adolescents with anorexia nervosa: A review of the literature. *International Journal of Eating Disorders, 37*(Suppl.), S52–S59.

Laessle, R. G., Uhl, H., & Lindel, B. (2001). Parental influences on eating behavior in obese and nonobese preadolescents. *International Journal of Eating Disorders, 30*(4), 447–453.

Lock, J., & le Grange, D. (2005). Family-based treatment of eating disorders. *International Journal of Eating Disorders, 37*(Suppl.), S64–S67.

Lock, J., le Grange, D., Agras, W. S., & Dare, C. (2001). *Treatment manual for anorexia nervosa: A family-based approach.* New York: Guilford Press.

Mayo Clinic (2006, March, 31). *Childhood obesity.* http://www.mayoclinic.com/health/childhood-obesity/DS00698/DSECTION=2. Author.

Mikhailovich, K., & Morrison, Paul (ba, Pgce,Graddip Coun, Phd). (2007). Discussing childhood overweight and obesity with parents: A health communication dilemma. *Journal of Child Health Care, 11*(4), 311–322.

O'Brien, K. M., & Vincent, N. K. (2003). Psychiatric comorbidity in anorexia and bulimia nervosa: Nature, prevalence, and causal relationships. *Clinical Psychology Review, 23*(1), 57–74.

Pike, K. M., Walsh, B. T., Vitousek, K., Wilson, G. T., & Bauer, J. (2003). Cognitive behavior therapy in the posthospitalization treatment of anorexia nervosa. *American Journal of Psychiatry, 160*, 2046–2049.

Rhee, K. (2008). Childhood overweight and the relationship between parent behaviors, parenting style, and family functioning. *The Annals of the American Academy of Political and Social Science, 615*, 12–37.

Rivinus, T. M., Drummond, T., & Combrinck-Graham, L. (1973). *A group-behavior treatment program for overweight children: The results of a pilot study*. Unpublished manuscript, University of Pennsylvania.

Rosen, J. C., Reiter, J., & Orosan, P. (1995). Assessment of body image in eating disorders with the body dysmorphic disorder examination. *Behaviour Research Therapy, 1*, 77–84.

Sanders, C. E. (1996). *The physiology and psychology of bulimia*. http://www.vanderbilt.edu/ans/psychology/health_psychology/bulimia.htm

Siegfried, Z., Berry, E. M., Hao, S., & Avraham, Y. (2003). Animal models in the investigation of anorexia. *Physiology & Behavior, 79*(1), 39–45.

Skrzypek, S., Wehmeier, P. M., & Remschmidt, H. (2001). Body image assessment using body size estimation in recent studies on anorexia nervosa. A brief review. *European Child & Adolescent Psychiatry, 10*(4), 215–221.

Stunkard, A. J. & Stellar, E. (Eds.) (1984). Eating and its disorders: *Research Publications, 62*(84), 259–260.

Summerbell, C. D., Ashton, V., Campbell, K. J., Edmunds, L., Kelly, S., & Waters, E. (2003). Interventions for treating obesity in children. *Cochrane Database of Systematic Reviews, 3*. Art. No.: CD001872. DOI: 10.1002/14651858.CD001872.

Telch, C. F., Agras, W. S., & Linehan, M. M. (2001). Dialectical behavior therapy for binge eating disorder. *Journal of Consulting and Clinical Psychology, 69*, 1061–1065.

Thackwray, D., Smith, M., Bodfish, J., & Meyers, A. (1993). A comparison of behavioral and cognitive-behavioral interventions for bulimia nervosa. *Journal of Consulting and Clinical Psychology, 61*(4), 639–645.

Treasure, J., Schmidt, U., Troop, N., Tiller, J., Todd, G., Keilen, M., & Dodge, E. (1994). First step in managing bulimia nervosa: Controlled trial of therapeutic manual. *BMJ, 308*, 686–689.

Waller, D., Fairburn, C., McPherson, A., Kay, R., Lee, A., & Nowell, T. (1996). Treating bulimia in primary care: A pilot study. *International Journal of Eating Disorders, 19*(1), 99–103.

Wheeler, M. E., & Hess, K. W. (1976). Treatment of juvenile obesity by successive approximation control of eating. *Journal of Behavior Therapy and Experimental Psychiatry, 7*, 235.

Wilfley, D. E., Agras, W. S., Telch, C. F., Rossiter, E. M., Schneider, J. A., & Cole, A. G., et al. (1993). Group cognitive-behavioral therapy and group interpersonal psychotherapy for the nonpurging bulimic individual: A controlled comparison. *Journal of Consulting and Clinical Psychology, 61*, 296–305.

Wilfley, D. E., Welch, R. R., Stein, R. I., Spurrell, E. B., Cohen, L. R., & Saelens, B. E., et al. (2002). A randomized comparison of group cognitive-behavioral therapy and group interpersonal psychotherapy for the treatment of overweight individuals with binge eating disorder. *Archives of General Psychiatry, 59*, 713–721.

Wilson, G., & Fairburn, C. (1993). Cognitive treatments for eating disorders. *Journal of Consulting and Clinical Psychology, 61*(2), 261–269.

Wilson, G. T., Grilo, C. M., & Vitousek, K. M. (2007). Psychological treatment of eating disorders. *American Psychologist, 62*(3), 199–216.

Wonderlich, S. A., Lilenfeld, L. R., Riso, L. P., Engel, S., & Mitchell, J. E. (2005). Personality and anorexia nervosa. *The International Journal of Eating Disorders, 37*(Suppl.), S68–S71.

11 Evidence-Based Practice with Children and Adolescents who Abuse Substances

11.1. INTRODUCTION

The number of children and adolescents with substance abuse problems should be of great concern to clinicians who may treat co-occurring emotional problems without knowing about serious secondary problems of substance abuse. Doran et al. (2004) report that about 1.1 million American adolescents (ages 12 through 17) met substance abuse treatment criteria in 2001, yet fewer than 100 000 received treatment. Tims et al. (2002) found that substance use before age 18 was associated with an eightfold greater likelihood of developing substance dependence in adulthood. Adults who began to use alcohol before age 15, according to Tims et al. (2002) are five times more likely to report previous-year alcohol dependence or abuse than those who began alcohol use at age 21 or older.

In terms of drug use, the rate of illicit drug use among youths 12–17 years of age was 9.9% in 2005; dependence or abuse of illicit drugs was 4.7%; and the rate of alcohol dependence or abuse was 5.5% (Substance Abuse and Mental Health Services Administration, 2005). Aranti (2008) reports that "Teenage girls now equal or outpace boys in alcohol consumption and drug use. Although boys are involved in more alcohol-related car accidents, girls are catching up" (p. A12).

In an editorial on illegal prescription drug use, the Arizona Republic (2008) reports that "One in five Arizona 12th graders used prescription drugs to get high and an alarming 10% of 8th graders had done the same" (p. B8). The Partnership on a Drug Free America (2006) reports that 1.6 million teens and young adults misused stimulants meant to treat attention-deficit hyperactivity disorder in 1 year. Among teenage males, who are most likely to use steroids, 1.8% of 8th graders, 2.3% of 10th graders, and 3.2% of 12th graders reported steroid use in 2003 (National Institute on Drug Abuse, 2004).

According to SAMSHA (2008), young people who take large doses of steroids over time risk serious health problems that may not appear until years later. In males, steroids can reduce the size of the testicles and the amount of sperm they can produce as well as increase breast growth. In females, steroids may disrupt the menstrual cycle and cause fertility problems. Steroids may also: (1) stunt growth in teens by causing the bones to mature too fast and fuse; (2) cause irreversible liver damage; (3) enlarge the heart muscles; (4) cause violent, aggressive mood swings; (5) cause or worsen acne; (6) contribute to heart disease and increase cholesterol and lipid levels; (7) create permanent stretch marks; (8) accelerate hair loss; and (9) cause muscles to ache. Teen girls risk additional side effects including excessive facial and body hair growth or male-pattern baldness, deepening of the voice and enlargement of the clitoris.

The Center for Substance Abuse Treatment (1999) reports an estimated 18% of drivers age 16–20 (or 2.5 million adolescents) drive under the influence of alcohol. Adolescents age 12–16 who have used marijuana are more likely at some point to have sold marijuana (24% versus less than 1%), carried a handgun (21% versus 7%), or been in a gang (14% versus 2 %) than youth who have never used marijuana. Adolescents who use marijuana weekly are six times more likely than nonusers to report they run away from home, five times more likely to say they steal from places other than home, and four times more likely to report they physically attack people. Adolescent substance abuse is associated with declining grades, absenteeism from school, and dropping out of school.

To summarize the harm done by substance abuse, using HHS data, Kann (2001) writes:

> *Alcohol and other drug use are among our nation's most pervasive health and social concerns, contributing to leading causes of death such as motor vehicle crashes, other injuries, homicide, suicide, cancer, and HIV infection and AIDS (U.S. Department of Health and Human Services, 2000). In addition, alcohol and other drug use contribute to social problems such as crime, lost workplace productivity, and lower educational achievement. Alcohol and other drug use among youth are common and contribute to health and social problems during adolescence, and are predictive of substance-related problems in adulthood. (Kann, 2001, p. 725)*

11.2. DIAGNOSTIC MARKERS OF SUBSTANCE ABUSE

The DSM-IV uses the following diagnostic markers to determine whether substance use is abusive: A dysfunctional use of substances causing impairment or distress within a 12-month period as determined by one of the following: (1) frequent use of substances that interfere with functioning and the fulfillment of responsibilities at home, work, school, etc.; (2) use of substances that impair functioning in dangerous situations such as driving or use of machines; (3) use of substances that may lead to arrest for unlawful behaviors; and (4) substance use that seriously interferes with relations, marriage, child rearing and other interpersonal responsibilities (APA, 1994, p. 182). Substance abuse may lead to slurred speech, lack of coordination, unsteady gait, memory loss, fatigue and depression, feelings of euphoria and lack of social inhibitions (APA, 1994, p. 197).

11.2.1. Short Tests

Miller (2001) reports that two simple questions asked of substance abusers have an 80% chance of diagnosing substance abuse: "In the past year, have you ever drunk or used drugs more than you meant to?" and, "Have you felt you wanted or needed to cut down on your drinking or drug abuse in the past year?" Miller reports that this simple approach has been found to be an effective diagnostic tool in three controlled studies using random samples and laboratory tests for alcohol and drugs in the blood stream following interviews.

Stewart and Richards (2000) and Bisson et al. (1999) suggest that four questions from the CAGE questionnaire are predictive of alcohol abuse. CAGE is an anachronism for Cut, Annoyed, Guilty, and Eye-Opener (see the questions below). Since many people deny their alcoholism, asking questions in an open, direct and non-judgmental way may elicit the best results. The four questions are:

> *(1)* ***Cut:*** *Have you ever felt you should cut down on your drinking? (2)* ***Annoyed:*** *Have people annoyed you by criticizing your drinking? (3)* ***Guilty:*** *Have you ever felt guilty about your drinking? (4)* ***Eye-Opener:*** *Have you ever had a drink first thing in the morning (eye-opener) to steady your nerves or get rid of a hangover? (Bisson et al., 1999, p. 717)*

Stewart and Richards (2000) write, "A patient who answers yes to two or more of these questions probably abuses alcohol; a patient who answers yes to one question should be screened further" (p. 56). Not everyone is as certain that the CAGE instrument, developed in the late 1970s to distinguish heavy from moderate drinkers, is an effective diagnostic tool. Bisson et al. (1999, May) write: "If the CAGE had any utility as an instrument informing on the prevalence or incidence of heavy drinking within the population, it would have discriminated between heavy and non-heavy drinkers. Our results show that this is not the case" (p. 720). The authors think the instrument is less than accurate because many people have a new awareness of alcoholism and have tried to do something to limit their alcohol use. Furthermore, the instrument asks about last year's alcohol consumption and since the subject may have changed his or her alcohol-related behavior, the answers may be misleading. Alcohol consumption has also decreased somewhat nationally. Consequently, a direct series of questions answered truthfully may fail to distinguish those who drink heavily from those who drink moderately because the responses of both groups may tend to be the same. This finding supports the notion that short questions may not be accurate in diagnosing substance abuse and that diagnosis requires an in-depth social, emotional, and medical history in which the guidelines of the DSM-IV provide direction for the types of historical and medical issues one might look for. Perhaps this lack of an in-depth history is why Backer and Walton-Moss (2001) found that fully 20–25% of all patients with alcohol-related problems were treated medically for the symptoms of alcoholism rather than for the condition itself (p. 13), and that a diagnosis of alcohol abuse was never made in almost one-fourth of all alcoholics seen for medical treatment.

11.2.2. Psychosocial Variables

Writing about female alcohol abuse, Backer and Walton-Moss (2001) report that,

> *Unlike men, women commonly seek help for alcoholism from primary care clinicians. Further, the development and progression of alcoholism is different in women than in men. Women with alcohol problems have higher rates of dual diagnoses, childhood sexual abuse, panic and phobia disorders, eating disorders, posttraumatic stress disorder, and victimization. Early diagnosis, brief interventions, and referral are critical to the treatment of alcoholism in women. (p. 13)*

The authors suggest the following diagnostic markers for female alcoholics: Since women metabolize alcohol differently than men, women tend to show signs of becoming intoxicated at a later age than men (26.5 versus 22.7), experience their fist signs of a recognition of alcohol abuse later (27.5 versus 25), and lose control over their drinking later in life (29.8 versus 27.2). The mortality rate for female alcoholics is 50–100% higher than it is for men. Liver damage occurs in women in a shorter period of time and with lower amounts of intake of alcohol. Backer and Walton-Moss (2001) also report that, "Female alcoholics have a higher mortality rate from alcoholism than men from suicide, alcohol-related accidents, circulatory disorders, and cirrhosis of the liver" (p. 15). Use of alcohol by women in adolescence is almost equal to that of male adolescents. The authors report that while men use alcohol to socialize, women use it to cope with negative moods and are likely to use alcohol in response to specific stressors in their lives.

Kuperman et al. (2001) report several risk factors for adolescent alcoholism, which include home problems, personal behavioral problems, and early use of alcohol. Home problems are considered problems with parental use and acceptance of alcohol and drugs, problems with family bonding and family conflict, ease in obtaining alcohol, a high level of peer use of alcohol, and positive peer attitudes toward alcohol and drug use. Personal behavioral problems include rebellious behavior against parents, gaining peer acceptance by drinking and other risky behaviors meant to impress peers, and self-treatment through use of alcohol and drugs for mental health and/or academic problems. Grant and Dawson (1997) report that early use of alcohol is a very strong predictor of life-long alcoholism and note that 40% of young adults aged 18–29 years who began drinking before the age of 15 were considered to be alcohol-dependent as compared to roughly 10% who began drinking after the age of 19. While Kuperman et al. (2001) suggest that these three domains are predictive of alcoholism, they also note that no one domain, by itself, can predict a diagnosis of alcoholism. In their study, all three domains were evident in adolescents who did not develop alcohol and drug problems and are idiosyncratic of a society in which many adolescents are rebellious and partake in risky behaviors. Nonetheless, the wise clinician will be aware that early and frequent use of alcohol has a fairly high probability of leading to prolonged alcohol use and will consider it as a screening and treatment issue.

Writing about the substance abuse problems of street youth, Smart and Ogborne (1994) note that street youth are more likely to be unemployed, on welfare, school drop-outs, on probation, recently incarcerated, estranged from their families, physically and sexually abused, depressed, and suffer from low self-esteem. Further, they are more likely to report eating problems, hyperactivity and attempted suicide. Street youth also reported using a wide range of drugs and more frequent use of illicit drugs. They were also more likely to describe themselves as both "alcoholic" and "drug addicted." Street youths were also more likely to report previous residential treatment for substance abuse and to have been in a detoxification center. Discharged street youth were likely to have dropped out of outpatient programs. Further, school drop-out rates were high. The average amount of time spent receiving outpatient services by both street youth and non-street youth was a very low three to three-and-a-half hours, suggesting that keeping youth in treatment is an ongoing problem. The authors write:

> *In general, the data suggest that for substance-abusing youth and especially those with street youth characteristics, many treatment episodes are brief and terminate prematurely. Although brief treatments and unplanned terminations do not necessarily represent treatment failures, the frequency of such events suggests the need for more experimentation in the delivery of youth services. This could include planned brief interventions, the use of outreach workers to maintain contact with drop-outs, as well as the establishment of long-term supportive residences for youth while they use other community resources. Of course, long-term follow-up should be a feature of any attempts to evaluate these and other innovations. (p. 1)*

11.2.3. Related Medical Problems

Stewart and Richards (2000) conclude that a number of medical problems may have their origins in substance abuse and may be indications of heavy alcohol and drug use. Head injuries and spinal separations, as a result of accidents, may have been caused by substance abuse. Because heavy drinkers often fail to eat, they may have nutritional deficiencies that result in psychotic-like symptoms, including abnormal eye movements, disorganization, and forgetfulness. Stomach disorders, liver damage, and severe heartburn may have their origins in heavy drinking, since alcohol destroys the stomach's mucosal lining. Fifteen percent of all heavy drinkers develop cirrhosis of the liver and many develop pancreatitis. Weight loss, pneumonia, muscle loss because of malnutrition, and oral cancer have all been associated with heavy drinking. The authors note that substance abusers are poor candidates for surgery. Anesthesia and pain medication can delay alcohol withdrawal for up to 5 days postoperatively. "Withdrawal symptoms can cause agitation and uncooperativeness and can mask signs and symptoms of other postoperative complications. Patients who abuse alcohol are at a higher risk for postoperative complications such as excessive bleeding, infection, heart failure, and pneumonia" (Stewart and Richards, 2000, p. 58).

The National Youth Network (2008) suggests that we think of substance abuse as three distinct levels of seriousness:

A. **Use:** The occasional use of alcohol or other drugs without developing tolerance or withdrawal symptoms when not in use.

B. **Abuse:** The continued use of alcohol or other drugs even while knowing that the continued use is creating problems socially, physically, or psychologically.

C. **Dependence:** At least three of the following factors must be present: (a) substance is taken in larger amounts or over longer periods of time than the person intended; (b) a persistent desire with unsuccessful efforts to control the use; (c) large periods of time spent obtaining, taking, or recovering from, the substance; (d) frequent periods of intoxication or detoxification, especially when social and major role obligations are expected (school, social situations, etc.); (e) continued use even while knowing that the continued use is creating problems socially, physically, and/or psychologically; (f) increased tolerance; (g) withdrawal symptoms; and (h) substance taken to relieve withdrawal symptoms.

Stewart and Richards (2000, February, p. 59) provide the following blood alcohol levels as measures of the impact of alcohol in screening for abuse:

- 0.05% (equivalent to one or two drinks in an average-sized person) – impaired judgment, reduced alertness, toss of inhibitions, euphoria.
- 0.10% – slower reaction times, decreased caution in risk taking behavior, impaired fine-motor control. Legal evidence of intoxication in most states starts at 0.10%.
- 0.15% – significant and consistent losses in reaction times.
- 0.20% – function of entire motor area of brain measurably depressed, causing staggering. The individual may be easily angered or emotional.
- 0.25% – severe sensory and motor impairment.
- 0.30% – confusion, stupor.
- 0.35% – surgical anesthesia.
- 0.40% – respiratory depression, lethal in about half of the population.
- 0.50% – death from respiratory depression. (Stewart, and Richards, 2000, p. 59).

11.3. BEST EVIDENCE FOR THE TREATMENT OF SUBSTANCE ABUSE

The author wishes to thank Pearson Education, Inc. for permission to reprint material from his book on the strengths perspective (Glicken, 2004, pp. 156–160) that relate to the treatment of substance abuse.

11.3.1. Short-term Treatment

Herman (2000) believes that individual psychotherapy can be helpful to substance abusers and suggests five situations where therapy would be indicated: (1) as an appropriate introduction to treatment; (2) as a way of helping mildly or moderately dependent drug abusers; (3) when there are clear signs of emotional problems such as severe depression, since these problems will interfere with the substance abuse treatment; (4) when clients progressing in 12-step programs begin to experience emerging feelings of guilt, shame, and grief; and (5) when a client's disturbed interpersonal functioning continues after a long period of sustained abstinence. Therapy might help prevent a relapse.

One of the most frequently discussed treatment approaches to addiction in the literature is brief counseling. Bien et al. (1993) reviewed 32 studies of brief interventions with alcohol abusers and found that, on the average, brief counseling reduced alcohol use by 30%. However, in a study of brief intervention with alcohol abusers, Chang et al. (1999) found that both the treatment and control groups significantly reduced their alcohol use. The difference between the two groups in the reduction of their alcohol abuse was minimal. In a study of 175 Mexican-Americans who were abusing alcohol, Burge et al. (1997) report that treated and untreated groups improved significantly over time, raising questions about the efficacy of treatment versus natural recovery, while in an evaluation of a larger report by *Consumers Reports* on the effectiveness of psychotherapy, Seligman (1995) notes that, "Alcoholics Anonymous (AA) did especially well, ... significantly bettering mental health professionals [in the treatment of alcohol and drug related problems]" (p. 10).

Bien et al. (1993) found that two or three 10–15 min counseling sessions are often as effective as more extensive interventions with older alcohol abusers. The sessions include motivation-for-change strategies, education, assessment of the severity of the problem, direct feedback, contracting and goal setting, behavioral modification techniques, and the use of written materials such as self-help manuals. Brief interventions have been shown to be effective in reducing alcohol consumption, binge drinking, and the frequency of excessive drinking in problem drinkers according to Fleming et al. (1997). Completion rates using brief interventions are better for elder-specific alcohol programs than for mixed-age programs (Atkinson, 1995) and late-onset alcoholics are also more likely to complete treatment and have somewhat better outcomes using brief interventions (Liberto and Oslin, 1995).

Miller and Sanchez (1994) summarize the key components of brief intervention using the acronym FRAMES: feedback, responsibility, advice, menu of strategies, empathy, and self-efficacy.

1. **Feedback:** Includes the patient's risk for alcohol problems, his or her reasons for drinking, the role of alcohol in the patient's life, and the consequences of drinking.
2. **Responsibility:** Includes strategies to help patients understand the need to remain healthy, independent and financially secure. This is particularly important when working with older clients and clients with health problems and disabilities.

3. **Advice:** Includes direct feedback and suggestions to clients to help them cope with their drinking problems and other life situations that may contribute to alcohol abuse.
4. **Menu:** Includes a list of strategies to reduce drinking and to cope with such high-risk situations as loneliness, boredom, family problems, and lack of social opportunities.
5. **Empathy:** Bien et al. (1993) strongly emphasize the need for a warm, empathic and understanding style of treatment. Miller and Rollnick (1991) found that an empathetic counseling style produced a 77% reduction in patient drinking, as compared with a 55% reduction when a confrontational approach was used
6. **Self-efficacy:** This includes strategies to help clients rely on their inner resources to make a change in their drinking behaviors. Inner resources may include positive points of view about themselves, helping others, staying busy, and good problem-solving and coping skills.

Some additional aspects of brief interventions suggested by Menninger (2002) are: drinking agreements in the form of agreed-upon drinking limits that are signed by the patient and the practitioner, ongoing follow-up and support, and appropriate timing of the intervention to the patient's readiness to change.

Babor and Higgins-Biddle (2000) discuss the use of brief interventions with people involved in "risky drinking" who are not as yet classified as alcohol dependent. Brief interventions are usually limited to 3–5 sessions of counseling and education. The intent of brief interventions is to prevent the onset of more serious alcohol-related problems. According to Babor and Higgins-Biddle (2000):

> *Most programs are instructional and motivational, designed to address the specific behavior of drinking with information, feedback, health education, skill-building, and practical advice, rather than with psychotherapy or other specialized treatment techniques. (p. 676)*

Higgins-Biddle et al. (1997) analyzed 14 random studies of brief interventions that included more than 20 000 risky drinkers. They report a net reduction in drinking of 21% for males and 8% for females. To improve the effectiveness of short-term interventions, Babor and Higgins-Biddle (2000) encourage the use of early identification of problem drinking, life-health monitoring by health and mental health professionals, and risk counseling that includes screening and brief intervention to inform and motivate potential alcohol abusers of the risk of serious alcohol dependence and to help change their alcohol use. This approach requires a high degree of cooperation among health and education personnel who are often loathe to identify very young people as having "at risk" alcohol problems because they fear that doing so will exacerbate the problem through public identification, and often believe that more moderate drinking will take place as the child matures.

Fleming and Manwell (1998) report that people with alcohol-related problems often receive counseling from primary care physicians or nursing staff in five or fewer standard office visits. The counseling consists of rational information about the negative impact of alcohol use, as well as practical advice regarding ways of reducing alcohol dependence and the availability of community resources. Gentilello et al. (1995) report that 25–40% of the trauma patients seen in emergency rooms may be alcohol dependent. The authors found that a single motivational interview, at or near the time of discharge, reduced drinking levels and re-admission for trauma during 6 months of follow-up. Monti et al. (1999) conducted a similar study with 18–19-year-olds admitted to an emergency room with alcohol-related injuries. After 6 months, all participants had decreased their alcohol consumption. However, "the group receiving brief intervention had a significantly lower incidence of drinking and driving, traffic violations, alcohol-related injuries, and alcohol-related problems" (Monti et al., 1999, p. 3).

Lu and McGuire (2002) studied the effectiveness of out-patient treatment with substance-abusing clients and came to the following conclusions: (1) the more severe the drug use problem before treatment was initiated, the less likely clients were to discontinue drug use during treatment when compared to other users; (2) clients reporting no substance abuse 3 months before admission were more likely to maintain abstinence than those who reported abstinence only in the past 1 month; (3) heroin users were very unlikely to sustain abstinence during treatment, while marijuana users were less likely to sustain abstinence during treatment than alcohol users; (4) clients with "psychiatric problem" were more likely to use drugs during treatment than clients without psychiatric problems; (5) clients with legal problems related to their substance abuse had reduced chances of improving during the treatment; (6) clients who had multiple prior treatments for substance abuse were less likely to remain abstinent during and after treatment; (7) more educated clients were more likely to sustain abstinence after treatment; and (8) clients treated in urban agencies were less likely to maintain abstinence than those treated rural agencies.

11.3.2. Longer-term Treatments

Walitzer et al. (1999) report that treatment attrition among substance abusers is such a pervasive problem in programs offering treatment services that it affects our ability to determine treatment effectiveness. Baekeland and Lundwall (1975) report drop-out rates for inpatient treatment programs of 28%, and that 75% of the outpatient alcoholic patients in their study dropped out of treatment before their fourth session. Leigh et al. (1984) report that of 172 alcoholism outpatients studied, 15% failed to attend their initial appointment, 28% attended only a session or two, and 19% attended only three to five times. In studying 117 alcoholism clinic admissions, Rees (1986) found that 35% of the clients failed to return after their initial visit and that another 18% terminated treatment within 30 days. To try and reduce the amount of attrition in alcohol treatment programs, Walitzer and Dermen (2002) randomly assigned 126 clients entering an alcohol treatment program to one of three groups to prepare them for the treatment program: a role induction (RI) session, a motivational interview (MI) session, or a no-preparatory session control group (CG). They found that clients assigned to the motivational interview "attended more treatment sessions and had fewer heavy drinking days during and 12 months after treatment relative to control group (p. 1161). Clients assigned to the motivational interview also were abstinent more days during treatment and in the first 3 months following treatment than the control group, but the difference, unfortunately, did not last for the remaining 9 months of follow up. Clients assigned to the role induction group did no better than the control group in any of the variables studied.

In describing the motivational interview, Walitzer and Dermen (2002) indicate that it consists of the following:

> *(a) Eliciting self-motivational statements; (b) reflective, empathic listening; (c) inquiring about the client's feelings, ideas, concerns, and plans; (d) affirming the client in a way that acknowledges the client's serious consideration of and steps toward change; (e) deflecting resistance in a manner that takes into account the link between therapist behavior and client resistance; (f) reframing client statements as appropriate; and (g) summarizing (p. 1164).*

Kirchner et al. (2000) considered the factors related to entry into alcohol treatment programs following a diagnosis of alcoholism. They found that many patients who might benefit from treatment were not referred by their medical providers because of a belief that treatment was not effective, even though a number of "well-designed and methodologically sound studies have repeatedly shown that treatment for alcohol-related disorders can be effective not only for reducing the consumption of alcohol but also for improving the patient's overall level of functioning" (p. 339). The authors also report that improved detection of alcoholism, the first step in the provision of services, is negatively influenced by a number of factors including younger age, non-Caucasian ethnicity, the severity of the alcohol use, lower socioeconomic status, and male gender. Drug and alcohol use to self-medicate for psychiatric disorders is also a key predictor of detection, as are alcohol-related medical problems such as liver disorders, high blood pressure, and adult onset diabetes. Herman (2000) reports that the reasons substance abusers enter treatment are usually external in nature and include legal problems with drug use (license suspension because of drunk driving), marital problems, work-related problems, medical complications caused by drug and alcohol abuse, problems with depression and anxiety that lead to self-medicating with alcohol and drugs, and referral by mental health professionals (a major reason women enter treatment programs.)

11.3.3. Treatment Strategies

Merrill et al. (2001) believes that the primary strategy in the treatment of substance abuse is to initially achieve abstinence. Once abstinence is achieved, the substance abuser can begin to address relationship problems that might interfere with social and emotional functioning. Merrill et al. (2001) believes that the key to treatment is to match the client with the type of treatment most likely to help. He suggests that the following phases exist in the treatment of substance abuse: *Phase 1*: Abstinence. *Phase 2*: Teaching the client coping skills to help prevent a relapse through cognitive-behavioral techniques that help clients manage stressful situation likely to trigger substance abuse. These may include recognizing cues that lead to substance abuse, managing external cues, avoiding peers who are likely to continue to abuse substances and encourage the client to do the same, and alternative behaviors that help the client avoid drug use. *Phase 3*: Since the underlying problems that contribute to substance abuse are often deeply internalized feelings of low self-worth, depression, and self-loathing, therapy should help the client deal with internalized pathologies that are likely to lead to relapse. The therapies that seem most effective in doing this are cognitive-behavioral therapies, the strengths approach, and affective therapies, including Gestalt therapy. Merrill suggests the use of psychodynamic therapy, but research evidence of the effectiveness of this form of treatment is not overly promising.

In a review of 30 years of research, the National Institute on Drug Abuse (1999) reports that the following are necessary elements of effective treatment of substance abuse:

> *(1) Treatment involves matching the patient to the correct treatment modality; (2) treatment is readily accessible; (3) treatment attends to the ancillary needs of the patient; (4) treatment is based on a comprehensive and regularly updated treatment plan; (5) treatment involves the patient remaining in treatment for an adequate period of time; (6) treatment assures the patient of receiving a sufficient amount of counseling; (7) treatment includes adjunctive pharmacotherapy, if necessary; (8) treatment is provided for coexisting mental disorders, if present; (9) treatment is provided beyond detoxification; (10) treatment accommodates patients that are mandated into treatment; (11) the treatment staff monitors the patient's drug use regularly; (12) an assessment is made for human immunodeficiency virus/acquired immune deficiency syndrome (HIV/AIDS) and other infectious diseases; and (13) multiple treatment episodes are provided for, if necessary. (Found in Lennox and Mansfield, 2001, p. 169)*

Other factors found to provide best evidence of treatment effectiveness include the following: Dahlgren and Willander (1989) compared women-only and mixed-gender treatment groups. Clients in the women-only group remained in treatment longer, had higher completion rates, and improved biopsychosocial rates compared with women who were in mixed-gender programs. Burtscheidt et al. (2002) studied the treatment effects of long-term treatment by comparing nonspecific supportive therapy with two different forms of behavioral therapy (coping skills training and cognitive behavioral therapy). One hundred twenty patents were randomly assigned to each of the three therapy approaches and were seen in treatment for 26 weeks with a follow-up period of 2 years. Patients receiving behavioral therapy showed consistently higher abstinence rates. Differences in treatment effectiveness between the two behavioral therapies could not be established. The study also established that cognitively impaired and severely personality disordered clients had less benefit from any of the therapies than clients not fitting into these two categories of dysfunction. The authors conclude that behavioral treatment had the best long-term effects and met high client acceptance, but that a great deal still needs to be done to develop even more effective behavioral therapies for clients who abuse substances.

Two family treatment approaches show evidence of helping. *Multisystemic treatment* (MST) has shown favorable short-term (Henggeler et al., 2000) and long-term (Henggeler et al., 2002) reductions in adolescent drug use. *Contingency management* (CM) (Donohue & Azrin, 2001) has produced promising results for substance-using adolescents. CM uses behavioral techniques to help youth; avoid situations associated with drug use; engage in pro-social activities incompatible with drug use; and change cognitions and feelings associated with drug use. Additionally, drug use is traced through frequent urine drug screens, and caregivers are empowered to reward abstinence and otherwise reinforce desired behavior change.

There is increasing evidence to suggest that the majority of youth referred for substance abuse treatment have at least one co-occurring mental health disorder. Rates of co-occurring conduct disorder with substance use disorder (SUD) have been estimated to range from 50% to 80% in clinical populations (Meyers et al., 1995; Milin et al., 1991). The research literature notes that HDHD, mood disorders and conduct disorders are most often reported to exist in conjunction with adolescence substance abuse (Bukstein et al., 1992; Deykin et al., 1992; Hovens et al., 1994).

Henggeler et al. (2002) suggest several reasons why finding best evidence for treatment effectiveness is particularly difficult for youth abusers. First, there are relatively few studies of the effectiveness in treating adolescent substance abuse. Second, most of the studies lack scientific rigor and fail to use control groups or take into consideration change brought about by maturation. Third, researchers tend to over-interpret favorable findings. For example, positive findings in psycho-social functioning may not be compared to actual substance abuse through drug screening, giving one the sense that treatment was successful when, in fact, drug abuse continued.

11.3.4. Natural Recovery

Granfield and Cloud (1996) estimate that as many as 90% of all problem drinkers never enter treatment and that many suspend problematic use of alcohol without any form of treatment (Hingson et al., 1980; Roizen et al., 1978; Stall and Biernacki 1989). Sobell et al. (1993) report that 82% of the alcoholics they studied who terminated their addiction did so by using natural recovery methods that excluded the use of a professional. In another example of the use of natural recovery techniques, Granfield and Cloud (1996) indicate that most ex-smokers discontinued their tobacco use without treatment (Peele 1989), while many addicted substance abusers "mature-out" of a variety of addictions, including heavy drinking and narcotics use (Snow 1973; Winick 1962). Biernacki (1986) reports that addicts who naturally stop their addictions use a range of strategies that include breaking off relationships with drug users, removing themselves from drug-using environments (Stall and Biernacki 1989), building new structures in their lives (Peele 1989), and using friends and family to provide support for discontinuing their substance abuse (Biernacki, 1986). Trice and Roman (1970) suggest that self-help groups with substance-abusing clients are particularly helpful because they tend to reduce personal responsibility with its related guilt, and help build and maintain a support network that assists in continuing the changed behavior.

Granfield and Cloud (1996) studied middle class alcoholics who used natural recovery alone without professional help or self-help groups. Many of the participants in their study felt that the "ideological" bases of many self-help programs were inconsistent with their own philosophies of life. For example, many felt that some self-help groups for substance abusers were overly religious, while other self-help groups believed in alcoholism as a disease, which suggested a lifetime struggle. The subjects in the study by Granfield and Cloud (1996) also felt that some self-help groups encouraged dependence on the group and that associating with other alcoholics would probably make recovery more difficult. In summarizing their findings, Granfield and Cloud (1996) report that:

> *Many [research subjects] expressed strong opposition to the suggestion that they were powerless over their addictions. Such an ideology, they explained, not only was counterproductive but was also extremely demeaning. These respondents saw themselves as efficacious people who often prided themselves on their past accomplishments. They viewed themselves as being individualists and strong-willed. One respondent, for instance, explained that "such programs encourage powerlessness" and that she would rather "trust her own instincts than the instincts of others." (Granfield and Cloud, 1996, p. 51)*

To further underscore the significance of natural healing, Waldorf et al. (1991) found that many addicted people with supportive elements in their lives (a job, family, and other close emotional supports) were able to "walk away" from their very heavy use of cocaine. The authors suggest that the "social context" of a drug user's life may positively influence his ability to discontinue drug use. Granfield and Cloud (1996) note that many of the respondents in their sample had a great deal to lose if they continued their substance abuse, and write,

> *The respondents in our sample had relatively stable lives: they had jobs, supportive families, high school and college credentials, and other social supports that gave them reasons to alter their drug-taking behavior. Having much to lose gave our respondents incentives to transform their lives. However, when there is little to lose from heavy alcohol or drug use, there may be little to gain by quitting. (Granfield and Cloud, 1996, p. 55)*

Humphreys (1998) studied the effectiveness of self-help groups with substance abusers by comparing two groups: one receiving in-patient care for substance abuse, and the other attending self-help groups for substance abuse. At the conclusion of the study, the average participant assigned to a self-help group (AA) had used $8840 in alcohol-related health care resources, as compared to $10 040 for the inpatient treatment participants. In a follow-up study, Humphreys (1998) compared outpatient services to self-help groups for the treatment of substance abuse. The clients in the self-help group had decreased alcohol consumption by 70% over 3 years, and consumed 45% less health care services (about $1800 less per person). Humphreys (1998) argues that, "From a cost-conscious point of view, self-help groups should be the first option evaluated when an addicted individual makes initial contact with professional services (e.g., in a primary care appointment or a clinical assessment at a substance abuse agency or employee assistance program)" (p. 16).

11.3.5. The strengths Perspective

Writing about the strengths perspective and the treatment of substance abuse, Moxley and Olivia (2001) conclude that recovery requires the client and the clinician to focus on the meaning of life and the higher purpose that binds us all together. The use of the strengths perspective to achieve this purpose does not deny the damage done by substance abuse or the pain it causes others. Furthermore, it does not deny the social conditions that often lead to substance abuse and the social forces that frequently disempower people who become addicted to substances. To achieve the goal of helping people with substance abuse problems find meaning in their lives, Moxley and Olivia (2001) write:

> *. . . [N]othing in life effectively helps people to survive even the worst conditions as the knowledge that one's life has meaning. A salient challenge is to ensure that individuals articulate their own perspectives concerning what the transpersonal means to them. But it is the responsibility of the transpersonal practitioner to offer people in recovery opportunities to awaken. (p. 259)*

Moxley and Olivia (2001, p. 260) suggest the following elements of the strengths perspective with clients who abuse substances:

1. The purpose of any human being is to fulfill a life goal that is constructive and vital to the advancement of humankind, of the environment, and of the universe.
2. The absence of opportunity induced by discrimination, stigmatization, and social marginalization can set conditions in which a career of chemical dependency can become a likely alternative.
3. People can gain insight when they come to understand the forces influencing their chemical dependency and when they realize that while they can blame these forces, they must also confront them and overcome them.
4. The transpersonal domain reminds people that nothing in life effectively helps people to survive even the worst conditions as the knowledge that one's life has meaning.

11.4. CASE STUDY: A BRIEF INTERVENTION AFTER AN ALCOHOL-RELATED CAR ACCIDENT

Robert is a 17-year-old high school student who was taken to the emergency room after his car spun out of control and hit an embankment. Three passengers in the car were slightly injured. Robert and his friends had been drinking "Ever clear," a 180-proof alcoholic beverage they purchased through an older friend. All four friends were highly inebriated and had walked a block and a half from a party they were attending to their car wearing tee-shirts in 40° below-zero weather. Robert sustained minor injuries. After he became sober enough in the emergency room to recognize the seriousness of the accident and that his blood alcohol level was in excess of 0.25%, three times the allowed drinking and driving level of 0.08%, he became antagonistic and withdrawn. His parents rushed to the hospital and were very concerned about Robert's behavior. His drinking was unknown to them, although Robert had begun drinking at age 10 and was regularly becoming intoxicated at weekend parties by age 13. Robert thought he was doing social drinking and felt that he was no different than his other friends. The accident, however, seemed to be a wake-up call to do something about his risky drinking.

A social worker and nurse met with Robert and his parents three times over the course of a 2-day stay in the hospital. They gave out information about the health impact of drinking and did a screening test to determine Robert's level of abusive drinking. They concluded that Robert was at very high risk of becoming an alcoholic since his drinking impaired his judgment, affected his grades, and was thought to be responsible for high blood sugar readings consistent with early onset diabetes and moderately high blood pressure. A psychosocial history taken by the social worker revealed that Robert had begun experimenting with alcohol at age 10 and was using it at home and with friends from age 13 on. He was drinking more than a quart of alcohol a week, some of it very high in alcohol content. Robert's driver's license was revoked by the court and, on the basis of the report made by the emergency room personnel, Robert was sent for mandatory alcohol counseling.

Robert is a reluctant client. He discounts his drinking problem, claiming that he drinks no more than his friends and that were it not for the accident, he would not be in counseling since he was not having any serious problems in his life. That is not altogether true, however. With an IQ of over 150, Robert's grades are mostly in the "D" range. He misses classes on a regular basis and often misses class in the mornings because of hangovers. His parents are having marital and financial problems and fail to supervise Robert closely. Furthermore, Robert has been fantasizing about harming his friends whom he thinks have been disloyal to him for reasons he cannot validate. "Just a feeling, ya know?" he told the therapist. Was the accident really an accident? "Sure," Robert says, "what else?" His therapist is not so certain. He has hints of Robert's antagonism toward other students and has heard Robert talk about dreams in which he harms others. Robert spends a great deal of time on the Internet and has assumed various identities, many of them harboring anti-social and violent intentions. The therapist believes that Robert is a walking time bomb of emotional distress and that his alcoholism, while robust, is just one way of self-medicating himself for feelings of isolation, low self-esteem, and rejection by parents and classmates.

After months of treatment during which time Robert would often sit in silence and stare at the therapist, he has begun to talk about his feelings and admits that he has continued drinking heavily. He also drives, although his license has been suspended. He is full of self-hate and thinks that he is doomed to die soon. He feels strong when he drinks, he told the therapist, and loves the peaceful feeling that comes over him as he gets drunk. Like his parents, he romanticizes his drinking and can hardly wait to have his first drink. Sometimes he drinks when he wakes up and often drinks rather than eats. He is aware that this cycle of drinking to feel better about himself can only lead to serious life problems, but does not think he is capable of stopping.

Robert's therapist asked Robert to help him do an Internet search to find the best approach to help Robert with his drinking problem. It seemed like a silly request to Robert since the therapist was supposed to be the expert, but Robert was intrigued and did as he was asked. When he met next with the therapist, Robert had printed out a number of articles suggesting ways of coping with adolescent alcoholism that seemed reasonable to him and to the therapist. From the work of Kuperman et al. (2001), they agreed that Robert had a number of problems that should be dealt with at home, with friends, and with his alcohol abuse. They decided that a cognitive-behavioral approach would work best with homework assignments and cognitive restructuring as additional aspects of the treatment. Robert was intrigued with an article he found on the strengths approach and showed the therapist an article by Moxley and Olivia (2001) they both found quite useful. Another article on self-help groups by Humphreys (1998) convinced them that a self-help group for adolescent alcohol abusers might also be helpful. Finally, Robert brought up the issue of working with his parents and it was decided that the family would be seen together to work on some of the problems they were having and to develop better communication skills.

Robert has been in treatment for over a year. He is applying himself in school and has begun thinking about college. His drinking has modified itself somewhat. Although he still drinks too much at times, he will not drive when he is drinking or engage in risky behavior. He feels much less angry and has developed new friendships with peers who do not drink or use drugs. The changes seem very substantial, but it is too early to know if the alcoholism is likely to display itself when he deals with additional life stressors. Robert is unsure and says that, "Yeah, it's all helping me but my head isn't always on straight and sometimes I do dumb stuff. I'm more aware of it now but I still do it. I'm getting along with my folks a lot better and my new friends are real friends, not drinking buddies. I don't know. I looked at some studies on the Internet and it looks like I have a pretty good chance of becoming an alcoholic. I like booze. It makes me feel good.

That's not a good sign, is it? And I'm still a pretty mad about a lot of things. I spend time on the Internet in chat rooms and it's pretty bizarre, sometimes, the things I say. But yeah, I know I'm better. I just hope it keeps up."

Robert's therapist said, "Robert has a good handle on himself. I wouldn't argue with anything he said. He has lots of potential but he also has enough problems to make me unwilling to predict the future. What I will say is that he works hard, is cooperative, and seems to be trying to work on some long-standing issues with his family and his perception of himself. I think that addictions are transitory and you never know when his desire to drink will overwhelm his desire to stay sober. The self-help group he is in keeps close tabs on his drinking and his new friends are a help. I had caution anyone who works with adolescents not to expect too much from treatment. I do want to applaud the professionals he worked with in the hospital. Even though the treatment was brief, it made a lasting impact on Robert to hear that he was considered an alcoholic, and it did bring him into treatment. That is exactly what you hope for in serious alcoholics who are in denial."

11.5. RESEARCH PROBLEMS AND BEST EVIDENCE

A major problem with the treatment of substance abuse is the lack of best evidence because of difficult research issues. Clifford et al. (2000) note that many research studies on the effectiveness of treatment for substance abuse have numerous methodological pitfalls and write, "It is recommended that treatment outcome studies be interpreted cautiously, particularly when the research protocols involved frequent and intensive follow-up interviews conducted across extended periods of time" (p. 741). As one example of the type of research error made in substance abuse research, Ouimette et al. (1997) compared 12-step programs such as AA with cognitive-behavioral programs and programs that combined both approaches. One year after completion of treatment, all three types of programs had similar improvement rates related to alcohol consumption. Participants in 12-step had more "sustained abstinence" and better employment rates than the other two programs, but Ouimette et al. (1997) caution the reader not to make more of these findings than is warranted because of nonrandom assignment of patients to the different treatment types. A careful look at many other substance abuse treatment studies suggests similar methodological concerns in a field where empirically based studies are essential to good treatment results.

11.6. SUMMARY

In this chapter on EBP and substance abuse, research findings are reported that suggest substantial disagreement regarding the effectiveness of certain types of treatment, particularly very brief treatment with high-risk abusers. However, promising research on natural recovery and self-help groups suggests that treatment effectiveness may be positive with these two approaches. Research issues are discussed which make the development of best evidence on the efficacy of all forms of treatment of substance abuse questionable, and the suggestion is made that before we can develop best evidence, more effective studies must take place that include adequate research designs and controls. A case study is provided that demonstrates the use of EBP with substance-abusing clients.

11.7. QUESTIONS FROM THE CHAPTER

1. Binge drinking is epidemic on many university campuses in the United States. Do you feel that binge drinking is a sign of potential for alcoholism?
2. Brief treatment of substance abuse flies in the face of what many people believe about the long-term addictive nature of alcohol and drug dependence. What is your view about the effectiveness of brief treatment?
3. Is it fair to criticize the lack of adequate research for self-help groups treating addictions? Should not we take at face value the overwhelmingly positive feedback from participants that they work very well?
4. The idea that people will walk away from their addictions when they are ready is contraindicated in studies of weight loss. In these studies, people cycle back and forth and fail to sustain weight loss. Might not the same thing be said about addictions to substances?
5. Focusing on positive behavior seems like a worthy way to treat substance abusers, but are not there dangerous behaviors (unprotected sex, date rape, automobile accidents) that need to be stopped immediately, and do not they require a type of "tough love"?

References

Aranti, L. (2008, February 11). *Girls' alcohol, drug use increasing*. The Arizona Republic, p. A12.

Atkinson, R. (1995). Treatment programs for aging alcoholics. In T. Beresford, E. & Gomberg (Eds.), *Alcohol and aging* (pp. 186–210). New York: Oxford University Press.

APA. (1994). p. 182.

Babor, T. F., & Higgins-Biddle, J. C. (2000, May). Alcohol screening and brief intervention: Dissemination strategies for medical practice and public health. *Addiction, 95*(5), 677–687.

Backer, K. L., & Walton-Moss, B. (2001, October). Detecting and addressing alcohol abuse in women. *Nurse Practitioner, 26*(10), 13–22.

Baekeland, F., & Lundwall, L. (1975). Dropping out of treatment: A critical review. *Psychological Bulletin, 82*, 738–783.

Bien, T. J., Miller, W. R., & Tonigan, J. S. (1993). Brief interventions for alcohol problems: A review. *Addictions, 88*(3), 315–335.

Biernacki, P. (1986). *Pathways from heroin addiction: Recover without treatment..* Philadelphia: Temple University Press.

Bisson, J., Nadeau, L., & Demers, A. (1999, May). The validity of the CAGE scale to screen heavy drinking and drinking problems in a general population. *Addiction, 94*(5), 715–723.

Bukstein, O. G., Glancy, L. J., & Kaminer, Y. (1992). Patterns of affective comorbidity in a clinical population of dually diagnosed adolescent substance abusers. *Journal of the American Academy of Child and Adolescent Psychiatry, 31*(6), 1041–1045.

Burge, S. K., Amodei, N., Elkin, B., Catala, S., Andrew, S. R., Lane, P. A., & Seale, J. P. (1997). An evaluation of two primary care interventions for alcohol abuse among Mexican-American patients. *Addiction, 92*(12), 1705–1716.

Burtscheidt, W., Wolwer, W., Schwartz, R., et al. (2002, September). Alcoholism, rehabilitation and comorbidity. *Acta Psychiatrica Scandinavica, 106*(3), 227–233.

Center for Substance Abuse Treatment. (1999). *Screening and Assessing Adolescents for Substance Use Disorders.* Treatment Improvement Protocol (TIP) Series, No. 31. DHHS Publication No. (SMA) 99-3282. Rockville, MD: Substance Abuse and Mental Health Services Administration.

Chang, G., Wilkins-Haug, L., Berman, S., & Goetz, M. A. (1999). Brief intervention for alcohol use in pregnancy: A randomized trial. *Addiction, 94*(10), 1499–1508.

Clifford, P. R., Maisto, S. A., & Franzke, L. H. (2000). Alcohol treatment research follow-up and drinking behaviors. *Journal of Studies on Alcohol, 61*(5), 736–743.

Dahlgren, L., & Willander, A. (1989). Are special treatment facilities for female alcoholics needed? Alcoholism. *Clinical and Experimental Research, 13*, 499–504.

Deykin, E. Y., Buka, S. L., & Zeena, T. H. (1992). Depressive illnesses among chemically dependent adolescents. *American Journal of Psychiatry, 149*, 1341–1347.

Donohue, B., & Azrin, N. H. (2001). Family behavior therapy. In E. F. Wagner, H. B. & Saldron (Eds.), *Innovations in adolescent substance abuse* (pp. 205–227). New York: Pergamon.

Doran, C. M., Shakeshaft, A. P., & Fawcett, J. E. (2004). General practitioners' role in preventive medicine: Scenario analysis using alcohol as a case study. *Drug and Alcohol Review, 23*, 399–404.

Editorial. The Arizona Republic (2008, Feb 11). *Prescription threat.* B 8.

Fleming, M. F., Barry, K. L., Manwell, L. B., Johnson, K., & London, R. (1997). Brief physician advice for problem alcohol drinkers: A randomized controlled trial in community-based primary care practices. *The Journal of the American Medical Association, 277*(13), 1039–1045.

Fleming, M., & Manwell, L. B. (1998). Brief intervention in primary care settings: A primary treatment method for at-risk, problem, and dependent drinkers. *Alcohol Research and Health, 23*(2), 128–137.

Gentilello, L. M., Donovan, D. M., Dunn, C. W., & Rivara, F. P. (1995). Alcohol interventions in trauma centers: Current practice and future directions. *The Journal of the American Medical Association, 274*(13), 1043–1048.

Glicken, M. D. (2004). *Using the strengths perspective in social work practice.* Boston, MA: Pearson Education, Inc..

Granfield, R., & Cloud, W. (1996, Winter). The elephant that no one sees: Natural recovery among middle-class addicts. *Journal of Drug Issues, 26*, 45–61.

Grant, B. F., & Dawson, D. A. (1997). Age at onset of alcohol use and its association with DSM-IV alcohol abuse and dependence: Results from the national longitudinal alcohol epidemiologic survey. *Journal of Substance Abuse, 9*, 103–110.

Henggeler, S. W., Schoenwald, S. K., Clingempeel, H. J., Rowland, M. D., & Cummmingham, P. B. (2002). *Serious emotional disturbance in children and adolescents: Multisystemic therapy*. New York: Guilford Press.

Henggeler, S. W., Pickrel, S. G., & Brondino, M. J. (2000). Multisystemic treatment of substance abusing and dependent delinquents: Outcomes, treatments, fidelity, and transportability. *Mental Health Services Research, 1*, 171–184.

Herman, M. (2000). Psychotherapy with substance abusers: Integration of psychodynamic and cognitive-behavioral approaches. *American Journal of Psychotherapy, 54*(4), 574–579.

Higgins-Biddle, J. C., Babor, T. F., Mullahy, J., Daniels, J., & Mcree, B. (1997). Alcohol screening and brief interventions: where research meets practice. *Connecticut Medicine, 61*, 565–575.

Hingson, R., Scotch, N., Day, N., & Culbert, A. (1980). Recognizing and seeking help for drinking problems. *Journal of Studies on Alcohol, 41*, 1102–1117.

Hovens, J., Cantwell, D. P., & Kiriakos, R. (1994). Psychiatric comorbidity in hospitalized adolescent substance abusers. *Journal of the American Academy of Child and Adolescent Psychiatry, 33*, 476–483.

Humphreys, K. (1998, Winter). Can addiction-related self-help/mutual aid groups lower demand for professional substance abuse treatment?. *Social Policy, 29*(2), 13–17.

Kann, L. (2001). Commentary. *Journal of Drug Issues, 31*(3), 725–727.

Kirchner, J. E., Booth, B. M., Owen, R. R., Lancaster, R. R., et al. (2000, August). Predictors of patient entry into alcohol treatment after initial diagnosis. *Journal of Behavioral Health Services & Research*, 27(3), 339–347, (p. 8).

Kuperman, S., Schlosser, S. S., Kramer, J. R., Bucholz, K., Hesselbrock, V., Reich, T., & Reich, W. (2001, April). Risk domains associated with an adolescent alcohol dependence diagnosis. *Addiction, 96*(4), 629–636.

Leigh, G., Ogborne, A. C., & Cleland, P. (1984). Factors associated with patient dropout from an outpatient alcoholism treatment service. *Journal of Studies on Alcohol, 45*, 359–362.

Lennox, R. D., & Mansfield, A. J. (2001, May). A latent variable model of evidence-based quality improvement for substance abuse treatment. *Journal of Behavioral Health Services & Research, 28*(2), 164–177.

Liberto, J. G., & Oslin, D. W. (1995). Early versus late onset of alcoholism in the elderly. *International Journal of Addiction, 30*(13–14), 1799–1818.

Lu, M., & McGuire, T. G. (2002). The productivity of outpatient treatment for substance abuse. *Journal of Human Resources, 37*(2), 309–335.

Menninger, J. A. (2002, Spring). Source assessment and treatment of alcoholism and substance-related disorders in the elderly. *Bulletin of the Menninger Clinic, 66*(2), 166A–184A.

Merrill, R. M., Salazar, R. D., & Gardner, N. W. (2001). Relationship between family religiosity and drug use behavior among youth. *Social Behavior & Personality: An International Journal*, 29(4), 347–357.

Meyers, M. G., Brown, S. A., & Mott, M. A. (1995). Preadolescent conduct disorder behaviors predict relapse and progression of addiction for adolescent alcohol and drug abusers. *Alcoholism: Clinical and Experimental Research, 19*, 1528–1536.

Milin, R., Halikas, J. A., Meller, J. E., & Morse, C. (1991). Psychopathology among substance abusing juvenile offenders. *Journal of the American Academy of Child and Adolescent Psychiatry, 30, 569–574.*

Miller, K. E. (2001). Can two questions screen for alcohol and substance abuse?. *American Family Physician, 64*, 1247.

Miller, W. R., & Rollnick, S. (1991). *Motivational interviewing: Preparing people to change addictive behavior*. New York: Guilford Press.

Miller, W. R., & Sanchez, V. C. (1994). Motivating young adults for treatment and lifestyle change.. In G. S. Howard, P. E. & Nathan (Eds.), *Alcohol Use and Misuse by Young Adults* (pp. 55–81). Notre Dame, IN: Univ. of Notre Dame Press.

Monitoring the Future Study: Overview of Key Findings. (2004). *National Institute on Drug Abuse, 2004*. http://ncadi.samhsa.gov/govpubs/phd726/

Monti, P. M., Colby, S. M., Barnett, N. P., et al. (1999). Brief intervention for harm reduction with alcohol-positive older adolescents in a hospital emergency department. *Journal of Consulting and Clinical Psychology, 67*(6), 989–994.

Moxley, D. P., & Olivia, G. (2001). Strengths-based recovery practice in chemical dependency: A transperson perspective. *Families in Society, 82*(3), 251–262.

National Institute on Drug Abuse. (1999). *Principles of drug addiction treatment: A Research-based guide*. Rockville, MD: National Institute on Drug Abuse. DHHS publication (ADM), 99–4180.

National Youth Network: Teenage Substance. Abuse retrieved Feb. 12, (2008) at http://www.nationalyouth.com/substanceabuse.html

Ouimette, P. C., Finney, J. W., & Moos, R. H. (1997). Twelve-step and cognitive-behavioral treatment for substance abuse: A comparison of treatment effectiveness. *Journal of Consulting and Clinical Psychology, 65*(2), 230–240.

Partnership for a drug Free America, The (March/April, 2006). *The Bulletin*. http://www.drugfree.org/Portal/About/Bulletins/March_April_2006

Peele, S. (1989). *The diseasing of America: Addiction treatment out of control*. Lexington, Mass: Lexington Books.

Rees, D. W. (1986). Changing patients' health beliefs to improve compliance with alcoholism treatment: A controlled trial. *Journal of Studies on Alcohol, 47*, 436–439.

Roizen, R., Cahalan, D., Lambert, E., Wiebel, W., & Shanks, P. (1978). Spontaneous remission among untreated problem drinkers. In D. & Kandel (Ed.), *Longitudinal research on drug use*. Washington, DC: Hemisphere Publishing.

SAMHSA's. (2008). *National clearinghouse for alcohol and drug information*. http://ncadi.samhsa.gov/govpubs/phd726/

Seligman, M. E. P. (1995). The effectiveness of psychotherapy: The consumers report study. *American Psychologist, 50*(12), 965–974.

Smart, R. G. & Ogborne, A. C. (1994, Fall), Street youth in substance abuse treatment: Characteristics and treatment compliance. *Adolescence*. http://findarticles.com/p/articles/mi_m2248/is_n115_v29/ai_16423348

Snow, M. (1973). Maturing out of narcotic addiction in New York City. *International Journal of the Addictions, 8*(6), 932–938.

Sobell, L., Sobell, M., Toneatto, T., & Leo, G. (1993). What triggers the resolution of alcohol problems without treatment?. *Alcoholism: Clinical and Experimental Research, 17*(2), 217–224.

Stall, R., & Biernacki, P. (1989). Spontaneous remission from the problematic use of substances. *International Journal of the Addictions, 21*, 1–23.

Stewart, K. B., & Richards, A. B. (2000). Recognizing and managing your patient's alcohol abuse. *Nursing, 30*(2), 56–60.

Substance Abuse and Mental Health Services Administration. (2005). *National household survey on drug use and health*. Rockville, MD: US Dept. of Health and Human Services, Office of Applied Studies.

Tims, F. M., Dennis, M. L., Hamilton, N. J., Buchan, B., Diamond, G., & Funk, R. (2002). Characteristics and problems of 600 adolescent cannabis abusers in outpatient treatment. *Addiction, 97*(Suppl. 1), 46–57.

Trice, H., & Roman, P. (1970). Delabeling, relabeling, and alcoholics anonymous. *Social Problems, 17*, 538–546.

Waldorf, D., Reinarman, C., & Murphy, S. (1991). *Cocaine changes: The experience of using and quitting*. Philadelphia: Temple University Press.

Walitzer, K. S., Dermen, K. H., & Connors, G. J. (1999). Strategies for preparing clients for treatment: A review. *Behavior Modification, 23*, 129–151.

Winick, C. (1962). Maturing out of narcotic addiction. *Bulletin on Narcotics, 6*, 1.

Further reading

National Institute of Alcohol Abuse and Alcoholism. (2000). *Alcohol alert*. NIAAA, Vol. 49.

12 Evidence-Based Practice with Gay, Lesbian, Bisexual and Transgender Children and Adolescents

12.1. INTRODUCTION

The author wishes to thank Sage Publications for permission to reprint portions of this chapter that first appeared in a book he wrote on resilience (Glicken, 2006, pp. 157–169).

Gay, lesbian, bisexual and transgender children and adolescents have an obvious set of traumas confronting them early in the lifespan. Being different in a society that is still homophobic and moralistic can have profound repercussions including being bullied in school, gay bashing, family rejection, job discrimination, and hate crimes. Many gay and bi-sexual children and adolescents suffer severe depressions as a result of homophobia, and experience a higher rate of suicide than the population at large. While we have moved to protect sexual orientation from legal discrimination, it occurs in great numbers, and the hidden and not so hidden conduct of all too many among us who bash and persecute gay and bi-sexual children and adolescents is a reminder of a long history of persecution of gays and bisexuals. But let us first be clear about sexual orientation and the way we are using it in this chapter.

The American Psychological Association (2005) defines sexual orientation as an "enduring emotional, romantic, sexual, or affectional attraction toward others. Sexual orientation exists along a continuum that ranges from exclusive heterosexuality to exclusive homosexuality and includes various forms of bisexuality" (p. 1).

In considering the development of identity and whether it suggests potential for emotional risk and reduced resilience, Elizur and Ziv (2001), describe the same-gender identity processes as follows:

1. **Self-definition:** The realization of same-gender feelings against the background of self and others' expectations for the development of heterosexuality breaks one's sense of belonging to a "reality" shared with the social-familial environment. The consolidation of an alternative identity narrative requires the working through of denials, pressures to conform to family expectations and the majority culture, internalized and external heterosexism, and fears of real and imagined consequences.

2. **Self-acceptance:** The development of acceptance helps to depathologize one's sense of self and to consolidate a positive gay identity. This is both an inner cognitive-emotional evolvement and an interpersonal process. Contact with others who share one's gender orientation is usually the primary means of developing self-acceptance. It helps to overcome the sense of isolation and stigmatization, and provides self-accepting role models. The sharing of one's identity with heterosexuals may complement the growth of acceptance.
3. **Disclosure:** This is an evolving process that encompasses both leaps of disclosure and continuous dialogues with others, during which the identity narrative is repeatedly reshaped and enriched with new meanings. Supportive relationships with other persons of same-gender orientation, feelings of acceptance by heterosexual significant others, including the family, and the level of tolerance and safety within one's social-cultural context influence the strategy and goals of disclosure (p. 131).

12.2. HARASSMENT, HOMOPHOBIA, AND VULNERABILITY

Human Rights Watch (2001) indicates that there are media and research reports that GLBT (gay, lesbian, bisexual and transgender) individuals experience high levels of anti-gay harassment, abuses, and violence. Transgender refers to those individuals who are male or female but regard themselves as actually being of the opposite sex. These reports may lead people to believe that only GLBT people experience anti-gay harassment, but adolescents targeted for harassment in public schools are mostly assumed to be homosexual. In fact, of the 5% of a school population in Seattle (Seattle Youth Risk Survey Results, 1995) who experienced anti-gay harassment, only 20% of the students were actually gay, demonstrating how homophobic behavior can affect even heterosexual adolescents.

From descriptions about their lives in public schools, many GLBT youth feel alone and fearful of being hated if others discover their sexual orientation. Many have no one to talk to about their feelings, desires, and problems. They usually do not know of peers who are gay or lesbian in their school or neighborhoods. A Canadian Public Health Association study (Health Canada, 1998) of youth living in large and small communities indicated that, "GLB youth almost universally experience a sense of isolation … [this happens to be] the most relentless feature in the lives of most gay, lesbian, bisexual and transgender youth. And the isolation is more profound than simply social and physical: it is also emotional and cognitive" (pp. 4–5).

SAMSHA (2001), a branch of National Institute of Mental Health writes, "Gay, lesbian, and bisexual youth experience significantly more violence-related behaviors at school and have higher rates of suicide attempts" (p. 1). The report continues, "Active homosexual and bisexual adolescents had higher rates of suicide attempts in the past year (27%) compared to youth with only heterosexual experience (15%). Students with same-sex experience were significantly more likely to be threatened with a weapon, to have property stolen or deliberately damaged, and to not go to school because of feeling unsafe" (p. 1). In describing the harm done by homophobia, Bidstrup (2000) writes:

> *There are the obvious murders inspired by hatred. In the U.S., they number in the dozens every year. Abroad, the numbers run to the hundreds to thousands, no one knows the precise number for sure, as in many countries, the deaths of homosexuals are not considered worth recording as a separate category.*
>
> *But there are other ways in which homophobia kills. There are countless suicides every year by gay men and lesbians, particularly youth, which mental health professionals tell us are not the direct result of the victim's homosexuality, but is actually the result of how the homosexual is treated by society. When one lives with rejection day after day, and society discounts one's value constantly, it is difficult to maintain perspective and realize that the problem is others' perceptions, not one's own, which is why suicide is several times as common among gay men as it is among straight men.*
>
> *Perhaps the highest price is paid by youth. The young person just emerging into adulthood who has begun to realize that he is different, and the difference is not approved of, finds acceptance of self particularly difficult. This is especially true when others perceive the young person as different, and persecute him as a result, with little effort made by authority figures to stop the torment. This is why gay youth commit suicide at a rate of about seven times that of straight youth. Yet it is surprising how often homophobes actually try to prevent intervention by teachers in the schools! (2004)*

According to Elizur and Ziv (2001), GLB youth are at much greater risk than the general population of youth for "major depressions, generalized anxiety disorders, conduct disorders, substance abuse and dependence, suicidal behaviors, sexual risk-taking, and poor general health maintenance (Fergusson et al., 1999; Lock & Steiner, 1999; Safren & Heimberg, 1999)" (p.125). The authors believe that sexual minority status is a significant risk factor for GLB adolescents' physical and mental health. The authors indicate that estimates of suicide attempts, for example, are far above adolescent norms: ranging from a figure of 30–42%.

Regarding adults, Elizur and Ziv (2001) note that available evidence indicates that sexual minorities experience increased psychological risk from experiences with stigma, discrimination, and violence predict psychological distress and dysfunction and that, "GLB survivors of hate crimes suffer from posttraumatic stress reactions and other negative mental health consequences that are often exacerbated by societal heterosexism" (p. 130). HIV-related symptoms and AIDS-related bereavement also contribute greatly to emotional distress. However, in all other ways, the authors found psychological adjustment between sexual minority and non-stigmatized samples to be the same.

In fact, disclosure of sexual orientation to families has been repeatedly found to be a risk factor for GLB youth (Savin-Williams, 1998). Those who had disclosed reported verbal and physical abuse by family members, and acknowledged more suicidality than those who had not "come out" to their families (D'Augelli et al., 1998). Therefore, it is not surprising that many youth tend to hide their sexual orientation, coming out first to peers and only later to siblings, mothers, and fathers, respectively (Savin-Williams, 1998). Full disclosure to parents, if it occurs, takes place after years of struggling with same-gender attractions.

Theuninck (2000) describes two primary sources of stress in the lives of GLBT individuals. External stressors include events that are largely independent of a person's perception of them such as physical and verbal insults and abuses. Internal stressors include internalized homophobia and the perception of a society that discriminates against gay people. Through internalized homophobia. Theuninck suggests that some GLBT individuals come to believe that homosexuality is illegitimate, a sickness, moral weakness, defect, or a deformation of self. This belief may lead to intense self-loathing, according to the author. Theuninck (2000) also believes that because of stigma, people come to fear that their sexuality will become known and that the ever-present possibility of being attacked or discriminated against in the course of daily life will increase.

Frankowski (2004) notes that non-heterosexual youth are at higher risk of dropping out of school, being forced out of their homes, and turning to life on the streets. Non-heterosexual youth are also more likely to have had sexual intercourse earlier than heterosexual youth, to have had more partners, and to have experienced sexual intercourse against their will, increasing their risk of STDs including HIV infection. Frankowski notes rates of 7% in HIV seroprevalence in 15–22-year-old males who have sex with males. Youth in high school who engage in same sex sexual activity report are more likely to attempt suicide, be victimized, and to abuse substances. According to Francowski, gay, lesbian, or bisexual school-based studies have found GLB adolescents are two to seven times more likely to attempt suicide, are two to four times more likely to be threatened with a weapon at school, and are more likely to engage in frequent and heavy use of alcohol, marijuana, and cocaine. It is important to note that these psychosocial problems are not attributable to homosexuality but are significantly associated with stigmatization of gender nonconformity, stress, violence, lack of support, dropping out of school, family problems, acquaintances' suicide attempts, homelessness, and substance abuse.

12.3. RESILIENCE IN GLBT CHILDREN AND ADOLESCENTS

While they accept the concept of resilience in GLB individuals, Rouse et al. (1999) believe that homophobia and gay bashing have an extraordinarily negative impact and that adolescents need love, care, and support from parents, educational personnel, close family friends, peers and other adults in the community. "People, opportunities, and atmospheres all add to the resilience equation. A resilient personality is not sufficient. It takes the person and his or her environment." (Rouse et al., 1999, p.)

Although many families may at first reject a child for their sexual identity, Savin-Williams (1998) found that families can add to the resilience of GLB youth because families evolve and may shift positions in an attempt to develop strategies to fight social stigma. The authors report that family support and assistance is a buffer for GLB adolescents against mental health problems associated with verbal abuse and gay bashing. The authors also report that the comfort of parents with the sexual identity of a GLB adolescent is a predictor of comfort with being gay. Smith and Brown (1997) found that once disclosure is made to parents, after an initial crisis, that family relationships often improve and, in some cases, improve to a better level than before the disclosure.

Elizur and Ziv (2001) report that "Following a particularly stressful adolescence, many GLB adults appear to make a rebound toward greater mental health and to achieve a level of psychological adjustment on par with heterosexual comparison groups, even though they continue to face unique stress factors" (p. 130). A significant aspect of later resilience is explained by family acceptance. In their study of GLB adults, the authors found support for the following propositions

> *(a) supportive families are more likely to be accepting of gay orientation; (b) family support has an effect on gay men's psychological adjustment that is partially mediated by family acceptance; and (c) the effects of family support on identity formation and family knowledge are fully mediated by family acceptance, while the effect of family acceptance on identity formation is partly mediated by family knowledge. Consistent with the resiliency model, these results suggest that families can play a positive role in the life of gay men, even in societies with traditional family values. As for identity formation, the acceptance of same-gender orientation by family members appears to be a particularly meaningful form of support (p. 135).*

While GLB and heterosexual persons alike develop their identities by struggling with issues that may be painful, denial, ambivalence and outright rejection of sexual identity increases the potential of rejection by family and community. Resilience can be reinforced when clients deal with feelings of "otherness" through self-exploration, discussions with others having similar issues, and certainly, through therapy. As the next story demonstrates, supportive parents and therapy can be very effective in helping GLB clients resolve feelings of "otherness."

12.4. EVIDENCE-BASED PRACTICE WITH GAY, LESBIAN, BISEXUAL AND TRANSGENDER CHILDREN AND ADOLESCENTS

Heffner (2003) lists six stages that many GLBT children and adolescents go through when dealing with their own sexual orientation that are relevant for human service professionals to know and to use in treatment. They are:

1. Identity awareness. The point at which the child or adolescent begins to realize he or she has feelings that are different from others and different from what they have been taught.

2. Identity comparison. The child or adolescent begins to explore his or her feelings alone and to compare them to the beliefs of society, parents, and peers.
3. Identity tolerance. During this stage, the child or adolescent may rebel against his or her feelings and attempt to deny them because of the stigma attached to being different.
4. Identity acceptance. After realizing that sexuality is a part of who they are, GLBT children and adolescents begin to embrace it, explore their feelings and desires, and start to find a place in the world where they are accepted and belong.
5. Identity pride. This stage often involves anger toward parents, society, religion, or other aspects of their world that tells them they are bad and immoral just because their feelings are directed toward the same sex. At this stage they accept and explore their sexuality and openly challenge others about their sexuality.
6. Identity synthesis. The final stage in which homosexuality becomes a part of who they are rather than the defining factor. Instead of being a gay man or lesbian, they begin to see themselves as parents, employees, leaders, teachers, supervisors, coaches, and volunteers who just happen to be gay. In the final stage, they are able to accept themselves more wholly rather than seeing their sexuality as separate from the rest of who they are.

Heffner (2003) suggests that when counseling young GLBT clients it is important to understand where they are in terms of their sexuality.

> *Those attempting to convert to a 'straight lifestyle' are likely in stage two or three. They have not yet accepted themselves as gay and have not likely experienced friendship and love from others who know their sexual orientation. Those in stages four and five are likely trying to reinvent themselves with this newfound acceptance. They have accepted their sexuality but have not yet learned to integrate this aspect of their life into their sense of self. In treatment, the strength these individuals feel should be embraced and treatment should be focused on what they can do, not to make the world accept them, but to show the world that they are worthy of acceptance.*
>
> *Individuals in stage six are often seen as no different from most clients we see in therapy. They have accepted their sexuality, have developed relationships, and don't see 'gay' as the issue, but rather as one of the many issues they deal with in an imperfect world. Being gay is often seen in a positive light. They can now begin to give back to others, become a mentor, volunteer, run for office, or otherwise use their whole self as a means to make the world a better place. Aside from issues arising from the first five stages above, treatment for homosexual clients should be no different than any other client. In terms of mood disorders, anxiety disorders, relationship concerns, stress, and sexual issues, homosexual clients present at about the same rate as their counterparts and treatment should not be any different although depression is significantly higher among gay adolescents and the suicide rate is double their straight counterpart. Suicidal ideation, depression, and anxiety are also higher among those who have not accepted their sexuality or who struggle for acceptance with friends and family because of their sexual orientation.*

In the following three cases, gay and lesbian youth discuss their experiences with life, therapy, and family with a discussion section after each case processing what was said.

12.5. CASE STUDY 1: THE STAGES OF ACCEPTANCE

"I think most gays are in some form of denial when they begin to suspect that they are gay. I mean, it's just about the worst thing that anyone can be for most teen-aged guys. I was not only in denial but I was homophobic. I played high school football and the worst thing you could say about someone was that they were 'queer' or a 'fag.' I said that to a lot of guys and kept the fact that I was having intense sexual fantasies about some of the guys on the team to myself. It was scary that I might be found out. I'd see guys in school who were very effeminate (we might say swishy now) and I'd tell myself that wasn't me, I wasn't one of those little sissy guys who looked and talked like a girl. I was an athlete and very macho. Still, the feelings I had for guys were very intense and I can remember having a crush on one of my teammates and feeling very foolish about it. A guy! It was disgusting. I started buying magazines with pictures of really buff men in them and masturbating to the pictures. I guess most of my friends were doing the same thing to pictures of women. It was my dad who found the pictures and asked me to chat about them."

"I told him that the pictures were for training so I could figure out the sort of body I wanted, but my dad wasn't buying it. Neither was I. Pretty soon I was blurting out all this stuff about how guys turned me on and how awful that made me feel. He wondered if girls did the same thing and I said, no, that they didn't. So we went to a counselor who specializes in this sort of thing and while I didn't want to be gay, and I mean I'd have done anything not to have been, I was, and I had to accept it."

"It took 2 years of therapy and some groups I went to with guys like me who were realizing they were gay, and hating it, to have my first sexual experience. It was wonderful and terrible and repulsive and sweet. I mean it was wonderful and it made me realize that I was gay and that it was just the way it was. If I accepted it and enjoyed the experience, I could be like anyone else. I could love someone, I could enjoy sex, and I could even be a couple."

"I'm ashamed to say I never told my friends in high school. I went to a college where no one from my school went. I met some great people, children and adolescents who were gay, and I learned a lot about how gays are as different in many ways as heterosexuals are. My mom and dad were wonderful about it. When I brought my first serious love relationships home for Thanksgiving, they were as excited about it as if it was a girlfriend. My brother, on the other hand has been a jerk and makes snide comments about it but screw him, he's always been a jerk. About 2 years after I started going to college I told a few of my good friends from high school and they treated my like I had leprosy. It's OK. I'm glad I've been open about it. I know people who marry and have kids, but are as gay as I am. It only leads to hurt feelings to be in denial. I belong to a gay church, and it's wonderful, and I've become involved in gay politics. I've been out drumming up support for gay marriage, which I think is something that will happen sooner than later."

"Do I wish I'd been heterosexual? You bet. It would have made my life easier. Am I comfortable with my gayness? Not entirely, but I'm getting there. I think gay people internalize negative stereotypes about gays that leave us with poor self-concepts. Do I think I could change and become straight? Of course not. I think you have to accept who you are and like yourself. My dad said something when we were having these long chats about being gay. He said that he always hoped for a strong, healthy child with great values. In that way he couldn't have asked for anything more than what he got in me. My being gay meant nothing to him because the son he loved was me, and it didn't matter, my being gay, and he meant it."

"Many of my friends have had bad experiences with their fathers when they come out. I know a number of guys who were disowned by their fathers and haven't seen them in years. I remember reading a story about a guy who was going to his parent's house to tell them that he was gay. He came from a very traditional culture and he figured that when he told them, he'd be disowned. He went into the house and began to bring up the subject, but his parents kept avoiding it until he finally realizes that they'd known all along and loved him, and that actually telling them that he was gay would break the facade, the charade they were playing, so they had this nice chat about the weather. His folks said they had a nice girl for him to meet and would he come for dinner that Sunday, and he did. He didn't want to change the rules of the game they were playing and, in that way, everyone maintained their integrity".

"I don't know if I like that story or not, but it's what you often hear. I'm pleased I didn't have to go through that sort of dishonesty and that I could be honest about it all. I think it made accepting myself a lot easier."

12.6. DISCUSSION

The storyteller is fortunate to have a father he trusted who was sensitive and caring and helped him deal with his initial anxiety about being gay. He sought professional help, with the support of his father that helped him deal with his negative feelings about being gay. As resistant as adolescents can be about therapy, his willingness to enter into long term therapy and become involved in groups with other gay young men having difficulty dealing with being gay were positive signs of his motivation to be happy in life and to be self-accepting.

He has exceptionally supportive parents. While coming out is sometimes difficult because of the strong negative reaction of parents, he has parents who have been supportive and loving, and it's helped him cope. He also took his time before he had a sexual experience and by that time was certain about his sexual orientation and felt comfortable with himself. He feels confident that hiding one's gayness will only lead to difficulty. This is a very mature and accurate perception on his part. Caldwell (2004) reports that once married gay and lesbian men and women come out about their sexual orientation, about 2/3 of the marriages end within 2 years. "Some estimates put the number of gays and lesbians who have or have had a straight spouse at around 2 million nationwide. However, with recent advances for gay rights, many married gay men are coming out and leaving their wives" (p. 56). However, as Caldwell indicates,

> *... there's a big price to be paid for coming out and ending a marriage. "A lot of times there is anger from the spouse and the children, and that has to be repaired over time," says Joni Lavick, director of mental health services at the Los Angeles Gay and Lesbian Center. "But at a certain point many of these men overcome their own internalized homophobia and can't live a lie anymore. The pressure of keeping a secret is so great that dealing with what is going to happen is less toxic than staying in the closet." (p. 56).*

He has developed a support group and uses a gay church congregation for affiliation and spirituality. He told childhood friends about his sexual orientation. While many were not accepting, he felt that coming out to his close friends was the appropriate thing to do, showing a high level of moral and ethical principles. Although he says that his brother has been a "jerk" about his sexual orientation, the storyteller is not fazed by it and continues to have a close relationship with other members of his family.

12.7. CASE STUDY 2: COMING OUT

"When I was growing up, I remember thinking that I'd never like to be married because I'd be married to a boy. Boys were great and I played a lot with them, but the idea of a romantic love with a boy seemed sort of repulsive. I knew for sure that I preferred girls by the time I was an adolescent. Not that it was easy for me to talk about because it wasn't. I grew up in a very traditional Catholic home and the idea of the oldest daughter being gay, it would have never flown. So I dated guys all through high school and being attractive, I guess, I had a lot of dates, none for more than a time or two. Making out was out of the question and word got around in high school that I wasn't about to put out so I never got asked to the prom or anything like that. It incensed my father who thought that I was being a good girl and that in our Catholic family, not being sexual before marriage was considered a positive quality. He was angry for me because he thought the guys were ignoring me because I wasn't easy."

"The truth was that I was having romantic fantasies about other girls and women. I had crushes and I knew from reading that I was probably gay. I hate the word Lesbian. It sounds like a disease. I tried to talk to my mother when I was around 15, but she was mortified and sent me to a priest who was even more mortified and told my father. My father hit the ceiling and sent me to a convent school out of town. I mean there were other girls who thought they were gay like me and it was where I had my first romantic and sexual experiences. The experiences were good and bad. Girls can be as shitty as guys when it comes to love and sex, and it took me some time to understand that there were female predators out there. But once I understood that and began to choose wisely, I've been very happy being gay. I mean it's what I am. Unfortunately, I've been estranged from my family and it hurts. I want to go home for Christmas and be with my family but there are always excuses why I can't come home. Aunt Mary needs my room or Cousin Ann is getting old and needs to be with us."

"I found a priest who does family reunifications and we met with my entire family. My father cried all through the meeting and wouldn't touch me. It was awful. He kept asking why God had done this and wasn't I a good enough Christian to know right from wrong and what the Bible says about unclean acts? To me it's not unclean, it's beautiful. Who are they to say such things? I went for therapy and it helped me a lot. I began to see it as their problem, not mine, and while I've kept the door open, they haven't walked through it."

"The therapy I went to was pretty wonderful. The therapist let me talk and was very supportive and positive. This was when I was an undergraduate at the college counseling center. The counselor I saw was pretty great. She asked me to do a lot of reading about Lesbians and even suggested some articles. What they had in common was the fact that many of them discussed the same struggle I was having with my family and urged readers not to give up. My therapist was very positive about me and reminded me that being gay was just a part of who I was. It didn't define me. I was, she said, a very accomplished and successful person who just happened to be gay. It made a lot of difference in the way I felt about myself to get such positive messages from someone I respected."

"I'm in graduate school now studying to be an architect. It's all I ever wanted to be. I had this fantasy of designing a house for my folks. Maybe I will some day. Right now I'm not in a relationship but I have good male and female friends, and I'm comfortable with who I am. It hurts sometimes when my family seems so down on me but recently my father wrote me a letter. I'd won an award for a design I did for a small affordable house and he said in his letter that he was very proud of what I'd done and that his heart was opening, through prayer, and he wanted to come, with my mom, and see my school and spend a weekend with me. He said to bring whomever I wanted to, I guess meaning a girlfriend. I'm not in a relationship right now so I brought 2 gay friends, a guy and girl, but said nothing about them. You could tell all through dinner that my folks were very confused. Were they or weren't they gay?"

"At the end of the weekend, which was great, my dad said he wanted to see me at Thanksgiving and Christmas and that my room was mine and always would be. It took almost 10 years for that to happen and while I was in a lot of pain, thank God it happened and we now have a real relationship, and it feels wonderful. You should always keep the door open and you should be optimistic, I guess, and you should know if you're gay that things like what happened to me are bound to happen. We're a very oppressive society toward people who are different."

12.8. DISCUSSION

As Elizur and Ziv (2001) have noted, families can both hurt and heal. Because a family has an initial strongly negative response to a young person's sexual identity doesn't mean that the relationship cannot improve. The author's write, "Consequently, coming-out to family is not a panacea, and it is neither good nor bad in itself. Rather, it is the quality of one's decision-making, the unfolding of disclosure as a process, and the fit between the configuration of disclosure and the familial/social environment that has repercussions for the consolidation of one's identity and psychological adjustment" (p. 128).

As Beeler and DiProva (1999) suggests, people who go through the process of coming out need to develop appropriate strategies. Therapists and friends can help develop this strategy but the main consideration is that the attempt to discuss sexual identity with parents and significant others should be done in a way that is authentic. The client was clearly authentic in her attempts to discuss her sexual identity with parents and others.

Even though her parents we're unresponsive to her attempts to discuss her sexual orientation with them and were, in fact, judgmental and rejecting, she left the door open to a family reunification. While it took almost 10 years to happen, it *did* take place and she and her family are in the process of healing old wounds from their earlier rejections.

Kline (1998) suggests that as important as healthy family support may be to the acceptance of self, consolidation of gay identity helps people discuss their sexual orientation with family and friends in a way that fosters support and acceptance. Our storyteller used the available literature and her own inquisitive nature to confirm for herself that she was gay. Once having confirmed and accepted that she was gay, she accepted herself in the face of considerable rejection and family withdrawal.

While our storyteller disclosed her sexual identity, Savin-Williams (1998) found that disclosure often brings with it verbal and physical abuse from family members. Many youth tend to keep their sexual orientation a secret and, unlike our storyteller who shows great resilience, "Full disclosure to parents, if it occurs, takes place after years of struggling with same-gender attractions" (Elizur and Ziv, 2001, p. 131.)

12.9. CASE STUDY 3: CONFRONTING HOMOPHOBIA

"Kids can be very cruel and they were very cruel to me when I was growing up. I was the scapegoat for every homophobic impulse anyone had when I was in school. I was beaten up a number of times and everything from having my locker trashed to having people put signs on my back that said 'Queer Here,' 'Beware of fag,' was done to me by the time I was 14. I didn't think I was gay and so it hurt all the more. I didn't think I was any different than any of the other boys in school."

"I started reading about gays when I was still in grade school. I was surprised to read that the descriptions of gay people were precisely what I felt about myself. I know it sounds naïve and maybe I was in denial, but what I felt about myself was what I thought everyone felt. By adolescence I knew that was complete nonsense and I could accept that I was gay, but the bullying and taunting were just making me miserable."

"My folks were working class people, not very sophisticated, and my dad told me to fight back, and I did. I hit a kid so hard who was taunting me about being gay that he was put in the hospital for observation. When the principal found out why, he seemed very embarrassed. I was suspended for a while but, believe me, the taunting and bullying stopped. I've never been one to think that gays should take gay bashing lightly. I don't. You listen to what other people say about you passively, and pretty soon you start believing it. What *crap* that is! I'm a gay guy with an MPA. I'm smart and able. I love my country and I'm a good person. To hell with letting others tell you what you're supposed to believe about yourself."

"My gay friends are intimidated by gay bashing. Well it *is* dangerous and scary. So we've taken up self-defense and when anyone bothers us, the stereotype of sissy men or girly boys, as our governor likes to call us, goes right out the window. You have to be tough to act tough, and while I see myself as a gentle person and I haven't hit anyone since that kid in high school, I have an inner belief that I can defend myself. It gives me a persona that even the dumbest homophobe knows means business. I hate the idea of gays feeling weak. It damages your self-esteem."

"My partner is a very tender guy. He's very emotional and he hurts when others hurt. He was in a bar with me a few weeks ago and someone said something so homophobic and full of malice, I thought I'd explode. My partner, who can bench press 350 pounds, just quietly told him that bashing was a sign of deep insecurity and rather than striking out against others because it made you feel more secure and powerful, to look inside so you could see the hurting, unloving person, full of sexual identity confusion and denial about your own attraction to gay men. I know it's pretty common stuff, but he said it in a way that took this guy back. Pretty soon the guy is telling my partner about his abusive dad and how his dad hated gays because he needed someone to hate, and he apologized. It was pretty terrific, that moment, and I cherish my partner for having the strength to be calm rather than getting angry. Where would that have led?"

"Maybe straights know that homophobia kills but it's so engrained in men and in the culture to fear us, that it's a real burden. I get depressed when I find out that there's been yet another gay killing. Isn't it enough that AIDS has almost done us in?"

"I wonder why homophobia is so strong in our culture. And I think it must have something to do with religion and the animosity religions have toward homosexuality. I also think that many men in our society worry about their masculinity and fear they won't cut it when it comes to being a man. The notion of machismo just seems extraordinarily homophobic and it's a concept that exists in every culture I know about. I wonder how many men, in their insecure and sometimes failing attempts to be real men, turn their anger at themselves outward so they can feel superior when inside they ache with insecurity. I don't know, but we gays are just like everyone else. If you got to know any of us, you'd see we don't have a secret society that's intent on world domination."

"I have a Jewish friend who told me that the club he'd just joined arrange a tennis match. The guy he played began talking about the World Zionist Conspiracy and, as an example, how Jews had ganged up on him when he ran for public office. My friend walked off the court and told the owner of the club about him. The owner just shrugged, so my friend contacted many of the Jewish members (there were a lot) and the guy was kicked out of the club or the owner risked losing our membership. Maybe that guy still believes in the International Zionist Conspiracy but at least he knows what happens when he's publicly anti-Semitic. I sense that the same thing operates with gays, that there's some primitive belief that we're contagious and that we carry the seeds of world destruction. It just can't be good for young gays to grow up with homophobia and I, for one, think the professional community has done all too little to combat it. I hear about counselors and therapists who go mum when clients say homophobic things. Being silent in the face of such bile only reinforces it. I agree with that 60s statement: if you aren't part of the solution, you're part of the problem."

12.10. DISCUSSION

Bullying in school led the storyteller to depression and a sense of isolation. The storyteller shows a rare ability to deal with the bullying he received by understanding its source and by reading about homophobia. To underscore the serious consequences of homophobic bullying, in a meta-analysis of the subject, Hawker and Boulton (2000) write, "peer victimization was most strongly related to depression. The results strongly suggest that" victims of peer aggression experience more negative affect, and negative thoughts about themselves, than other children" (Hawker and Boulton, 2000, p. 451).

He understands that certain male behaviors, often called machismo, are sometimes associated with homophobia. In defining machismo, Baca Zinn (1980) writes that it is "the male attempt to compensate for feelings of internalized inferiority by exaggerating masculinity" (p. 20). Mirande (1977) describes the behaviors associated with machismo: "The macho male demands complete deference, respect and obedience not only from his wife but from his children as well" (p. 749). Perhaps the term machismo is more easily understood as "traditional." Explaining machismo in this way, Chafetz (1974) writes, "the masculine sex role for [traditional men] is generally described by reference to the highly stereotyped notion of machismo. In fact, a strong emphasis on masculine aggressiveness and dominance may be characteristic of most groups in the lower ranges of the socioeconomic ladder" (p. 59). But to attribute homophobia only to this group of men is a mistake. Homophobia is present in a number of children and adolescents who are well educated, sophisticated, and who would never think of themselves as "traditional."

The story of his partner's resolution of a homophobic encounter suggests a very evolved way of dealing with anger, one he admires and respects. Although he sounds fairly belligerent, he has elegant ways of coping with his anger. He also understands that his level of achievement in life and the homophobic responses he endures are quite separate from his self-identity as a person. He has a very positive opinion of himself and tells us "You listen to what other people say about you passively, and pretty soon you start believing it. What *crap* that is! I'm a gay guy with an MPA. I'm smart and able. I love my country and I'm a good person. To hell with letting others tell you what you're supposed to believe about yourself."

He doesn't believe in being passive in the face of homophobia and remarks, "I hate the idea of gays feeling weak. It damages your self-esteem." While he isn't confrontational to the point of a fight, he does believe in being physically and emotionally strong as one important way of coping with homophobia. And he understands the origins of homophobia, which not only makes him strong but also knowledgeable.

He accurately accesses a criticism of the helping professions when he comments that therapist often let clients share homophobic feelings and beliefs without trying to change those beliefs. Sandage and Hill (2001) agree and suggest that modern psychology has no model of the civic virtues that promote healthy individual and community behavior. In fact, they believe that much of psychology and perhaps most of the helping professions have no model of the positive values that should be stressed with our clients or the necessary constructive social behaviors that will lead to an increased sense of social responsibility and healthier community life.

12.11. SUMMARY

This chapter discusses the resilience of gay, lesbian, bi-sexual and transgender children and adolescents. Three stories discuss difficult issues facing GLBT individuals including homophobia, coming out about their sexual orientation, and family rejection. Homophobia is a serious problem resulting in gay bashing, depression, and higher levels of suicide among GLBT individuals. Clearly, much of the difficulty faced by GLBT individuals can be explained by external pressures and attitudes that are sometimes internalized by GLBT clients and may challenge new ways of coping with issues related to their gender identity. A more accepting and understanding society would go a long way toward reducing psychosocial problems experienced by GLBT children and adolescents in America.

12.12. QUESTIONS FROM THE CHAPTER

1 In discussing former President Bill Clinton, conservative writer Ann Coulter said that Clinton's numerous affairs were an attempt to prove that he was not gay. What do you think of her analysis?
2 At its core, homophobia is about hatred. Why do you think so much hatred exists against GLBT men and women in America?
3 Treatment of GLBT youth seems more about helping them overcome prejudice and discrimination than dealing with their mental health. Might one say the same about men and women of color and other groups where society often creates dysfunction by its pathological attitudes?
4 How might one help families with negative attitudes toward their GLBT children overcome those negative attitudes?
5 Getting back to Ann Coulter, do you think that her comment about Bill Clinton demonstrates her own dysfunctional attitudes toward gender issues? If so, what might those attitudes be?

References

American Psychological Association (2005). The Help Line. Found on the Internet May 14, 2005 at: http://helping.apa.org/articles/article.php?id=31.

Baca Zinn, M. (1980). Gender and ethnic identity among Chicanos. *Frontiers, 2*, 18–24.

Beeler, J., & DiProva, V. (1999). Family adjustment following disclosure of homosexuality by a member: Themes discerned in narrative accounts. *Journal of Marital and Family Therapy, 25*, 443–459.

Caldwell, J. (2004). Gay men, straight lives. *Advocate, 924*, 55–58.

Chafetz, J. S. (1974). *Masculine/feminine or human*. E.E. Ithica, Ill: Peacock Publishers, Inc.

D'Augelli, A. R., Hershberger, S. L., & Pilkington, N. W. (1998). Lesbian, gay, and bisexual youth and their families: Disclosure of sexual orientation and its consequences. *American Journal of Orthopsychiatry, 68*, 361–371.

Elizur, Y., & Ziv, M. A. (2001, Summer). Family support and acceptance, gay male identity formation, and psychological adjustment: A path model. *Family Process, 40*, 125–144.

Fergusson, D. M., Horwood, L. J., & Beautrais, A. L. (1999). Is sexual orientation related to mental health problems and suicidality in young people?. *Archives of General Psychiatry, 56*, 876–880.

Frankowski, B. L. (2004, June 6). Pediatrics, *113*(6), 1827–1832.

Glicken, M. D. (2006). *Learning from resilient people: Lessons we can apply to counseling and psychotherapy*. Thousand Oaks, CA: Sage.

Hawker, D. S. J., & Boulton, M. J. (2000). Twenty years' research on peer victimization and psychosocial maladjustment: a meta-analysis review of cross-sectional studies. *Journal of Child Psychology and Psychiatry, 41*(4), 441–455.

Health Canada. (1998). Suicide in Canada: Update of the Task Force on Suicide in Canada. Ottawa: Mental Health Division, Health Services Directorate, Health Programs and Services Branch, Health Canada.

Heffner, C. L. (2003, August 12).Counseling the Gay and Lesbian Client: Treatment Issues and Conversion Therapy. AllPsych at http://allpsych.com/journal/ counseling-gay.html.

Human Rights Watch. (2001). Hatred in the Hallways: Violence and Discrimination Against Lesbian, Gay, Bisexual and Transgender Students in U.S. Schools. New York/ Washington: Human Rights Watch. Found on the Internet April 13, 2005 at: http://www.hrw.org/reports/2001/uslgbt/.

Kline, R. B. (1998). *Principles and practice of structural equation modeling*. New York: Guilford Press.

Lock, J., & Steiner, H. (1999). Gay, lesbian, and bisexual youth risks for emotional, physical, and social problems: Results from a community-based survey. *Journal of the American Academy of Child and Adolescent Psychiatry, 38*, 297–304.

Rouse, K. A. G., Longo, M., Trickett, M. (1999). Fostering resilience in children. *Bulletin* 875-99. The Ohio State University, p. 883. Internet: http://ohioline.osu.edu/b875/ - Citation from "Definition of resilience": http://ohioline.osu.edu/b875/b875_1.html.

Safren, S. A., & Heimberg, R. G. (1999). Depression, hopelessness, suicidality, and related factors in sexual minority and heterosexual adolescents. *Journal of Consulting and Clinical Psychology, 67*, 859–866.

SAMSHA. (2001).The CMHS Approach to Preventing Violence. United States Department of Health and Human Services. Found on the Internet May 14, 20-05 at: http://alt.samhsa.gov/grants/content/2002/YouthViolence/need.htm.

Sandage, S. T., & Hill, P. C. (2001). The virtue of positive psychology: The repprochment and challenge of an affirmative postmodern perspective. *Journal of Theory of Social behavior, 31*(3), 241–260.

Savin-Williams, R. C. (1998). The disclosure to families of same-sex attractions by lesbian, gay, and bisexual youths. *Journal of Research on Adolescence, 8*, 49–68.

Seattle Youth Risk Survey Results. (1995). Information made available by the Safe Schools Coalition of Washington (1996, 1999). Summaries of Youth Risk Behavior Survey: Table 4 (p. 10) and Table 6 (p. 15), Reis B, Saewyc E (1999). *Eighty-Three Thousand Youth*. Internet: PDF Download at http://www.safeschoolscoalition.org/safe.html.

Smith, R. B., & Brown, R. A. (1997). The impact of social support on gay male couples. *Journal of Homosexuality, 33*, 39–61.

Theuninck, A. (2000). *The traumatic impact of minority stressors on males self-identified as homosexual or bisexual*. Master's of Arts (Psychology) Dissertation, University of the Witwatersrand, Johannesburg.

Further reading

D'Augelli, A. R., & Hershberger, S. L. (1993). Lesbian, gay, and bisexual youth in community settings: Personal challenges and mental health problems. *American Journal of Community Psychology, 21*, 421–449.

Mirande. (1979). A reinterpretation of male dominance in the Chicano family. *Family Coordinator, 28*, 473–497.

13 Evidence-Based Practice and Attention Deficit Hyperactivity Disorder (ADHD)

13.1. INTRODUCTION

The author wishes to thank Ms. Joan Bourne, one of my wonderful MSW students for permission to include some of her material written for a research class for parts of this chapter.

Attention deficit hyperactivity disorder (ADHD) is a neurobiological disorder in which children exhibit abnormal levels of inattention, impulsivity, hyperactivity, academic underachievement and behavioral problems affecting between 3% and 18% of school-aged children (Barzman et al., 2004; Findling et al., 2006). Prevalence estimates vary greatly among sources. Powell et al. (2003) state that 3–5% of children in the United States have some form of ADHD. However, Barzman et al. (2004) place the prevalence rates somewhere between 4% and 12% of children 6–12 years old in the non-referred community. Barzman et al. (2004) estimate that as many as 70% of children diagnosed with ADHD also have one or more co-morbid disorder, including depression, oppositional defiance disorder (ODD), conduct disorder (CD), and learning disabilities (LD). Children with ADHD may exhibit abnormal levels of inattention, impulsivity, hyperactivity, academic underachievement, and behavioral problems (Barzman et al., 2004).

13.2. DIAGNOSING ADHD

The Diagnostic and Statistical Manual of Mental Disorders (DSM IV-TR; American Psychiatric Association, 2000) differentiates between three subtypes described as primarily inattentive, hyperactive, or a combination of the two. A diagnosis of subtype is determined by the existence of six or more criteria for the previous 6 months on the inattentive or hyperactive-impulsive scales. If criteria are met for both inattentive and hyperactive-impulsive subtypes, a diagnosis of ADHD combined type is made (DSM IV-TR; American Psychiatric Association, 2000). Symptoms must be present in at least two settings, for at least 6 months, cause significant clinical impairment, and begin before age seven. The symptoms typically are descriptive of behaviors in school or playground settings and reflect developmentally inappropriate behavior in children. Inabilities to appropriately interact in social, academic, and occupational settings can lead to impaired social relationships, depression, low self-concept, antisocial behavior, drug use, and educational and occupational disadvantages (Barzman et al., 2004). Various studies on the effects of ADHD have found that children with ADHD are at higher risk for grade retention in school, placement in special education, dropping out of high school, and lower than expected rates of post-secondary education (Barzman et al., 2004).

To assess whether a child has ADHD, several critical questions need to be answered: Are these behaviors excessive, long-term, pervasive and do they occur more often than in other children the same age? Are they a continuous problem, not just a response to a temporary situation? Do the behaviors occur in several settings or only in one specific place such as the playground or in the schoolroom? The child's pattern of behavior is compared against a set of criteria and characteristics of the disorder as listed in the DSM-IV-TR (National Institute of Health, 2006).

For an attention deficit diagnosis, six (or more) of the following symptoms of inattention must have persisted for at least 6 months to a degree that is maladaptive and inconsistent with developmental levels: (1) inattention leading to careless mistakes in schoolwork and other functions; (2) inattention in play activities; (3) seeming inability not to listen when spoken to; (4) failure to follow through on assignments, instructions and chores in a way not consistent with ODD; (5) difficulty organizing tasks or activities; (6) avoidance of or a dislike for tasks that require sustained mental effort; and (7) a tendency to be easily distracted, neglectful or frequently losing objects (American Psychiatric Association, 1994, p. 80).

For a diagnosis of hyperactivity–impulsivity, six (or more) of the following symptoms must have persisted for at least 6 months to a degree that is maladaptive and inconsistent with developmental levels: (1) fidgets or squirms in seat; (2) leaves his or her seat in classroom or in other situations in which remaining seated is expected; (3) often runs or climbs excessively in situations in which it is inappropriate (in adolescents this may be limited to subjective feelings of restlessness); (4) often has difficulty playing or engaging in leisure activities quietly; (5) is often "on the go" or acts as if "driven by a motor;" (6) often talks excessively, blurts out answers before questions have been completed, has difficulty awaiting his or her turn; and (7) often interrupts or intrudes on the conversations or games of others (American Psychiatric Association, 1994, p. 80).

Males are currently diagnosed two four times more often than females (Trout et al., 2007). There is considerable debate over whether higher prevalence rates in males are due to a neurobiological feature of the male brain, confusing typical male behavior with ADHD, or a decreased likelihood that ADHD symptoms are recognized in females. The controversy continues when the issue of correctly diagnosing and treating children with ADHD is considered. Diagnoses are usually determined by the child's pediatrician and are based primarily on parent and teacher reports (Barzman et al., 2004). Assessment information is obtained from parents and teachers through assessment forms that ask the parent or teacher to describe their child or student's observed behavior. Some pediatricians may perform physical exams, order lab tests and/or check the child's hearing. Sometimes educational and/or psychological testing is done to rule out other possible disorders or identify co-morbid disorders (Davis et al., 2008). Junod et al. (2006) found few gender differences in school impairment. Although girls in their study were less likely to have ADHD than boys, the researchers found that their impairments were just as severe, and possibly more severe than for boys with ADHD.

Goodenough (2003) argues that ADHD has a straightforward diagnosis if children are properly assessed, but that cases of ADHD have been reported in children who can play video games for hours on end or whose symptoms completely disappear when parents make simple changes in their style of responding to the child. If the disease were real in these children diagnosed with ADHD, it would not simply disappear or go into remission so easily. Good enough believes that we have become intolerant of children who have short attention spans or who seem overly energetic, many of whom are gifted and impatient because they want to move on to more challenging activities. He concedes that ADHD exists, but that the increase in reported cases of 500 000 children in 1985 to 7 000 000 children in 2003 is due to parental and teacher overreactions, pressure by the drug companies to sell more medications, and a general case of hysteria by the society. He does admit, however that education has played a role in the increase and that more parents and teachers are aware of the symptoms of ADHD and want children to be helped. He points out that ADHD has increased in places like Australia but that the increase in prescribed medication rose 400% between 1984 and 2001, while in the United States the increase was on the order of 1300% during the same period. Unless there are unique factors creating more ADHD in the United States, diagnosis and treatment of the problem should be constant. He believes that in countries like Australia only the very difficult cases of ADHD are prescribed medication, while in the United States medication is used in mild or non-existent cases and that the docile nature of the child given medication is proof in itself that the condition exists. It is a situation, he believes, that has long-term negative consequences for children who do not have the disorder but are on medication anyway.

13.3. PSYCHOSTIMULANTS

Davis et al. (2008) indicate that current treatments for ADHD using medications have a number of unwanted side effects, including decreased appetite, headaches, insomnia, asthma, and abdominal pain. There has also been research into reports of cardiac complications in patients taking psychostimulant medications. Other medications have been linked to psychiatric risks, such as medication-induced psychosis, hallucinations, and even suicidal ideations (Young, 2006). The Harvard Mental Health Letter (2006) notes that the medications dextroamphetamine and methylphenidate (MPH) are the only proven treatments for ADHD. However, the effects of the medications last only as long as the patient continues to take them. These medications, particularly MPH, have serious possible adverse effects and significant risks.

The Harvard Mental Health Letter (2006) reports that an FDA panel voted to issue a black box warning regarding the cardiovascular risks of MPH following numerous entries into the Adverse Events Reporting System database. This black box warning was the most severe action that could be taken short of banning the medication, and would include a warning directly on prescription label. Later, a second FDA panel voted to cancel the proposed black box warning, but strengthened warnings that persons with high blood pressure or heart defects should not take MPH. Stimulants are known to raise blood pressure and heart rate, leading to increased cardiovascular risk. An additional risk of the stimulants used to treat ADHD is that they can produce a cocaine-like high if crushed and snorted, although this concern has been addressed via extended-release formulas and a recently approved skin patch that delivers the medication more gradually, thus eliminating the euphoric sensation or "high," making them much less susceptible to misuse.

The U.S. Food and Drug Administration (2007) issued an advisory in 2007 regarding possible side effects of all drugs given approval by the FDA to treat ADHD. The advisory read:

> *An FDA review of reports of serious cardiovascular adverse events in patients taking usual doses of ADHD products revealed reports of sudden death in patients with underlying serious heart problems or defects, and reports of stroke and heart attack in adults with certain risk factors.*
>
> *Another FDA review of ADHD medicines revealed a slight increased risk (about 1 per 1,000) for drug-related psychiatric adverse events, such as hearing voices, becoming suspicious for no reason, or becoming manic, even in patients who did not have previous psychiatric problems.*
>
> *FDA recommends that children, adolescents, or adults who are being considered for treatment with ADHD drug products work with their physicians or other health care professional to develop a treatment plan that includes a careful health history and evaluation of current status, particularly for cardiovascular and psychiatric problems (including assessment for a family history of such problems. (p. 1)*

Rostain (2006) notes that initial medication treatment for ADHD begins with either methylphenidate or amphetamine with increasing dosage to optimal levels as needed. If the child experiences a partial response or is non-responsive to the medication, using another stimulant is recommended. If this fails to help, atomoxetine is used in place of a stimulant. If the response is not satisfactory, combining atomoxetine with a stimulant is recommended. Following this, bupropion or a tricyclic antidepressant is substituted for atomoxetine. As a last step, the addition of an a-agonist (guanfacine or clonidine) is advised. If there is still no satisfactory clinical response, a consultation with a specialist in ADHD pharmacology may be in order. A further discussion of non-responsiveness to medication may be found in the case study at the end of this chapter.

13.4. PSYCHOSOCIAL INTERVENTIONS

DuPaul and Weyandt (2006) examined three major types of school-based interventions with ADHD, including behavioral, academic, and social. They found relatively strong evidence to support the use of behavioral interventions in reducing disruptive and off-task behaviors, while evidence for academic and social interventions was weaker. The authors found that found that less than 10% of ADHD school-aged students could accurately state the rules for their classroom when interviewed, suggesting that active teaching and enforcement of classroom rules are a possible behavioral strategy to improve ADHD symptoms in the classroom.

Cole et al. (2005) studied the use of behavioral techniques with a small sample of ADHD children attending a summer camp and found positive results. Fox et al. (2005) found that neurofeedback is a potentially effective alternative treatment for ADHD in improving attention span, reducing impulsivity, controlling hyperactive behaviors, and producing long-term change. However, Fox et al. admit that it could take up to 60 sessions, or 6 months of treatment, for long-term relief of symptoms and that this form of treatment is initially very expensive. Because the long-term effects seem very positive, it may be less expensive than other forms of treatment, including psychostimulant medications. Heinreich et al. (2007) had similar success using neurofeedback. Overall however, as Trout et al. (2007) found in their review of research studies of non-medicinal treatments for ADHD, there are severe limitations on the number of research studies, making it difficult to determine whether psychosocial interventions work.

Kendall (1998), and Kendall and Shelton (2003) interviewed parents of ADHD children who indicated that raising a child with ADHD was a long-term process often marked by frequent disruptions caused by the variability in symptoms and performance characteristic ADHD. Family members noted seven types of disruption: aggression, uncontrolled hyperactivity, emotional and social immaturity, learning difficulties and poor school performance, negative interactions with peers, family conflict, and difficult relations with members of their extended family. Outlasting the disruption was found to be primary goal for parents in their attempts to manage the disruptions and their consequences so that the child and the family might experience the best possible outcome. The process of managing disruptions required families to make sense of the disorder by realizing that something was wrong which required them to understand the chronic nature of ADHD and the possibility that their child might not be as successful in adulthood as they had first hoped. Often parents felt guilty about the child's difficulties but in time managed to cope with the child and the disruptions in their lives in a way that ultimately made them much more empathic.

Parents caring for children with ADHD must manage stress and feelings of inadequacy rarely experienced by most parents. Family members require supportive help that recognizes and builds on their strengths. As Kendall (1998) noted, "A comprehensive family approach must be taken ... and it should emphasize services for the entire family rather than concentrating on the treatment of the disorder" (p. 855).

The MTA study (1999) included 579 elementary school boys and girls with ADHD, who were randomly assigned to one of four treatment programs: (1) medication management alone; (2) behavioral treatment alone; (3) a combination of both; or (4) routine community care. All of the children were reassessed regularly throughout the 14-month study period by teachers and parents who rated the children on hyperactivity, impulsivity, inattention, symptoms of anxiety and depression, as well as social skills. The children in two groups (medication management alone and the combination treatment) were seen monthly on a half hour medication visit. The prescribing physician spoke with the parent, met with the child, and sought to determine any concerns that the family might have regarding the medication or the child's ADHD-related difficulties. The physicians in the medication-only group did not provide behavioral therapy but did advise the parents when necessary concerning any problems the child might have.

In the behavior treatment-only group, families met up to 35 times with a behavior therapist, mostly in group sessions. These therapists also made repeated visits to the schools to consult with the children's teachers and to supervise a special aide assigned to each child in the group. In addition, children attended a special 8-week summer treatment program where they worked on academic, social, and sports skills, and where intensive behavioral therapy was delivered to assist children in improving their behavior.

Children in the combined therapy group received the same assistance that the medication-only group received, as well as all of the behavior therapy treatments. In routine community care, the children saw the community-treatment doctor of their parents' choice one to two times per year for short periods of time, although the community-treatment doctor did not have any interaction with the teachers.

The results of the study indicated that long-term combination treatments and the medication-management alone were superior to intensive behavioral treatment and routine community treatment. In some areas of functioning including anxiety, academic performance, oppositionality, parent–child relations, and social skills, the combined treatment was usually superior. A real advantage of combined treatment for those who are concerned about unwanted side effects of medication was that children could be successfully treated with lower doses of medicine, compared with the medication-only group.

Chronis et al. (2006) conducted a comprehensive review of the effectiveness of psychosocial treatments with ADHD. A number of studies found that manualized parent training resulted in reduced parental stress and improvements in social behavior among children. Behaviorally based classroom interventions using daily report cards and contingency management programs were found to improve classroom conduct and academic performance. Academic interventions including task and instructional modification, homework assistance, peer tutoring, computer-assisted instruction, and strategy training also seemed to help children with ADHD. Barkley (2000) compared behavior management training, problem solving, communication training, and structural family therapy and found comparable improvements in such functional measures as parent–child communication and conflict resolution, internalizing and externalizing symptoms, and parent-reported school adjustment. Group-based training for parents of adolescents with ADHD was also shown to have promising results.

Johnston et al. (2008) studied mothers with children who had severe symptoms of ADHD and asked about their preference for behavioral treatment over the use of psychostimulants. Because many of the mothers had been successfully involved in behavioral parent groups to learn strategies for helping their ADHD child, the parents preferred behavioral treatment, but also said that when the two were compared, psychostimulants were more effective. In explaining this finding, the authors write:

> *Regardless of the reasons for the discrepancy in acceptability and effectiveness ratings, it does suggest that parents of children with ADHD face a dilemma as they navigate treatment decision-making for their children. They must reconcile their perception of medication as a less acceptable treatment with knowledge that it also is likely to be an important component of effective treatment for their children. Combining behavioral and medication treatments may offer some alleviation of this conflict, by allowing parents to access the advantages of both treatments; however, combined treatments are unlikely to eliminate parents' concerns regarding the unacceptability of medication. (Johnston et al., 2008, p. 30)*

Suggestions for parents when relating to their ADHD child are: (1) follow a specific schedule for all activities – from waking up to doing homework to bedtime; (2) keep rules and consequences simple and easy to understand; (3) keep directions clear and brief. Ask the child to repeat directions back to you; (4) reward appropriate behavior; (5) closely supervise the child and observe his behavior with friends because he or she may need help in learning appropriate social behavior; (6) focus on the child's effort and reward small accomplishments; (7) be sure to have the child follow a healthy and well-balanced diet and encourage a regular exercise routine; and (8) use "reminder" language to overcome short-term memory problems and be certain to keep language positive.

13.5. CASE STUDY: WHEN MEDICATION DOES NOT WORK

Jimmy Anderson is a bright outgoing 7-year-old in second grade. He has many of the symptoms of ADHD and finds it difficult to sit still or focus on schoolwork. At home he cannot stick with video games or TV programs for more than a few minutes. He sleeps badly and while he is an agreeable and responsible little boy his behavior is becoming a problem at school and at home. Jimmy was diagnosed with attention-deficit/hyperactivity disorder, combined type (Code 314.01, DSM-IV, p. 80; American Psychiatric Association, 1994). This diagnosis is given when a child has more than six symptoms of inattention and more than six symptoms of hyperactivity–impulsivity that have lasted at least 6 months. The diagnosis came after a thorough medical workup by a team of ADHD specialists at a nearby university teaching hospital. The parents are confident that it is a correct diagnosis. Jimmy was placed on a psychostimulant and had immediate relief. The parents and teacher reported excellent improvement for the first 6 months of treatment.

Gradually, however, the change in behavior began to disappear and Jimmy's old behavior began to return. Concerned that the medication was not working or that the diagnosis was incorrect, the parents brought Jimmy back for a second evaluation. The team examined Jimmy again and decided that he had medication-resistant ADHD, and the only options were to increase the dosage of his current medication or to try a different psychostimulant and introduce behavior modification. The parents wondered about the other medications, since they had been told the medication they were given initially had the best treatment results with the fewest known side effects over time. The team admitted that the next class of medications, while approved for ADHD, had some potential side effects including cardiovascular problems. The hospital *did* have a behavior modification program for Jimmy and his parents and suggested they might want to try using that program with Jimmy if trying different medications with troubling side effects concerned them. In the meantime they thought raising the dose on his current medication might be an alternative, since Jimmy was on a low dose and a higher dose might help. Side effects with the higher dose were nominal but one always had to worry about them. The team proposed monthly medical evaluations to make certain there were no heart problems or evidence of serious emotional problems as a side effect of the medication. The parents agreed to the higher dose of his current medication and the behavior modification program.

We often think that medication always works with ADHD, but Owens et al. (2003) found that only 62% of the patients in the best outcome groups (medication management or combined treatment) had an excellent response as defined by reaching normal or near-normal levels of behavior. Owens et al. (2003, p. 544) found a link between drug resistant ADHD and the existence of the following co-morbid symptoms in ADHD children and depression and anxiety in parents:

> *Among children in the optimal treatment groups, having parents with even mild depression dropped the excellent response rate down to 45%. The investigators identified five moderator-defined groups of children receiving either combined or medication-management treatment:*
>
> *Group A (low initial ADHD severity, low parental depression) had 73% excellent responders.*
>
> *Group B (low initial ADHD severity, high parental depression) had 59% excellent responders.*
>
> *Group C (high initial ADHD severity and high IQ, high parental depression) had 48% excellent responders.*

> *Group D (high initial ADHD severity, low parental depression) had 48% excellent responders.*
>
> *Group E (high initial ADHD severity and low IQ, high parental depression) had 10% excellent responders.*
>
> *The clinical implications are clear: parental depression needs to be addressed when it is present, and when ADHD symptoms are severe, additional treatment approaches (as yet unidentified in published studies) may need to be used in order to maximize the chances for success.*

The parents and Jimmy were seen by a human service professional on the staff of the behavioral program at the hospital. In an extended interview it became apparent that Jimmy's parents were having marital problems as a result of disagreements over the best approach to managing Jimmy's ADHD as well as the stress of dealing with his symptoms over a number of years. The husband wanted to use tough love and the mother wanted to use support and encouragement. As Jimmy's symptoms decreased initially, Jimmy became much more aware of his parent's marital problems, felt responsible, and believed that they were planning to divorce because of him. His anxiety went up dramatically and the worker wondered if the lack of improvement in his ADHD symptoms was partially the result of increased anxiety. This information was given to the treatment team who recommended individual treatment for Jimmy to deal with his anxiety and marital counseling for the parents in addition to the behavioral program in the hospital.

Jimmy's medication was increased slightly, and with short-term individual cognitive-behavioral therapy and marital therapy for the parents in addition to the behavioral program (a weekend program of 4 h each Saturday lasting 6 months), Jimmy's ADHD is in full remission and his school behavior has improved along with his grades. The parents told the worker:

"We were confounded by Jimmy's behavior. We thought we were just being bad parents but the diagnosis helped a lot. The medication is essential but the therapy and behavioral program have made all the difference. Jimmy is acting like what we thought a normal kid should act like. His attention span is good and he isn't jumping all over the place. We see the doctor every week in the behavioral program just to make certain everything's going well and that we're doing the right things with him. Our marriage is a lot better than it was. We've begun to understand that parents have a handful with their ADHD kids and most of the parents in the program have had the same marital problems we have. We've since joined a support group and find it very helpful in recognizing the stress related to having and helping an ADHD child. We think Jimmy's a great kid and we look forward to a time when he outgrows his ADHD but if that doesn't happen, we think we'll have a successful and happy child who goes into adulthood and does just fine."

13.6. SUMMARY

This chapter discusses ADHD and the concerns many people have over the growing numbers of children diagnosed with the problem, and the use of medications with potentially serious side effects. Limits on the efficacy of medication for ADHD was noted with the added problem of co-morbid conditions in children and/or parents a limiting factor in the effectiveness of medication. Research on psychosocial interventions, while promising, are too limited at present and much more research needs to be done on the efficacy of psychosocial interventions as an adjunct to medication and as the primary treatment without the use of medication.

13.7. QUESTIONS FROM THE CHAPTER

1. The numbers of children diagnosed with ADHD and using medication is just another example of how we limit childhood behavior. If we left kids alone to grow up without all this medical nonsense, would we see that just a few kids really have ADHD?
2. Why do we need to diagnose everything? When I was growing up there were a lot of kids who were developmentally behind but in time they did just fine. Should not we give kids more room to grow up and develop instead of always seeing problems that probably go away in time?
3. Does the fact that a third of all ADHD children on medication do not improve prove that they really do not have ADHD?
4. Should not the serious side effects of psychostimulants make it imperative that we develop and research the effectiveness of new psychosocial interventions?
5. It is hard to explain ADHD as just simply a condition of the brain without recognizing the fact that many children with ADHD have co-morbid conditions. Is not it more likely that the co-morbid conditions create the ADHD symptoms and that treatment should focus on the co-morbidity and less on the ADHD?

References

ADHD update: New data on the risks of medication (2006). *Harvard Mental Health Letter, 23*(4), 3–5.

American Psychiatric Association (APA). (1994). *Diagnostic and statistical manual of mental disorders* (4th ed.). Washington, DC, USA: American Psychiatric Association.

American Psychiatric Association. (2000). *Diagnostic and Statistical Manual of Mental Disorders* (4th ed.). Washington, DC: American Psychiatric Association, [Text revision].

Barkley, R. A. (2000). *Taking charge of ADHD*. New York: The Guilford Press.

Barzman, D. H., Fieler, L., & Sallee, F. R. (2004). Attention-deficit hyperactivity disorder diagnosis and treatment. *Journal of Legal Medicine, 25*(1), 23–38.

Chronis, A. M., Jones, H. A., & Raggi, V. L. (2006). Evidence-based psychosocial treatments for children and adolescents with attention-deficit/hyperactivity disorder. *Clinical Psychology Review, 26*, 486–502.

Cole, E. K., Pelham, W. E., Gnagy, E. M., Burrows-MacLean, L., Fabiano, G. A., Chacko, A., et al. (2005). A controlled evaluation of behavioral treatment with children with ADHD attending a summer treatment program. *Journal of Emotional & Behavioral Disorders, 13*(2), 99–112.

Davis, W. B., Patel, N. C., Robb, A. S., McDermott, M. P., Bukstein, O. G. Jr., Pelham, W. E., et al. (2008). Clonidine for attention-deficit/hyperactivity disorder: II. EGG changes and adverse events analysis. *Journal of the American Academy of Child & Adolescent Psychiatry, 47*(2), 189–198.

DuPaul, G. J., & Weyandt, L. L. (2006). School-based intervention for children with attention deficit hyperactivity disorder: Effects on academic, social, and behavioural functioning. *International Journal of Disability, Development & Education, 53*(2), 161–176.

Findling, R. L., Quinn, D., Hatch, S. J., Cameron, S. J., DeCory, H. H., & McDowell, M. (2006). Comparison of the clinical efficacy of twice-daily ritalin and once-daily equasym™ XL with placebo in children with attention deficit/hyperactivity disorder. *European Child & Adolescent Psychiatry, 15*(8), 450–459.

Fox, D. J., Tharp, D. F., & Fox, L. C. (2005). Neurofeedback: An alternative and efficacious treatment for attention deficit hyperactivity disorder. *Applied Psychophysiology & Biofeedback, 30*(4), 365–373.

Goodenough, P. (2003, April 18). *Ritalin debate: Some experts doubt existence of ADHD*. CNSNews.com Pacific Rim Bureau Chief http://www.cnsnews.com/Culture/Archive/200304/CUL20030418a.html

Heinreich, H., Gevensleben, H., & Strehl, U. (2007). Annotation: Neurofeedback – train your brain to train behaviour. *Journal of Child Psychology & Psychiatry, 48*(1), 3–16.

Johnston, C., Hommersen, P., & Seipp, C. (2008, March). Parent characteristics. *Behavior Therapy, 39*(1), 22–32.

Junod, R. E., DuPaul, G. J., Jitendra, A. K., Volpe, R. J., & Cleary, K. S. (2006, April). Classroom observations of students with and without ADHD: Differences across types of engagement. *Journal of School Psychology, 44*(2), 87–104.

Kendall, J. (1998). Outlasting disruption: The process of reinvestment in families with ADHD children. *Qualitative Health Research, 8*(6), 839–857.

Kendall, J., & Shelton, K. (2003). A typology of management styles in families with children with ADHD. *Journal of Family Nursing, 9*(3), 257–280.

MTA Cooperative Group (1999). A 14-month randomized clinical trial of treatment strategies for attention-deficit hyperactivity disorder (ADHD). *Archives of General Psychiatry, 56*, 1073–1086.

National Institute of Health (2006). *Attention deficit hyperactivity disorder*. URL of this page: http://www.nimh.nih.gov/publicat/adhd.cfm

Owens, E. B., Hinshaw, S. P., & Arnold, L. E. (2003). Which treatment for whom with ADHD? Moderators of treatment response in the MTA. *Journal of Consulting and Clinical Psychology, 71*, 540–552.

Powell, S., Welch, E., Ezell, D., Klein, C. E., & Smith, L. (2003). Should children receive medication for symptoms of attention deficit hyperactivity disorder?. *PJE Peabody Journal of Education, 78*(3), 107–115.

Rostain, A. L. (2006). Treatment resistance in youths with ADHD and co-morbid conditions. *Psychiatric Times, 24*(12).

Trout, A. L., Ortiz Lienemann, T., Reid, R., & Epstein, M. H. (2007). A review of non-medication interventions to improve the academic performance of children and youth with ADHD. *Remedial & Special Education, 28*(4), 207–226.

U.S. Food and Drug Administration. (2007). FDA directs ADHD drug manufacturers to notify patients about cardiovascular adverse events and psychiatric adverse events. P07-26 February 21, 2007. http://www.fda.gov/bbs/topics/NEWS/2007/NEW01568.html

Young, D. (2006). Experts advise med guides for ADHD drugs. *American Journal of Health-System Pharmacy, 63*(9), 794.

Further reading

Barkley, R. A., Fischer, M., Edelbrock, C. S., & Smallish, L. (1990). The adolescent outcome of hyperactive: An 8-year prospective follow-up study. *Journal of the American Academy of Child and Adolescent Psychiatry, 29*, 546–557.

14 Pervasive Developmental Disorders: Autism, Asperger's Syndrome, and Pervasive Developmental Disorder-Not Otherwise Specified

14.1. INTRODUCTION

The term pervasive developmental disorders (PDD) was first used in the 1980s to describe a class of disorders that have the following characteristics in common: Severe and pervasive impairments in social interaction, imaginative activity and verbal and nonverbal communication skills; and a limited number of interests and activities that tend to be repetitive. Five disorders are identified under the category of pervasive developmental disorders: (1) autistic disorder, (2) Rett's disorder, (3) childhood disintegrative disorder, (4) Asperger's syndrome, and (5) pervasive developmental disorder-not otherwise specified, or PDD-NOS (DSM-IV-TR, 2000). The two most common PDDs, autism and Asperger syndrome, will be discussed in detail later in the chapter. Two less common PDSs and the category of PPD-not otherwise specified will be discussed briefly as follows:

1. **Rett's disorder:** Rett's disorder is diagnosed primarily in females. Development proceeds in a normal fashion over the first 6–18 months at which point there is loss of abilities in gross motor skills such as walking and moving, followed by an obvious loss in abilities such as speech, reasoning, and hand use. The repetition of gestures or movements such as constant hand-wringing or hand-washing (Moeschler et al., 1990) is an important clue to diagnosing Rett's disorder. Poorly coordinated gait and impaired language development are also present.
2. **Childhood disintegrative disorder:** Childhood disintegrative disorder is a very rare disorder typified by at least 2 years of normal development followed by regression in multiple areas of functioning (such as the ability to move, bladder and bowel control, and social and language skills) following a period of at least 2 years of apparently normal development. By definition, childhood disintegrative disorder can *only* be diagnosed if the symptoms are preceded by *at least* 2 years of normal development and the onset of decline is prior to age 10 (American Psychiatric Association, 1994).
3. **Pervasive developmental disorder-not otherwise specified (PPD-NOS):** Children with PDD-NOS either do not fully meet the criteria of symptoms clinicians use to diagnose

any of the four specific types of PDD and/or do not have the *degree* of impairment described in any of the above four PDD specific types. The DSM-IV indicates that this category should be used:

> *... when there is a severe and pervasive impairment in the development of social interaction or verbal and nonverbal communication skills, or when stereotyped behavior, interests, and activities are present, but the criteria are not met for a specific Pervasive Developmental Disorder, Schizophrenia, Schizotypal Personality Disorder, or Avoidant Personality Disorder." (American Psychiatric Association, 1994, pp. 77–78)*

The confusion over this term stems from the intent of the DSM-IV, which was not to be used as a checklist but, rather, as a guideline for diagnosing pervasive developmental disorders. There are no clearly established guidelines for measuring the severity of a person's symptoms. Therefore, the line between autism and PDD-NOS is blurry (Boyle, 1995). Additionally, some professionals consider "autistic disorder" appropriate only for those who show extreme symptoms in every one of several developmental areas related to autism. Other professionals are more comfortable with the term autistic disorder and use it to cover a broad range of symptoms connected with language and social dysfunction. Therefore, an individual may be diagnosed by one practitioner as having autistic disorder and by another practitioner as having PDD-NOS. As one will note, treatment for any of the PPDs is similar.

The Yale Developmental Disabilities Clinic provides the following case example of a child diagnosed with PDD-NOS.

> *Leslie was the oldest of two children. She was noted to be a difficult baby who was not easy to console but whose motor and communicative development seemed appropriate. She was socially related and sometimes enjoyed social interaction but was easily over-stimulated. She was noted to exhibit some unusual sensitivities to aspects of the environment and at times of excitement exhibited some hand flapping. Her parents sought evaluation when she was four years of age because of difficulties in nursery school. Leslie was noted to have problems with peer interaction. She was often preoccupied with possible adverse events. At evaluation she was noted to have both communicative and cognitive functions within the normal range. Although differential social relatedness was present, Leslie had difficulty using her parents as sources of support and comfort. Behavioral rigidity was noted, as was a tendency to impose routines on social interaction. Subsequently Leslie was enrolled in a therapeutic nursery school where she made significant gains in social skills. Subsequently she was placed in a transitional kindergarten and did well academically, although problems in peer interaction and unusual affective responses persisted. As an adolescent she describes herself as a 'loner' who has difficulties with social interaction and who tends to enjoy solitary activities. (p. 1)*

14.2. AUTISM

The U.S. Centers for Disease Control and Prevention (2007), in the largest US study of childhood autism to date, found that about one in 150 children have the disorder – a higher prevalence than previous national estimates. The autism rate was found to be about 6.6 per 1000, a higher rate than the agency had estimated a year earlier when it thought the prevalence rate was about 5.5 in 1000. As this chapter will note, however, there is considerable confusion over what constitutes autism and whether the diagnostic indicators are applied correctly.

Autism is a pervasive development disorder (PDD), a group of illnesses that involve delays in the development of many basic skills, most notably the ability to socialize or form relationships with others, as well as the ability to communicate and to use imagination (including fantasy play). Children with these disorders often are confused in their thinking and generally have problems understanding the world around them (WEBMD, 2006).

In addition to problems with social interaction, imagination and communication, children with autism also have a limited range of interests. Many children with autism (nearly 75%) also have mental retardation. In many cases, children with autism are unable to emotionally bond with their parents or other family members.

14.3. SYMPTOMS OF AUTISM

The symptoms of autism typically appear before a child is 3 years old and last throughout life. Children with autism can display a wide range of symptoms, which can vary in severity from mild to disabling. General symptoms that may be present to some degree in a child with autism include:

- Difficulty with verbal communication, including problems using and understanding language.
- Inability to participate in a conversation, even when the child has the ability to speak.
- Difficulty with non-verbal communication, such as gestures and facial expressions.
- Difficulty with social interaction, including relating to people and to his or her surroundings.
- Inability to make friends and preferring to play alone.
- Unusual ways of playing with toys and other objects, such as only lining them up a certain way.
- Lack of imagination.
- Difficulty adjusting to changes in routine or familiar surroundings, or an unreasonable insistence on following routines in detail.
- Repetitive body movements or patterns of behavior, such as hand flapping, spinning and head banging.
- Preoccupation with unusual objects or parts of objects.

14.4. THE WARNING SIGNS THAT A CHILD MAY HAVE AUTISM

Babies develop at their own pace, some more quickly than others. However, an evaluation for autism should be made if any of the following apply:

- The child does not babble or coo by 12 months of age.
- The child does not gesture, such as point or wave, by 12 months of age.
- The child does not say single words by 16 months.
- The child does not say two-word phrases on his or her own (rather than just repeating what someone else says) by 24 months.
- The child has lost any language or social skills (at any age).

14.5. THE CAUSES OF AUTISM

The exact cause of autism is not known, but research has pointed to several possible factors, including genetics (heredity), certain types of infections, and problems occurring at birth. Recent studies strongly suggest that the condition may be passed on from parents to children. Researchers are looking for clues about which genes contribute to this increased vulnerability. In some children, environmental factors may also play a role. Studies of people with autism have found abnormalities in several regions of the brain, which suggest that autism results from a disruption of early brain development while still in utero. Other theories suggest that (a) the body's immune system may inappropriately produce antibodies that attack the brains of children causing autism, (b) abnormalities in brain structures cause autistic behavior, and (c) children with autism have abnormal timing of the growth of their brains. Early in childhood, the brains of autistic children grow faster and larger than those of other children. Later, when a child's brain gets bigger and better organized, the brains of autistic children grow more slowly.

A study of families in Sweden with children born between 1977 and 2003 involved 1227 children diagnosed with autism who were compared with families of nearly 31 000 children who did not have autism. The study concluded that having a schizophrenic parent or a mother with psychiatric problems roughly doubled a child's risk of being autistic. The study also found higher rates of depression and personality disorders among mothers, but not fathers. The association between a child's autism and mental illness in the parent was strongest with schizophrenia, and was less powerful when the mother suffered from depression or personality disorders. There was little association between autism and parental addiction to alcohol or drugs or some other types of mental illness.

To date there is no convincing evidence that any vaccine can cause autism or any kind of behavioral disorder. A suspected link between measles, mumps, rubella (MMR) vaccine and autism has been suggested by some parents of children with autism. Typically, symptoms of autism are first noted by parents as their child begins to have difficulty with delays in speaking after age one. MMR vaccine is first given to children at 12–15 months of age. Therefore autism cases with an apparent onset within a few weeks after MMR vaccination may be coincidental. A California study found that autism rates have been steadily rising since 1995, even with the elimination of mercury in MMR vaccinations in 2001 (MSN.COM, 2007). Rates for children born in 1993 were 0.03 per 1000, but for children born in 2003 the rates had risen to 1.3 per 1000. The study concluded that something must be at play to drive rates up so dramatically, but that vaccinations were not responsible and urged continued research.

14.6. EVIDENCE-BASED PRACTICE IN THE TREATMENT OF AUTISM

There currently is no cure for autism, but treatment may allow for relatively normal development in some children and reduce many undesirable behaviors. The outlook depends on the severity of symptoms, the age at which treatment is started and the availability of supportive resources for the child and his or her family. Symptoms in many children improve with intervention or as the children age. Some people with autism are able to lead normal or near-normal lives. However, many children with autism do not develop enough functional and communication skills to live independently as adults. The outlook is better for children with higher levels of intelligence who are able to communicate with language. Children with autism generally benefit most from a highly structured environment and use of routines. Treatment for autism may include a combination of the following:

- *Special education*: Education is structured to meet the child's unique educational needs.
- *Behavior modification*: This includes strategies for supporting positive behavior and decreasing problem behavior by the child.
- *Speech, physical or occupational therapy*: These therapies are designed to increase the child's functional abilities.

There are no medications currently approved to treat autism, but medications may be used to treat specific symptoms, such as anxiety (nervousness), hyperactivity and behavior that may result in injury. A recent study found that a drug often used to treat schizophrenia in adults, called Risperdal, might benefit children with autism. Hoffman et al. (2005) found that children with autism have breathing difficulties when they sleep. Helping the child breathe better can, according to the authors, reduce daytime symptoms of autism. The authors write:

> *Children's sleep-disordered breathing and parasomnias may be seen as negatively affecting their sleep duration and, in turn, their sleepiness during the day. Consistent with the deleterious effects of sleep deprivation on behavior and performance demonstrated in other populations of children (e.g., NIH, 2003), these sleep-deprived children evidence increased autistic symptomology*

> *during the day. Although future research is needed to confirm the relationships obtained in the present study, this interpretation suggests that treatments developed to address sleep problems for children with autism (here, their breathing problems and parasomnias) may permit them to sleep longer and, thereby, contribute to a decrease in their daytime behavior problems. (p. 198)*

14.7. ASPERGER'S SYNDROME

The term Asperger's syndrome (AS) is a widely misunderstood and misused diagnostic term. Incorrectly applied to a number of otherwise normal people who may be shy, socially awkward, or heavily invested in subjects (we often incorrectly think of geeks as having AS), this section deals with the research on correct diagnosis of AS and its relationship to other disorders.

Asperger's syndrome (AS) is a form of PDD characterized by two primary areas of deficit: (a) social interaction (e.g., gaze avoidance; failure to develop normal peer relations; failure to spontaneously share enjoyment, interest, and achievements; lack of social or emotional reciprocity) and (b) restricted repetitive and stereotyped patterns of behavior, interests, and activities (e.g., stereotyped and repetitive motor mannerisms, rigid adherence to nonfunctional routines, persistent preoccupation with parts of objects) (American Psychiatric Association [APA], 2000).

Children with AS also have difficulty inferring the emotions of others from facial and body language (Baron-Cohen et al., 2002). These social difficulties severely limit the child's ability to develop and maintain appropriate social relationships. In contrast to the substantial cognitive and language deficits characterized by autism, children with AS experience no unusual delays in cognition or language (APA, 2000). Additional symptoms of AS include the following (NAMI, North Carolina, 2008):

- Severe difficulty with social interactions; socially naïvety, inappropriate and awkward behavior.
- Repetitive, narrow and unusual patterns of behavior and interests.
- No clinically-significant delays in language or cognition, unlike classic autism.
- Appearance of clumsiness or delayed motor development.
- Appearance of eccentricity to other children.
- Behavior of a loner, but intense desire to be included by other children and to be sociable, but lack of appropriate social skills.
- Frequent difficulty with written language.
- Hypersensitivity to light, touch, noise, or smell.
- Lack of conversational reciprocity, unless explicitly taught.

Rutherford et al. (2002) note that, to correctly diagnose AS, a child requires impairment in social interaction, and repetitive and stereotyped behaviors and interests, without significant delay in language or cognitive development. Diagnosis is most commonly made between the ages of 4 and 11. The authors state that before a correct diagnosis can be made, a complete assessment should involve a multidisciplinary team that observes the child across multiple settings, and includes neurological and genetic assessments, as well as tests for cognition, psychomotor function, verbal and non-verbal strengths and weaknesses, style of learning, and skills for independent living. An incorrect diagnosis can lead to medications that result in unwanted side effects or lack of needed services.

Tryon et al. (2006) caution that many children with AS are initially misdiagnosed with attention-deficit hyperactivity disorder (ADHD). The authors suggest that before a diagnosis of Asperger's syndrome is given, other conditions that must be considered include "the schizophrenia spectrum, ADHD, obsessive compulsive disorder, depression, semantic pragmatic disorder, nonverbal learning disorder, Tourette syndrome, stereotypic movement disorder and bipolar disorder" (p. 2). Tryon et al. (2006) note that AS has been misdiagnosed more frequently in recent years,

> *... partly as a residual diagnosis for children of normal intelligence who do not have autism but have social difficulties. There are questions about the external validity of the AS diagnosis, that is, it is unclear whether there is a practical benefit in distinguishing AS from HFA and from PDD-NOS; the same child can receive different diagnoses depending on the screening tool (p. 2).*

Baron-Cohen (2000) wonders if we should even use the diagnosis of AS since it implies a disability where one might not exist. Baron-Cohen (2000) wonders if what we call commonly AS is just a variant of normal behavior in a society that is obsessed with diagnosing every fluctuation of childhood behavior.

14.8. ASPERGER'S DISORDER OR HIGH-LEVEL AUTISM?

The validity of Asperger's syndrome as a diagnosis separate and distinct from autism remains an ongoing issue in the literature. Using the *DSM-IV* criteria for autism, Eisenmajer et al. (1996) and Howlin (2000) among a host of researchers, have shown that most, if not all, children diagnosed with AS actually meet *DSM-IV* criteria for autism. Much of the current literature (Ozonoff et al., 2000) indicates that Asperger's syndrome is at the high-functioning or mild end of the autism continuum. In fact, one of the early Asperger's syndrome researchers now writes, "Asperger syndrome and high-functioning autism are not distinct conditions".

Tryon et al. (2006) argue that "According to the *DSM-IV*, if an individual meets criteria for autism, the individual cannot have Asperger's disorder" (p. 2). Tryon et al. (2006) studied a sample of children diagnosed with AD, and using the *DSM-IV-TR* criteria ruled out Asperger's disorder in 85% of the cases and could not be confirmed in the other 15%. The author's believe there is "mounting empirical evidence that Asperger's disorder is high-functioning autism and that

Asperger's disorder should be deleted from the next version of the *DSM*. High and low-functioning autism would continue to be indicated" (p. 6). According to the *DSM-IV-TR*, a child can still have autism even without language or cognitive delays. A diagnosis of autism takes precedence over Asperger's syndrome. The authors note that "If a child meets *DSM-IV-TR* autism criteria, the child cannot have Asperger's disorder" (p. 6).

14.9. EVIDENCE-BASED PRACTICE IN THE TREATMENT OF ASPERGER'S DISORDER

Lopata et al. (2006) describe their research in which skill streaming was used with children diagnosed with Asperger's syndrome. The following components are the basis of the nine-step skill streaming procedure:

1. Define the skill.
2. Model the skill.
3. Establish trainee skill need.
4. Select role player.
5. Set up the role play.
6. Conduct the role play.
7. Provide performance feedback.
8. Assign skill homework.
9. Select next role player (Goldstein et al., 1997, p. 37).

For a more complete description of each step, see Goldstein et al. (1997) and McGinnis and Goldstein (1997). Lopata et al. (2006) report the following results of their study:

> *These results appear to provide tentative support for interventions that incorporate cognitive-behavioral strategies targeting social skills deficits for children with AD. In the present study, parents and staff reported a significant increase in social skills across the program. This result is consistent with prior assertions and findings that cognitive and cognitive-behavioral techniques represent a promising approach to social skills development in children with AD (e.g., Attwood, 2000; Gray, 1998; Marks et al., 1999; Myles and Simpson, 2001).*

Much of the existing literature suggests that behavioral-cognitive techniques that teach social skills and strategies for interpreting and managing social situations are most likely to work with AS children. Attwood (2000) reports the benefits of behavioral-cognitive approaches to strengthen pro-social behaviors and reduce maladaptive behaviors. Simpson and Myles (1998) suggest that firm rules and expectations are liked by AS children because they want consistency and predictability in their lives. Additionally, AS children require instruction and practice in understanding and responding to non-verbal behavior. Little (2002) believes that a major problem with AS children is their literal interpretation of language and their inability to understand abstractions. Practice in these areas can be very helpful to AS children. Little also believes that helping children expand their areas of interest can be helpful, but research using social skills interventions are inconclusive and efficacy of these approaches are not known at present. In evaluating our current level of knowledge regarding best interventions with AS children, Lopata et al. (2006) write:

> *Although a number of authors have proposed explanations and treatment models, sound empirical research is virtually nonexistent (McLaughlin-Cheng, 1998). Of particular importance is the development of validated programs that significantly improve social skills and peer relationships (Greenway, 2000). In addition, Krasny et al. (2003) reported that few programs and curricula designed to facilitate social skills development within group settings are available. Research on the treatment of AD is critical because these children are at risk for additional psychiatric issues, including attention-deficit/hyperactivity disorder, depression, Tourette's syndrome, and psychotic symptoms (Wing, 1981). (p. 238)*

14.10. CASE STUDY: ASPERGER'S OR NORMAL BEHAVIOR?

Tim is an 8-year-old third grader who was recently diagnosed with Asperger's syndrome. He has some of the characteristics of AS such as being a bit socially awkward and a bit clumsy but is otherwise a fairly normal child. His father says that he was just like Tim when he was a child and continues to be a poor athlete and a bit socially awkward, but is otherwise just fine. Tim's mother thinks the problem is much more serious and notes that Tim is a loner, has no friends, and that his eccentricities are apparent to everyone. She believes that having a diagnosis of AS will lead to treatments that will help Tim overcome these troubling problems, and points to her sister's son who was considered a normal child with some eccentricities but now at 18 is drug addicted, has terrible temper problems, and in any practical way is non-functioning.

Tim has been going to a group for children with AS where social skills are taught. Tim would rather be at home working on his computer or putting together intricate models of buildings. He says that the kids in the group are "really weird" and that he is the only normal kid in the group and the kids resent him. His father sides with Tim but his mother says the groups are helping, and that Tim's social skills are improving and he is made a friend at school. Tim counters that he has lots of friends at school but because of the distance Tim lives from the school (he has bused 15 miles to school), his friends cannot come to visit but Tim e-mails them and they all seem, like Tim, to be interested in science and things Tim's mother calls "nerdy."

The conflict between mother and father over Tim has created marital problems, which the husband thought were serious enough to seek professional help. The father asked his therapist to see Tim for an evaluation. What she saw troubled her. Tim was certainly a bit socially awkward, eccentric and a bit shy but otherwise pretty normal. She thought it would be stretching the term

Asperger's to give him such a diagnosis and asked how he was give the diagnosis of AS in the first place? She was told that the parents took him to their pediatrician and his wife kept mentioning AS until the physician said that it was possible he had AS but that Tim should be seen by specialists who knew much more about it than he did. They never took him to a specialist and the possibility of AS was enough for Tim's mother to confirm the diagnosis. She was reading a good deal of material on the Internet and was now convinced Tim had AS.

Tim's father urged his wife to see the therapist, and they decided to go as a family. The mother admitted that her sister's son scared her and that she had wondered if Tim would be like him, and if maybe the problem was genetic. She also said that she had been depressed during her pregnancy and had taken antidepressives, which she now thinks may have given Tim AS. Finally, she said her brother was like Tim when he was a child and he ended up profoundly mentally ill and had to be institutionalized when he was 15. She did not want the same thing to happen to Tim.

Tim sat quietly and listened. Finally, he said, "Mom, I'm a little different than some of the kids but I'm OK. They like me at school because I'm smart and I can do stuff a lot of the kids can't do. I'm pretty bad at sports, like dad was but I'm just a kid. I'm OK. I don't like the group because the kids there are really weird and it makes me feel weird to be with them. I just want to be with my friends, and to do the stuff I like to do at home. If you'd drive my friends to our house you'd see how nice they are."

With some work with mom and some support from dad, Tim's mother began to see that she was creating a diagnosis for Tim that may have been incorrect. She took Tim out of the group, did meet his friends who now come to house often, and believes that Tim is a little different than most kids but the difference is OK and he will be fine.

The therapist told me, "The problem with having so much information available is that parents are doing a lot of incorrect diagnosing without having their children seen professionally, although I have to say that too many professionals are diagnosis happy and want to leave parents with something to explain their child's behavior, even if it's incorrect. We have professionals in our community who see AS everywhere just as 15 years ago they saw sexual abuse in every child they saw. The determinates of AS are quite clear and Tim doesn't have AS. He's a normally eccentric boy and giving him an AS diagnosis will follow him throughout his life. It's one of the worst things you can do to a child. I respect Tim's mother's concern, but a diagnosis by Internet is always something to worry about."

14.11. SUMMARY

This chapter discusses pervasive developmental problems with special attention to autism and Asperger's syndrome and the significant but unexplained increases in PDD. The chapter suggests that Asperger's syndrome is really high-level autism. Treatment options are summarized and a case of misdiagnosis is provided demonstrating that many conditions, normal and more serious, explain social awkwardness and many of the symptoms of Asperger's syndrome. Careful attention to the diagnostic indicators of PDD is recommended before a diagnosis is given.

14.12. QUESTIONS FROM THE CHAPTER

1. Is not there something more positive for young people about being given a diagnosis of Asperger's rather than calling it high-level Autism? Does not the word autism conjure up a much more severe disorder?
2. Do you fault Tim's mother in the case study for wondering if Tim had AS and for doing as much reading on the subject as she could? Would you prefer a parent to be very involved in the health of their child or to leave things to professionals.
3. Do not you think that being given a diagnosis of AS or AD locks you into diagnosis for life and becomes a self-fulfilling prophecy?
4. When I was growing up I knew a few kids with Asperger's but since we did not know the term at the time we just thought they were different and sort of eccentric and nerdy. Is not that better than using a word that conjures up such a negative view of children?
5. A study noted in the chapter suggests that parents with emotional problems have a higher risk of their child developing AD and AS. Do you think this is a genetic indicator of potential for a developmental problem or do these parents have difficulty bonding with children or using healthy parental behaviors that cause the child's AD and AS?

References

American Psychiatric Association. (1994). *Diagnostic and statistical manual of mental disorders* (4th ed.). Washington, DC: Author.

American Psychiatric Association. (2000). Diagnostic criteria for 299.80 Asperger's Disorder (AD), *Diagnostic and Statistical Manual of Mental Disorders*, *4*, text revision. (DSM-IV-TR).

Attwood, T. (2000). Strategies for improving the social integration of children with Asperger's syndrome. *The National Autistic Society, 4*(1), 85–100.

Autism, http://www.webmd.com/content/article/60/67141.htm?printing=true WEBMD 11-24-06.

Baron-Cohen, S. (2000). Is Asperger syndrome/high-functioning autism necessarily a disability?. *Development and Psychopathology, 12*(3), 489–550.

Baron-Cohen, S., Wheelwright, S., Lawson, J., Griffin, R., & Hill, J. (2002). The exact mind: Empathizing and systemizing in autism spectrum conditions. In U. & Goswami (Ed.), *Handbook of childhood cognitive development* (pp. 491–508). Malden, MA, USA: Blackwell Publishers.

Boyle, T., (1995). *Diagnosing autism and other pervasive development disorders* [*excerpt from Autism: Basic information* (3rd ed., pp. 6–7)]. Ewing, NJ: The New Jersey Center for Outreach & Services for the Autism Community, Inc. (COSAC).

Eisenmajer, R., Prior, M., Leekam, S., Wing, L., Gould, J., Welham, M., & Ong, B. (1996). Comparison of clinical symptoms in autism and Asperger's disorder. *Journal of the American Academy of Child and Adolescent Psychiatry, 35*, 1523–1531.

Goldstein, A. P., McGinnis, E., Sprafkin, R. P., Gershaw, N. J., & Klein, P. (1997). *Skill-streaming the adolescent: New strategies and perspectives for teaching prosocial skills* (Rev. ed.). Champaign, IL: Research Press.

Gray, C. (1998). Social stories and comic strip conversations with students with Asperger syndrome and high-functioning autism. In E. Schopler, G. Mesibov, L. J. & Kunce (Eds.), *Asperger syndrome or high-functioning autism?* (pp. 167–198). New York: Plenum Press.

Greenway, C. (2000). Autism and Asperger's syndrome: Strategies to promote prosocial behaviors. *Educational Psychology in Practice, 16*(3), 469–486.

Hoffman, D. C., Sweeney, D. P., Gilliam, J. E., Apodaca, D. D., Lopez-Wagner, M. C., & Castillo, M. M. (2005, Winter). Sleep problems and symptomology in children with autism. *Focus on Autism and Other Developmental Liabilities, 20*(4), 194–200.

Howlin, P. (2000). Outcome in adult life for more able individuals with autism or Asperger's syndrome. *Autism: The International Journal of Research and Practice, 4*(1), 63–84.

Krasny, L., Williams, B. J., Provencal, S., & Ozonoff, S. (2003). Social skills interventions for the autism spectrum: Essential ingredients and a model curriculum. *Child and Adolescent Psychiatric Clinics of North America, 12*, 107–122.

Little, C. (2002). Which is it? Asperger's syndrome or giftedness? Defining the differences. *Gifted Child Today Magazine, 25*(1), 58–63.

Lopata, C., Thomeer, M. L., Volker, M. A., & Nida, R. E. (2006, Winter). Effectiveness of a cognitive-behavior treatment on social behaviors of children with Asperger disorder. *Focus on Autism and Other Developmental Disabilities, 21*(4), 237–244.

Marks, S. U., Schrader, C., Levine, M., Hagie, C., Longaker, T., Morales, M., et al. (1999). Social skills for social ills: Supporting the social skills development of adolescents with Asperger's syndrome. *Teaching Exceptional Children, 32*(2), 56–61.

McGinnis, E., & Goldstein, A. P. (1997). *Skillstreaming the elementary school child: New strategies and perspectives for teaching prosocial skills* (Rev. ed.). Champaign, IL: Research Press.

McLaughlin-Cheng, E. (1998). Asperger syndrome and autism: A literature review and meta-analysis. *Focus on Autism and Other Developmental Disabilities, 14*(4), 234–245.

Moeschler, J., & Gibbs, E. Jr., Graham, J. (1990). *A summary of medical and psychoeducation aspects of Rett syndrome*. Lebanon, NH: Clinical Genetics and Child Development Center.

Myles, B. S., & Simpson, R. L. (2001). Understanding the hidden curriculum: An essential social skill for children and youth with Asperger syndrome. *Intervention in School and Clinic, 36*(5), 279–286.

NAMI, North Carolina. Asperger's Syndrome Fact Sheet http://www.naminc.org/CFS%20ASPERGERS.htm

Ozonoff, S., South, M., & Miller, J. (2000). DSM-IV-defined Asperger's syndrome: Cognitive, behavioral and early history differentiation from high-functioning autism. *Autism, 1*, 29–46.

Rutherford, M. D., Baron-Cohen, S., & Wheelwright, S. (2002). Reading the mind in the voice: A study with normal adults with Asperger syndrome and high-functioning autism. *Journal of Autism and Developmental Disorders, 32*(3), 189–194.

Simpson, R. L., & Myles, B. S. (1998). Aggression among children and youth who have Asperger's syndrome: A different population requiring different strategies. *Preventing School Failure, 42*(4), 149–153.

Tryon, P. A., Mayes, S. D., Rhodes, R. L., & Waldo, M. (2006, Spring). Can Asperger's disorder be differentiated from autism using DSM-IV Criteria?. *Focus on Autism and Other Developmental Disabilities, 21*(1), 2–6.

U.S. Centers for Disease Control and Prevention. (2007). WEBMD 11-24-06 http://www.webmd.com/content/article/60/67141.htm?printing=true.

Wing, L. (1981). Asperger's syndrome: A clinical account. *Psychological Medicine, 11*, 115.

Further reading

Autism cases still on rise after vaccine change. New Calif. finding refutes link between thimerosal and disorder, study says MSNBC.com (Jan 7, 2008). http://www.msnbc.msn.com/id/22542677/. Retrieved Jan 7, 2008.

Pervasive Developmental Disorders Fact Sheet 20 (FS20). (1998). *Resources updated, October 2003* National Dissemination Center for Children with Disabilities. http://www.nichcy.org/pubs/factshe/fs20txt.htm

Reuters. (2008, May 5) *Child's autism linked to parents' mental illness.* http://www.msnbc.msn.com/id/24465288. Author.

Yale Developmental Disabilities Clinic (2008). *Pervasive Developmental Disorder-Not Otherwise Specified (PDD-NOS).* http://www.med.yale.edu/chldstdy/autism/pddnos.html

Simpson, R. L., & Myles, B. S. (1998). Aggression among children and youth who have Asperger's syndrome: A different population requiring different strategies. *Preventing School Failure, 42*(4), 149–153.

Tryon, P. A., Mayes, S. D., Rhodes, R. L., & Waldo, M. (2006, Spring). Can Asperger's disorder be differentiated from autism using DSM-IV criteria? *Focus on Autism and Other Developmental Disabilities, 21*(1), 2–6.

U.S. Centers for Disease Control and Prevention (2007).

Wing, L. (1981). Asperger's syndrome: A clinical account. *Psychological Medicine, 11*, 115–129.

Further Reading

[illegible]

15 Evidence-Based Practice with Serious Emotional Problems of Children and Adolescents

15.1. INTRODUCTION

This chapter will focus on serious emotional problems of childhood and adolescence including borderline personality disorder, which often has its origins in childhood, child and adolescent schizophrenia, and because of its serious nature and its relationship to high suicide and co-occurring disorders such as substance abuse, bi-polar disorder.

15.2. BORDERLINE PERSONALITY DISORDER

Before we discuss borderline personality disorder (BPD), it might be helpful to briefly summarize the larger category of personality disorders, since BPD is part of the family of personality disorders.

15.2.1. Personality Disorders

One of the most difficult problems facing clinicians is the treatment of clients diagnosed with a personality disorder. In the popular mind, personality disorders suggest major treatment problems. The DSM-IV (APA, 1994) does not help matters when it defines a personality disorder as:

> *...[A]n enduring pattern of inner experience and behavior that deviates markedly from the expectations of the individual's culture. This pattern is manifested in two (or more) of the following areas: (1) In ways of perceiving self, others and events; (2) in the range, intensity, liability and appropriateness of the response; (3) in interpersonal functioning and; (4) in impulse control. The enduring pattern is inflexibly and impairment in many important areas of functioning that can usually be traced back to early childhood and is of a long duration, and is not caused by a mental or physical disorder or brain trauma (p. 633).*

This discouraging list of problems has generally made many therapists leery of working with clients who have what the DSM-IV calls "Cluster B" personality disorders. Personality disorders are placed into three clusters by the DSM-IV. "Cluster A" includes "Paranoid, Schizoid and Schizotypal Disorders. People with this disorder often appear odd or eccentric" (APA, 1994, p. 629).

Clients with "Cluster B Personality Disorders" (also termed severe Personality Disorders), often appear dramatic, emotional, or erratic and have major difficulties in establishing and maintaining adequate social relationships due to their emotionally labile and impulsive behavior (APA, 1994, p. 630). Cluster B Personality Disorders include individuals with "Borderline, Antisocial, Histrionic, and Narcissistic Personality Disorders" (APA, 1994, p. 630). Cluster C "includes Avoidant, Dependent and Obsessive Compulsive Personality Disorders. Individuals with this Disorder often appear anxious or fearful" (APA, 1994, p. 630).

Establishing the number of people with severe personality disorders in the population is difficult because of the diversity of diagnostic criteria used (Stone, 1993). Drake and Vaillant (1985) estimate the prevalence in the population as one percent with borderline personality disorders, and a lifetime risk of antisocial personality disorder of just under three percent, with a fourfold increase in risk among men (Robins et al., 1991).

15.3. BORDERLINE PERSONALITY DISORDER

Clients with BPD (DSM-IV Code# 301.83) have all of the elements of a personality disorder but have five or more of the following symptoms: (a) A pattern of unstable relationships; (b) an unstable self-image or identity; (c) self-destructive impulsivity; (d) suicidal behavior; (e) irritability, anxiety and severe swings in mood; (f) chronic feelings of emptiness; (g) difficulty controlling anger; and (h) transient paranoid ideations or dissociative symptoms (APA, 1994, p. 654). Clients with BPD may also experience numerous unfulfilling relationships, sexual acting out, behavior which sometimes appears to demonstrate signs of mental illness, and severe ongoing depression and/or anxiety. Completed suicides in BPD are 8–10% (DSM-IV, APA, 1994, p. 651).

The Cornell Psychotherapy Program (2008) describes clients with BPD as unable to tolerate levels of frustration most people tolerate and who lack the ability to cope when they become upset. The report goes on to say that:

> *The one word that best characterizes borderline personality is "instability." Their emotions are unstable, fluctuating wildly for no discernible reason. Their thinking is unstable – rational and clear at times, quite psychotic at other times. The effect upon others of all this trouble is profound: family members never know what to expect from their volatile child, siblings, or spouse, except they know they can expect trouble: suicide threats and attempts, self-inflicted injuries, outbursts of rage and recrimination, impulsive marriages, divorces, pregnancies and abortions; repeated starting and stopping of jobs and school careers, and a pervasive sense, on the part of the family, of being unable to help (p. 1).*

Craig (2001) believes that clients with BPD can be distinguished from histrionic personality disorder and major depressive disorder by their "self-destructiveness, chronic emptiness and loneliness, and sensitivity to criticism and rejection"

(p. 2). Patients with BPD may have paranoia and delusions, although the episodes are usually transient and normally do not have the eccentric qualities associated with schizotypal personality disorder (Craig, 2001).

Frey (1999) describes clients with BPD as unstable, prone to wide mood swings, inclined to experience frequent relationships that are very intense but troubled, impulsive, and experiencing confusion about important life issues. This sense of confusion about life issues may suggest severe confusion about self-identity. Frey notes that people with BPD frequently cut or burn themselves and often threaten or actually attempt suicide. Many of these clients have experienced severe childhood abuse or neglect. Frey reports that roughly two percent of the general population has BPD, and that 75% are female (Frey, 1999, p. 3).

Zanarini (2000) indicates that although the cause of BPD is unknown, studies show that many, but not all, individuals with BPD report a history of abuse, neglect, or separation as young children and that 40–71% of BPD patients report having been sexually abused, usually by a non-caregiver. Researchers believe that BPD results from a combination of individual vulnerability to environmental stress, neglect or abuse as young children, and a series of events that trigger the onset of the disorder as young adults. Adults with BPD are also considerably more likely to be the victim of violence, including rape and other crimes. This may result from both harmful environments as well as impulsivity and poor judgment in choosing partners and lifestyles.

In several quantitative studies, the origins of BPD found in borderline children include physical and sexual child abuse and neglect, separation from parents (Bemporad et al., 1982; Kestenbaum, 1983), as well as serious parental psychopathology including depression, substance abuse, or antisocial personality (Goldman et al., 1993). In a study of latency-aged children showing signs of BPD, Guzder et al. (1999) found that 34% of the children in their sample had actual reports of sexual abuse made by adults who had knowledge of the abuse. The authors suggest that in seeing a relationship between sexual abuse and BPD, it is also true that many abused children have little parental supervision and that lack of supervision could also relate to the development of BPD. Children with the symptoms of BPD go on to exhibit the same symptoms as adults at a very high rate (Guzder et al., 1999).

The prevalence of BPD, according to the DSM-IV is "2% of the general population, 10% of those seen in mental health clinics, and about 20% of the psychiatric patients. Borderline Personality Disorder ranges from 30% to 60% of the clinical population with Personality Disorder" (APA, 1994, p. 652).

Paris (2008) reports that BPD usually begins in adolescence or youth and that about 80% of patients are women. BPD is usually chronic, and severe problems often continue to be present for many years. About one out of ten patients eventually succeed in committing suicide. However, in the 90% who do not kill themselves, borderline pathology tends to "burn out" in middle age, and most patients function significantly better by the ages of 35–40. The mechanism for this improvement is unknown. However, other disorders associated with impulsivity, such as antisocial personality and substance abuse, also tend to burn out around the same age. While the mainstay of treatment for BPT has been cognitive psychotherapy that may reduce suicidal and impulsive behavior within a year of treatment, Paris (2008) reports that about two thirds of clients with BPD drop out of treatment within two months. In noting the difficulty of treating BPD, Paris writes, "The chaos that characterizes borderline patients makes them difficult cases for therapists. A patient with BPD may be continuously suicidal for months or years. Moreover, many of the same problems that patients have with other people arise in their relationships with helping professionals" (p. 1).

In a study of the treatment of BPD, Bateman and Fonagy (1999) studied 38 borderline patients in a psychoanalytically oriented partial hospital program with a similar group of controls. They found a reduction in suicide attempts from 95% on admission to 5.3% after 18 months. Some promising results for patients with anti-social personality disorder emerged from a study of opiate addicts (Woody et al., 1985) in which 110 male patients with opiate addiction received either paraprofessional drug counseling alone or counseling plus professional psychotherapy (either supportive-expressive or cognitive-behavioral). Those in the study who had antisocial personality disorders with an Axis 1 diagnosis of depression made significant improvement in both symptoms and employment. Antisocial personality disordered clients without depression showed little improvement as a result of psychotherapy. Koerner and Linehan (2000) report that group and individual psychotherapy are at least partially effective for many patients. They also note that within the past 15 years, a new psychosocial treatment termed dialectical behavior therapy (DBT) was developed specifically to treat BPD, and this technique has promising results in treatment studies.

Lehman (2003) believes that "[T]herapists often have intense, unproductive emotional reactions to patients with borderline personality disorder because borderline patients engage in self-injurious behavior and suicide attempts and perceive these acts as manipulative and attention seeking" (p. 29). These negative perceptions often result in stigmatizing clients with BPD. To be effective, therapists must maintain a positive treatment alliance with clients and communicate often with other professionals involved with the client to prevent "splitting," a reaction that occurs when clients pit one therapist against the other. Treatment approaches that seem best suited for effective work with the BPD client are cognitive therapy and dialectic behavior therapy with serotonin selective reuptake inhibitors, and mood stabilizers added when drug therapy is recommended (Lehmann, 2003, p. 29).

15.4. BI-POLAR DISORDER IN CHILDREN AND ADOLESCENTS

Papolos and Papolos (1999) suggest that children with early-onset bipolar disorder rarely fit the pattern of bipolar disorder in adults. Early-onset bipolar disorder may present a wide range of symptoms from mild to extreme that may begin as early as infancy and include irritability, unpredictability, hyperactivity and attention problems, conduct problems, social problems, childhood depression, eating disorders, self-mutilation, and suicidal ideation. State et al. (2002) found that a third of the children who initially seem to be suffering from depression, as defined by frequent crying, loss of interest in enjoyable activities, changes in appearance (e.g., lack of self-care), increased irritability, changes in sleeping patterns (e.g., too much or too little sleep), and increased social withdrawal later develop the symptoms of bipolar disorder.

Wozniak et al. (1995) found that severe irritability is often a predominant mood in *children* meeting the criteria for mania, with an increase in behaviors such as increasing silliness, grandiose ideas (e.g., that they can teach better than the teacher), racing thoughts, difficulty explaining ideas, bizarre hallucinations, and outrageous comments. State et al. (2002) report mixed states and rapid cycling in over 70% of the *children* diagnosed with early-onset bipolar disorder. In a mixed state the child may be agitated, constantly restlessness and often feeling worthlessness and self-destruction. Geller et al. (1998) defined rapid cycling as a very fast change between depressive and manic symptoms. Kovacs and Pollock (1995) report that children with early onset bipolar disorder may exhibit symptoms we often associate with ODD and CD in children and adolescents. Geller and Luby (1997) found that approximately 22% of children and 18% of adolescents with bipolar disorder demonstrated features of CD, such as poor judgment and grandiose behaviors, as indicators of early-onset bipolar disorder. Papolos and Papolos (1999) found self-mutilation and suicidal ideations common symptoms even in children as young as four years of age.

The current controversy over the numbers of children with bipolar disorder may in part be due to a difference of opinion in diagnosis. A diagnosis of bipolar disorder requires distinct manic episodes, during which one's mood is altered, sleep and activity patterns change and children are constantly irritable. Sometimes clinicians may diagnose irritable children with bipolar disorder based on outbursts that occur during extreme frustration, but are too short in duration to meet the necessary criteria for a manic episode. Often these children are more appropriately diagnosed with ADHD or OCC than bipolar disorder. In response to data showing that bipolar disorder among children and adolescents has increased more rapidly as a diagnosis than in adults. NIMH (2007) states that "[i]t is likely that this impressive increase reflects a recent tendency to over-diagnose bipolar disorder in young people, a correction of historical under-recognition, or a combination of these trends. Clearly, we need to learn more about what criteria physicians in the community are actually using to diagnose bipolar disorder in children and adolescents and how physicians are arriving at decisions concerning clinical management" (p. 1). However, the NIMH report goes on to say that:

> *A forty-fold increase in the diagnosis of bipolar disorder in children and adolescents is worrisome. We do not know how much of this increase reflects earlier under-diagnosis, current over-diagnosis, possibly a true increase in*

> *prevalence of this illness, or some combination of these factors. However, these new results confirm what we are hearing increasingly from families who tell us about disabling, sometimes dangerous psychiatric symptoms in their children. This report reminds us of the need for research that validates the diagnosis of bipolar disorder and other disorders in children and the importance of developing treatments that are safe, effective, and feasible for use in primary care (p. 1).*

Regardless of who may be correct, a search of the literature confirmed that as much as we disagree about the existence of bipolar disorder in children, there is strong disagreement about treatment. Use of medication is advised in a number of articles but there were few if any well done pieces of research to support the use of medication in other than very difficult-to-manage cases of extreme mania and depression. Even then, researchers wonder whether the medications were having the desired impact or if positive changes were more a result of maturation and other bio-social changes. A number of researchers worried that we had too little information about side effects, which could, over time, be problematic. Groopman (2007) found that medical researchers are so concerned about the misuse of powerful psychotropic drugs with children that they worry that the side effects might cause a number of children to become obese diabetics with involuntary movements. Although it is important we correctly diagnose and treat children who really have the destabilizing symptoms of bipolar disorder, with their extreme changes in mood and the potential for deep depression resulting in suicidal attempts, it is also important that we not use the label of bipolar disorder with children who are sometimes moody or show excessive exuberance. These children may just be demonstrating normal changes in development that balance themselves out as the child develops.

The Harvard Mental Health Letter (2007) believes that whether or not children who are diagnosed with bipolar disorder take medication for the illness, psychotherapy can help in ways that are helping adults with the disorder. Supportive therapy often provides "sympathy, reassurance, and strategies for managing everyday problems" (p. 3). Psychodynamic therapy may help older children and adolescents "explore their present and past personal relationships, their psychological development, and how they defend against uncomfortable feelings" (p. 3). With cognitive-behavioral therapy, younger clients can "examine and re-examine their thoughts and ways of interpreting experience and help them observe and change their behavior" (p. 3) and the cognitive errors often made because of the disorder. Younger clients can be helped to learn better social skills and problem-solving approaches and learn to rehearse them if they sense a relapse coming on. Going to bed and getting up at the same times as a sleep regimen can help prevent episodes of mania. Some bipolar children benefit from tutoring for learning disabilities and time lost from classes while coping with the disorder. Parents can benefit from specialized help to understand and cope with the erratic behavior associated with bipolar disorder and should be encouraged to read the literature and discuss it with professionals and members of support groups. These support groups may be found through the Child and Adolescent Bipolar Foundation and other self-help groups.

Prien and Potter (1990) report that 25–50% of their adolescent clients were non-compliant with their medication regimens, causing relapses of symptoms in 90% of their clients over an 18-month period. The authors indicate that support groups are often helpful with adult clients in maintaining compliance and may be helpful with children and adolescents as well. Fristad et al. (2003) developed a manual-based psycho-educational approach (The Multi Family Psychoeducation Group program: MFPG), which shows promise with bipolar children and adolescents and their families. The goals of treatment are to help the child and his or her family understand the symptoms of bipolar disorder and the best evidence for treatment, as well as to improve the management of manic and depressive symptoms, improve peer relations, and to learn to respond to the child rather than to his or her symptoms. Kendall et al. (1998) have shown that manual-based programs such as the MFPG can be used creatively and with considerable flexibility.

15.5. CHILDHOOD SCHIZOPHRENIA

Remschmidt et al. (1994) report that schizophrenia is rarely seen in childhood, especially before the age of 12, and is less than one sixteenth as common as the adult-onset type (Harvard, 1997). Tolbert (1996) reports that one in 10 000 children will develop the disorder, and that generally it occurs in late adolescence but can also strike young children. About 50% of the children with childhood schizophrenia will experience serious neuropsychiatric symptoms (Taylor, 1998). Asarnow et al. (1994) report that 61% of children with early-onset childhood schizophrenia maintained the same diagnosis throughout adolescence and young adulthood. Eggers and Bunk (1997) indicate that early onset schizophrenia results in high levels of social disability. The researchers found that no gender differences exist in the average age of onset.

Young schizophrenic children often experience psychotic episodes, behavioral problems, developmental lags, and language and motor delays well before the development of actual psychosis. About 30% of these children will demonstrate symptoms of pervasive developmental disorder such as posturing, rocking, and arm flapping, and may present as anxious, confused, or disruptive (Harvard, 1997). Children with schizophrenia fail to develop normal relationships, problem-solving skills, the ability to do abstract reasoning, or age-appropriate self-care. Although there is no intellectual impairment, there are cognitive impairments which make it difficult for children to learn (Taylor, 1998). Additional symptoms may include poor grades despite strong efforts, excessive worrying or anxiety, hyperactivity; nightmares, persistent disobedience and/or aggressive behavior, and frequent temper tantrums.

Spencer and Campbell (1994) reported that children between five and a half and and 11.75-years old had shared their auditory hallucinations in very specific terms with others, and described them as usually being auditory and persecutory or command in nature. Visual hallucinations also may be present (Werry, 1992). Russell (1994) reports that the development of the psychosis is gradual, without the sudden onset so common in adolescence and adults. The gradual onset of symptoms, or the prodromal phase, appears early in the child's development and gradually increases in intensity.

Although symptoms of childhood schizophrenia and pervasive developmental disorder may be similar, Tolbert (1996) reports that PPD has an onset before age three and, unlike childhood schizophrenia, retardation is common. Tolbert (1996) reports that 25% of all autistic children have seizures, unlike children with schizophrenia. Tolbert (1996) also notes that Rett's disorder, Asperger's disorder, obsessive compulsive disorders, psychotic mood disorders, and childhood disintegrative disorder must be ruled out, as well as organic conditions such as metabolic disorders, delirium, epilepsy, and neurodegenerative disorders, before a diagnosis of childhood schizophrenia can be given, and then it should only be made by taking into consideration maturation requiring a period of observation while the child is drug free.

15.6. ADOLESCENT ONSET SCHIZOPHRENIA

Haines (2005) notes that the onset of schizophrenia peaks in males during their late teens to mid-twenties, while the age of onset in women is somewhat later. While rare in children, schizophrenia is not rare in teens. Warning signs may be present for months and even years before the onset of full-blown symptoms. These initial or prodromal symptoms include increasing withdrawal, disorganization, declines in schoolwork, social functioning with flat affect, and the occasional unprovoked outbursts. Early signs may also include odd thoughts or beliefs and episodes of garbled language.

Haines (2005) reports that full-blown schizophrenia includes delusions (bizarre, strongly-held false beliefs), hallucinations (sensing something that is not there), disorganized speech and behavior, voices that compel behavior, flat affect, apathy, paranoia, social withdrawal, and very disorganized and confused thinking. Adolescent schizophrenics often use drugs and alcohol as a way to self-medicate.

According to Hollis (2000) the impact of child and adolescent onset schizophrenia is long-lasting. Hollis (2000) studied the psychosocial functioning of children and adolescents over an 11-year period following diagnosis. Sixty percent of the subjects left school without having graduated, although 22% did graduate, some with high levels of achievement. The employment record for the subjects studied was almost non-existent. Almost half the subjects had no social contact with anyone other than professionals or close relatives, while only 14% socialized with friends. Only one subject had a reciprocal love relationship, and none had married or had a stable partner. Hollis believes that the 11-year study suggests that the diagnosis of childhood and adolescent onset schizophrenia is a stable diagnosis with long-term impact and argues for early diagnosis and appropriate treatment as soon after the diagnosis as possible. Hollis (2000) writes:

> *These findings should give clinicians greater confidence in making an early diagnosis of schizophrenia in children and adolescents. The very poor prognosis described here for child- and adolescent-onset schizophrenia suggests that early and aggressive treatment, special education, and support for families should begin as soon as possible after onset of psychosis (p. 1658).*

Turner and Salzer (2006) asked consumers of services with a diagnosis of schizophrenia what they value most in treatment. More important than medication, consumers of services said that bonding with providers and a positive supportive relationships were most helpful to them, particularly in light of the fact that the authors found that 74% of the subjects discontinued their initial medications within an 18-month period. The bond provided between consumer and professional would help reduce problems with medication compliance or help determine which medication worked best. Consumers were atheoretical when describing treatment approaches but used words like "non-threatening" and "friendly" when describing what they looked for in treatment. The authors also found that clients want to be included in all decision-making regarding their treatment. Half of the subjects spoke to the importance of strong case management services and a third noted the importance of determining which medication worked best for them. High turnover rates that one hears of regarding mental health professionals and case managers cannot be a positive sign for future client satisfaction with services. These high turnover rates need to be addressed if these and other studies like them have any meaning.

In reviewing the effectiveness of psychosocial treatments for first episode schizophrenia, Penn et al. (2005) note that most of the deteriorating effects of the disorder occur within the first five years of a diagnosis of schizophrenia, and that psychosocial interventions can help medicate some of the harm caused by the disorder. The researchers found that interventions may positively influence social functioning, as well as time spent in the hospital and the likelihood of hospital readmission. Cognitive therapy was found to improve symptoms and quality of life but was ineffective in preventing relapse and rehospitalization. Research on the effectiveness of group and family therapy was mixed, according to the authors, with some studies showing positive benefits and others showing minimal benefits. All the studies reported on had serious methodological problems or very small samples that made forming conclusions difficult. While some studies of intervention show positive initial improvement, most of the improvement diminishes with time. The authors believe that this suggests longer-term intervention with more controlled research was necessary to determine the benefits of combinations of psychosocial interventions over time.

Several studies of early psychosocial show promise. Tarrier et al. (2004) found that in an 18-month follow up, both cognitive behavior therapy and supportive counseling were significantly better than routine care in reducing symptoms. Jackson et al. (1998) found that cognitive psychotherapy for early psychosis promoted adjustment to the illness, helped individuals resume developmental tasks, and focused on overall recovery, in addition to targeting secondary morbidity (i.e., depression, anxiety). At the end of treatment, the patients receiving cognitively oriented psychotherapy performed significantly better than the control group on measures of insight and attitudes toward treatment, adaptation to illness, quality of life, and negative symptoms, but they significantly outperformed the group unwilling to take part in the study only with respect to adaptation to illness. Neither study was able to reduce relapse rates or rehospitalization, but Penn et al. (2005) believe these initial positive results will have a long-term positive impact and that longitudinal studies which follow people over the course of the life span are needed to determine long-term effectiveness of early interventions.

Zhang et al. (1994) randomly assigned 83 outpatients with first-episode psychosis to 18 months of family therapy and routine care or to routine care alone. Family therapy emphasized identification of warning signs of relapse, stress management, the importance of attributing maladaptive behavior to the illness, communication skills training, and a reduction of criticism. The results showed much lower rates of hospital readmissions and fewer days spent in the hospital. The researchers found that patients not receiving the family intervention were 3.5 times more likely to be readmitted to the hospital during the study period as the patients who did receive family therapy. Patients receiving family therapy who were not rehospitalized had improved symptoms and social functioning. Lehtinen (1993) had similar positive outcomes, including fewer hospital admissions, less time spent in the hospital, and a reduction in symptoms. Both studies were done in countries outside of the United States.

15.7. THE STIGMA OF MENTAL ILLNESS

Markowitz (1998) reports that people with mental illness are "more likely to be unemployed, have less income, experience a diminished sense of self, and have fewer social supports" (p. 335). Part of the reason for this finding may be a function of the stigma attached to mental illness. Markowitz (1998) goes on to note that "[m]entally ill persons may expect and experience rejection in part because they think less of themselves, have limited social opportunities and resources, and because of the severity of their illness" (p. 343). Markowitz also notes that the impact of anticipated rejection of mentally ill people is largely caused by "discriminatory experiences" in which the person observes an employer perceiving potential problems based solely on a diagnostic label and not on the person's actual behavior. This perception of rejection compounds feelings of low self-worth and depression (Markowitz, 1998).

Manfred-Gilham et al. (2002) studied social and vocational barriers to participation in treatment for mentally ill patients as one reason for treatment attrition. They concluded that the more realistically workers prepared clients for barriers they might encounter in the community, the more likely clients were to continue on with their treatment regimen. The authors write, "We have some evidence from Kazdin et al. (1997) that therapists' perceptions of barriers predicted client treatment continuation more strongly than did the client's own self-report" (p. 220). Manfred-Gilham et al. (2002) go on to note that there is a strong link between the strategies used by the worker to prepare the client for barriers in their lives and the client's ability to resolve those barriers.

Carpenter (2002) suggests that mental health services have been developed with the belief that mental illness is a chronic disease requiring continual care and supervision. She notes that the DSM IV (1994) still indicates that schizophrenia will result in progressive deterioration and cautions readers that complete remission of symptoms is rare. However, research studies fail to support the concept of long-term chronicity in patients diagnosed with mental illness. Carpenter (2000) reports that most people with a diagnosis of schizophrenia or other serious mental illness experience "either complete or significant remission of symptoms, and work, have relationships, and otherwise engage in a challenging and fulfilling life" (Carpenter, 2002, p. 89). In a study of over 500 adults diagnosed with schizophrenia, Huber et al. (1975) found that over one-fifth of the sample experienced complete remission and over two-fifths experienced significant remission of symptoms. In a 40-year follow-up study, Tsuang et al. (1979) found that 46% of those diagnosed with schizophrenia had no symptoms or had only non-incapacitating symptoms. The Vermont Longitudinal Study, (Harding et al., 1986a, 1986b), a 20–25-year follow-up study of former state hospital patients, found that 72% of the people diagnosed with schizophrenia had only slight or no psychiatric symptoms. Despite these very optimistic findings, Carpenter (2002) writes:

> *...[T]he premise of chronicity continues to be widely accepted in the mental health system, and dismal prognoses continue to be communicated to people with psychiatric disabilities (Kruger, 2000). These prognoses leave little room for a sense of hope on the part of those labeled with mental illness and, as such, may become a self-fulfilling prophecy (Jimenez, 1988). The consumer-survivor recovery movement has sought to restore that hope with an innovative perspective on the meaning and course of psychiatric disability (Kruger, 2000) (Carpenter, 2002, p. 89).*

15.8. THE CONSUMER-SURVIVOR RECOVERY MOVEMENT

This discussion of the consumer-recovery movement first appeared in a book by the author on the strength's perspective (Glicken, 2004, pp. 173–174). The author thanks Pearson Education, Inc. for permission to reprint this material.

Carpenter (2002) defines the consumer-survivor recovery movement as one that assumes that people with psychiatric disabilities can and will recover. Recovery is defined as a process of achieving self-management through increased responsibility for a person's own recovery. This process is aided by a sense of hope provided by the person's professional, family, and support systems. Carpenter (2002) also indicates that "the consumer-survivor definition of the experience of psychiatric disability is as much about recovery from the societal reaction to the disability as it is about recovery from the disability itself" (p. 90). Anthony (1993) believes that recovery from mental illness is aided by what he calls, "recovery triggers" that include sharing with patients, their families, and the community the research indicating that many people with psychiatric problems do, in fact, recover. Another trigger involves information about the availability of services and treatment options such as self-help groups and alternative treatment approaches. Using a strengths oriented assessment approach also helps in recovery and is a strong antidote to the medical model that perceives the person as pathological and often ignores significant growth and change. The experience of Nobel Prize winner John Nash (Nasar, 1998), who had a gradual remission from many years of mental illness, is a reminder that people change with time and that remission of symptoms, if not outright cures of mental illness, are often possible.

Chinman et al. (2001) suggest that one way of improving treatment results and decreasing recidivism is through the mutual support of other mentally ill clients. According to the authors, mutual support groups reduce hospitalization rates, the amount of time spent in hospitals, symptoms, and number days spent in the hospital. Additionally, support groups improve quality of life and self-esteem, and contribute to better community reintegration of clients with severe psychiatric disorders (Davidson et al., 1999; Kyrouz and Humphreys, 1996; Reidy, 1992). Mutual support groups provide acceptance, empathy, a feeling of belonging to a community, necessary information to help with management of social and emotional problems, new ways of coping with problems, and role models who are coping well. Chinman et al. (2001) report that "[m]utual support also operates through the 'helper-therapy' principle that suggests that by helping one another, participants increase their social status and self-esteem (Riessman, 1965)" (p. 220).

Beyond mutual support groups, Chinman et al. (2001) suggest that there is growing evidence that consumer-run services may prove to be very effective in helping clients with mental illnesses (Davidson et al., 1999). They write:

> *Consumer providers are sometimes better able to empathize, to access social services, to appreciate clients' strengths, to be tolerant and flexible, to be patient and persistent, to be aware of and respond to clients' desires, and to be able to create supportive environments which can foster recovery and the restoration of community life (Dixon et al., 1994). Other studies found that a consumer-run case management service yielded equivalent outcomes to those generated by a conventional case management team (Felton et al., 1995) (Chinman et al., 2001, p. 220).*

Writing about the treatment of severe depression, O'Connor (2001) believes that we often fail to recognize that what keeps people depressed is their own view of their depression as ongoing, untreatable, and hopeless. These cognitive definitions of people's depression, in time, become self-definitions, which reinforce the depression and keep it from improving. To help his patients cope with their depressions, O'Connor (2001) provides them with "aphorisms" about depression that he believes serve as a way of changing long held beliefs about their depression and about themselves. While cognitive in nature, the aphorisms O'Connor provides are also strengths based. Several aphorisms that seem particularly relevant to a book on the strengths perspective are: "(1) If I change what I do, I can change how I feel; (2) Change can come from anywhere; (3) I am more than my depression" (p. 517). These aphorisms are "assertions about the nature of depression and recovery from it, which help patients move toward taking an active role in questioning how the condition affects them" (p. 507). O'Connor goes on to say that "aphorisms [are] statements that perform an action simply by being spoken" (p. 512).

15.9. CASE STUDY: EVIDENCE-BASED PRACTICE WITH A BORDERLINE PERSONALITY DISORDERED ADOLESCENT CLIENT

This case first appeared in modified form in a book the author wrote on evidence-based practice (Glicken, 2005, pp. 134–138). The author thanks Sage Publications for permission to reprint this material.

Loni Morrison is a 17-year-old senior in high school referred for residential treatment after her fourth suicide attempt and hospitalization in four months. Loni has been diagnosed with BPD since age 12 when she began a long series of disastrous relationships with much older men, alcohol and drug abuse, deep depressions often resulting in nearly fatal suicide attempts, and other symptoms of BPD that have caused her a great deal of sorrow. Loni is a very talented artist and is just beginning to show her works at private galleries. She is also brilliant, and superficial contact with her would indicate that this highly intelligent and creative person is much healthier than her history would suggest. Loni is currently on anti-depressive medication and has been in therapy since age 12 with a number of therapists. She usually leaves therapy after a few sessions, believing that the therapists do not understand her well enough to help.

Her last four suicide attempts have been a response to a love interest who, once knowing Loni well, was unwilling to deal with her labile and irrational demands and expectations. He felt that Loni needed constant attention and reassurance and he was deeply troubled by her depressions and suicide attempts. Loni does not know what to do to get him back in her life and often feels that life is so hopeless that it is not worth living. Her suicide attempts are increasingly serious, and the last attempt would have been fatal had a friend not stopped by her house and, finding the door locked and sensing something was wrong, summoned the police.

Loni is highly depressed, often uncommunicative, and sits in the facility with a blank look on her face. After the initial first three days of hospitalization, during which she was placed on high levels of antidepressants to stabilize her and to reduce the threat of suicide, the medication dosage was reduced and her therapist was able to speak to her. Loni told her that she had little confidence in therapy, has had very poor experiences with therapists, recognizes that she has serious emotional problems, and does not feel optimistic that therapy will be helpful. Her depressions are worsening and the desire to end her life and to put herself out of the continuing misery she feels is becoming overwhelming. "I get up in the morning and I feel hopeless," she said. "I look at my paintings and I want to rip them up and throw them away. People say they're good but they seem artificial and dishonest to me. No one in my personal life can deal with my jealousy or my need to love and be loved. They think I'm oppressive. The therapists I've gone to give up on me right away. I can see it in the way they look at me. My parents don't talk to me anymore and my friends don't either. I feel alone and hopeless. The kind thing to do would be to let me get on with my plan to kill myself."

The therapist told Loni that these were serious problems that she didn't take lightly, but she felt there were many things that could be done to help Loni and urged her to go to the facility's library and do research on her condition using the available literature and the Internet. The therapist gave her a number of websites and thought that she might find other sources on the Internet regarding the best treatment for the symptoms Loni was experiencing. They would meet again the next day and discuss what Loni had found. While Loni thought the therapist was nice, she also wondered why she wasn't talking about the suicide attempt and the emotional pain Loni was in, and decided that the therapist was a "cold fish," but that she'd play along with her anyway.

Much to Loni's surprise, there were a number of very interesting studies that suggested treatments far different than the ones she'd had in the past. When she met with the therapist the next day, she brought the promising studies along and entered into a discussion of the best evidence for treating Loni's problems. The therapist urged Loni to continue searching for best evidence over the next few days, and when she had at least 10 studies that seemed in agreement, that they would establish a treatment regimen based upon the best evidence available in the literature. Several days later, they did just that. The plan they agreed upon was written and signed by Loni, the therapist, and the director of the facility. The plan was as follows:

1. Loni had to sign a "no suicide" contract. Once having signed it she was committed to sharing suicidal feelings with the staff and to enter into emergency treatment to prevent any suicide attempts.
2. Loni had to keep a record of the relationship between highly labile emotions and events in her life. She was to use that record in discussions with her therapist so they could construct patterns that led to dangerous emotions that might then lead to destructive behaviors.

3. She was to stop self-medicating by using drugs and alcohol and was to keep a record of her daily emotional life so that drug treatment could be monitored and evaluated. This also involved frequent use of psychological tests to evaluate her levels of depression and self-destructive thinking.
4. The focus on helping Loni was to contain dangerous behaviors and move toward stability in her life. This precluded love relationships until she was better prepared to handle them.
5. She was to write a letter to her parents asking if they might have contact with her and that meeting with them might hopefully lead to an improvement in her condition. She had never asked her parents to be part of her treatment before because she thought they were the cause of her problems.
6. She was to attend and be actively involved in group treatment and patient-management efforts. This meant establishing a helping involvement with other patients in the facility.
7. She was to begin her artwork again and the facility would set up an area for her to continue painting. She was not to destroy any work but would instead solicit feedback from others she respected and use that feedback in the development of her talent.
8. If she progressed in treatment, the facility had bungalows on the grounds where she could live more independently, although she would have the same treatment regimen as she presently had.
9. If treatment was successful and she no longer felt suicidal or worried about self-destructive or dangerous behaviors, plans would be made for her to live off the grounds but to be involved in the program on a daily basis. Therapy would continue.
10. Her progress would be constantly evaluated and any concerns she had about treatment, including the relationship with her therapist, would be discussed. She would agree to individual and group treatment even though she had concerns about both. It was her responsibility to share those concerns and to be involved in making the needed changes to improve the effectiveness of her therapy.
11. The facility agreed to make Loni a full partner in her treatment.

Loni stayed in the facility for six months before returning to independent living. The last two months were spent in a bungalow on the grounds of the facility. After leaving the facility and establishing independent living, she has been attending the facility's day program for eight months now. She has not attempted suicide since entering the facility, although she's had days when she is highly depressed. She self-medicates occasionally but not to the degree she did before her treatment began. She has a good working relationship with the therapist and staff. She can be difficult and manipulative at times, but always recognizes the behavior, apologizes, and tries to work on feelings and issues that may have led to the behavior. She is painting, enjoys moderate success, and has begun a relationship quite unlike those she was involved in prior to treatment. The young man in her life grew up with a borderline sister and understands and empathizes with Loni's emotional turmoil. He is supportive, encouraging, but also knows when to be up front with Loni. They attend a couples group and have found it helpful in resolving problems that would have ended the relationship for Loni in the past.

Loni has no illusions about her life. She understands that just as people have medical conditions that need constant monitoring, she has an emotional condition that requires monitoring and treatment. Keeping a daily log, attending the day program, working in a stable therapeutic relationship, and maintaining close contact with a psychiatrist to make certain her medications are working have all been helpful. In evaluating her treatment, Loni said: "I have no illusions. I'm a troubled person and I'll always be a troubled person. What the program did was to stabilize me and give me a sense of family. I love the people in the program as if they really were my family. I've been able to reestablish some contact with my real family, but years of trouble make it hard for us to get past a certain point. This program is expensive and it has allowed me to work, and paint, and try to pay back the facility. I'll be doing that all my life, and it's worth it. I know that others like me without money wouldn't have had the chance to get such wonderful treatment and I'm thankful I had my parents and their excellent insurance. I hate the label of being a borderline, but I am, and it's good that I can read the research and be involved in my treatment. Every day is a struggle and I don't know if I'd be honest to say that I'm over the hump. I feel better and I'm doing better. All I can do is to keep a watchful eye on myself and trust the people I work with to help me when I go off the deep end. You never know when that might happen and every day I pray that it won't."

In adding to Loni's evaluation of her situation, her therapist said: "Loni has come a long way, but she's absolutely right that every day is a challenge. This program seems to work for people with Loni's symptoms but it's a terribly expensive program and it offers no long-term solutions. We keep up on the latest research, constantly evaluate the effectiveness of our work, believe that clients should be in a cooperative relationship when it comes to their treatment, and learn from our successes and our failures. We spend a great deal of time in staff meetings poring over the literature and taking seriously our responsibility to use the best available evidence in treating our clients. The new research is exciting and hopeful, but we move cautiously. People with BPD have very high rates of suicide. One suicide attempt throws the staff into a long period of self-evaluation about whether we're doing the best we can for our clients."

15.10. SUMMARY

This chapter discusses three types of serious emotional problems in children and adolescents: Bi-polar disorder, schizophrenia and borderline personality disorder. Concerns were raised about the numbers of children who may be incorrectly diagnosed with bi-polar disorder and childhood schizophrenia and often unproven use of adult medications with potentially serious side effects. A case study suggested a treatment strategy with an adolescent experiencing borderline personality disorder.

15.11. QUESTIONS FROM THE CHAPTER

1 The case study of Loni proposes a treatment regimen out of most people's level of affordability. How might the same treatment be integrated into programs that are far less expensive and affordable for most clients with BPD?
2 Do you believe the use of labels with highly negative connotations such as those associated with personality disorders may assume a lifetime diagnosis with little likelihood of change? If that is the case, what might be some harmful outcomes of incorrectly assuming that an initial diagnosis will last throughout the life cycle?
3 How could anyone even think it is possible that 3- or 4-year-old could have childhood schizophrenia when studies suggest that schizophrenia almost never occurs in children that young?
4 Most children behave oddly from time to time. Do not you think we should focus on normal behavior instead of abnormal behavior and in that way say to children and their parents that it is OK to act differently from time to time and that it is only when different behavior becomes a problem that we should worry about it?
5 It is hard to understand how anyone could become psychotic unless there is some brain or biochemical malfunction. Do you think life traumas like war, abuse, and emotional maltreatment can cause children to become psychotic?

References

American Psychiatric Association. *Diagnostic and statistical manual of mental disorders.* 4th ed. Washington: APA, 1994.

Anthony, W. A. (1993). Recovery from mental illness: The guiding vision of the mental health service system in the 1990's. *Psychosocial Rehabilitation Journal, 16*, 12–23.

Asarnow, J. R., Thompson, M. C., & Goldstein, M. J. (1994). Childhood onset schizophrenia: A follow-up study. *Schizophrenia Bulletin, 20*, 599–617.

Bateman, A., & Fonagy, P. (1999). The effectiveness of partial hospitalization in the treatment of borderline personality disorder: a randomized controlled trial. *American Journal of Psychiatry, 156*, 1563–1569.

Bemporad, J. R., Smith, H. E., Hanson, G., & Cicchetti, D. (1982). Borderline syndromes in childhood: Criteria for diagnosis. *American Journal of Psychiatry, 139*, 596–601.

Carpenter, J. (2002). Mental health recovery paradigm: Implications for social work. *Health & Social Work, 27*(2), 86–94.

Chinman, M. J., Weingarten, R., Stayner, D., & Davidson, L. (2001). Chronicity reconsidered: Improving person-environment fit through a consumer-run service. *Community Mental Health Journal, 37*(3), 215–229.

Craig, D.Y. (2001). Managing borderline personality disorder. *Patient Care, 23*, 60–64.

Davidson, L., Chinman, M., Moos, B., Weingarten, R., Stayner, D. A., & Tebes, J. K. (1999). Peer support among individuals with severe mental illness: A review of the evidence. *Clinical Psychology: Science and Practice, 6*, 165–187.

Dixon, L., Krauss, N., & Lehman, A. L. (1994). Consumers as service providers: The promise and challenge. *Community Mental Health Journal, 30*, 615–625.

Drake, R. E., & Vaillant, G. E. (1985). A validity study of Axis II of DSM III. *American Journal of Psychiatry, 142*, 553–558.

Eggers, C., & Bunk, D. (1997). The long-term course of childhood-onset schizophrenia: A 42-year follow up. *Schizophrenia Bulletin, 23*, 105–117.

Felton, C. J., Stastny, P., Shern, D., Blanch, A., Donahue, S. A., Knight, E., & Brown, C. (1995). Consumers as peer specialists on intensive case management teams: Impact on client outcomes. *Psychiatric Services, 46*, 1037–1044.

Frey, R. J. (1999). Personality disorders. *Gale Encyclopedia of Medicine*. http://www.findarticles.com/cf_0/g2601/0010/2601001049/p1/article.jhtml?term = treating + personality + disorders.

Fristad, M. A., Goldberg-Arnold, J. S., & Gavazzi, S. M. (2003). Multifamily psychoeducation groups (MFPG) in the treatment of children with mood disorders. *Journal of Marital and Family Therapy, 29*(4), 491–504.

Geller, B., & Luby, J. (1997). Child and adolescent bipolar disorder: A review of the past 10 years. *Journal of the American Academy of Child and Adolescent Psychiatry, 36*, 1168–1176.

Geller, B., Williams, M., Zimmerman, B., Frazier, J., Beringer, L., & Warner, K. L. (1998). Prepubertal and early adolescent pibolarity differentiate from ADHD by manic symptoms, grandiose delusions, ultra-rapid or ultradian cycling. *Journal of Affective Disorders, 51*, 81–91.

Glicken, M. D. (2004). *Using the strengths perspective in social work practice*. Boston, MA: Pearson Education, Inc.

Glicken, M. D. (2005). *Improving the effectiveness of the helping professions: An evidence based approach to practice*. Thousand Oaks, CA: Sage.

Goldman, S. J., D'Angelo, E. J., & DeMaso, D. R. (1993). Psychopathology in the families of children and adolescents with borderline personality disorder. *American Journal of Psychiatry, 150*, 1832–1835.

Groopman, J. (2007, April 9). What's normal?. *New Yorker, 83*(7), 28–33.

Guzder, J., Paris, J., Zelkowitz, P., & Feldman, R. (1999, February). Psychological risk factors for borderline personality in school age children. *Journal of the American Academy of Child and Adolescent Psychiatry, 38*, 206–212.

Haines, C. (2005) Warning Signs of Schizophrenia http://www.webmd.com/ content/article/60/67138.htm?printing=true.

Harding, C. M., Brooks, G. W., Ashikaga, T., Strauss, J. S., & Breier, A. (1986a). The Vermont longitudinal study of persons with severe mental illness: I. Methodology, study sample, and overall status 32 years later. *American Journal of Psychiatry, 144*, 718–725.

Harding, C. M., Brooks, G. W., Ashikaga, T., Strauss, J. S., & Breier, A. (1986b). The Vermont longitudinal study of persons with severe mental illness: II. Long-term outcome of subjects who retrospectively met DSM-II criteria for schizophrenia. *American Journal of Psychiatry, 144*, 727–735.

Hollis, C. (2000). Adult outcomes of child- and adolescent-onset schizophrenia. Diagnostic stability and predictive validity. *Am J. Psychiatry, 157*, 1652–1659.

Huber, G., Gross, G., & Schuttler, R. (1975). A long-term follow up study of schizophrenia: Psychiatric course of illness and prognosis. *Acta Psychiatrica Scandinavica, 52*, 49–57.

Jackson, H., McGorry, P., Edwards, J., Hulbert, C., Henry, L., Francey, S., Maude, D., Cocks, J., Power, P., Harrigan, S., & Dudgeon, P. (1998). Cognitively-oriented psychotherapy for early psychosis (COPE): preliminary results. *British Journal of Psychiatry Supplement, 33*, 93–100.

Jimenez, M. A. (1988). Chronicity in mental disorders: Evolution of a concept. *Social Casework, 69*, 627–633.

Kazdin, A. E., Holland, L., Crowley, M., & Breton, S. (1997). Barriers to treatment participation scale: Evaluation and validation in the context of child outpatient treatment. *Journal of Child Psychology and Psychiatry, 38*(8), 1051–1062.

Kendall, P. C., Chu, B., Gifford, A., Hayes, C., & Nauta, M. (1998). Breathing new life into a manual: Flexibility and creativity with manual-based treatments. *Cognitive and Behavioral Practice, 5*, 177–198.

Kestenbaum, C. J. (1983). The borderline child at risk for major psychiatric disorder in adult life. In K. R. & Robson (Ed.), *The borderline child* (pp. 49–82). New York: McGraw Hill.

Koerner, K., & Linehan, M. M. (2000). Research on dialectical behavior therapy for patients with borderline personality disorder. *Psychiatric Clinics of North America, 23*(1), 151–167.

Kovacs, M., & Pollock, M. (1995). Bipolar disorder and comorbid conduct disorder in childhood and adolescence. *Journal of the American Academy of Child and Adolescence, 34*, 715–723.

Kruger, A. (2000). Schizophrenia: Recovery and hope. *Psychiatric Rehabilitation Journal, 24*, 29–37.

Kyrouz, E., & Humphreys, K. (1996). Do psychiatrically disabled people benefit from participation in self-help/mutual aid organizations? A research review. *The Community Psychologist, 29*, 21–25.

Lehman, C. (2003, January 17). Clinicians strive to avert frustration with BPD patients. *Psychiatric News, 38*(2), 29.

Lehtinen, K. (1993). Need-adapted treatment of schizophrenia: a five-year follow-up study from the Turku project. *Acta Psychiatrica Scandinavica, 87*, 96–101.

Manfred-Gilham, J. J., Sales, E., & Koeske, G. (2002). Therapist and case manager perceptions of client barriers to treatment participation and use of engagement strategies. *Community Mental Health Journal, 38*(3), 213–221.

Markowitz, F. E. (1998). The effects of stigma on the psychological well-being and life satisfaction of persons with mental illness. *Journal of Health & Social Behavior, 39*(4), 335–347.

Nasar, S. (1998). *A brilliant mind: the life of mathematical genius and Nobel Laureate John Nash*. New York: Simon and Schuster.

O'Connor, R. (2001). Active treatment of depression. *American Journal of Psychotherapy, 55*(4), 507–530.

Papolos, D. F., & Papolos, J. (1999). *The bipolar child: The definitive and reassuring guide to childhood's most misunderstood disorder*. New York: Broadway Books.

Paris, J. (2008). Borderline personality disorder: What is it, what causes it? How can we treat it? http://www.jwoodphd.com/borderline_personality_disorder.htm.

Penn, D. L., Waldheter, M. A., Perkins, D. O., Mueser, K. T., & Lieberman, J. A. (2005, December). Psychosocial treatment for first-episode psychosis: A research update. *American Psychiatric Association, 162*, 2220.

Prien, R. R., & Potter, W. Z. (1990). NIMH workshop on treatment of bipolar disorder. *Psychopharmacology Bulletin, 26*, 409–427.

Reidy, A. (1992). Shattering illusions of difference. *Resources, 4*, 3–6.

Remschmidt, H. E., Schultz, E., Martin, M., Warnke, A., & Trott, G. (1994). Childhood-onset schizophrenia: History of the concept and recent studies. *Schizophrenia Bulletin, 20*, 727–745.

Riessman, F. (1965). The helper-therapy principle. *Social Work, 10*, 27–32.

Robins, L. N., Tipp, J., & Przybeck, T. (1991). Antisocial personality. In L. N. Robins, D. A. & Regier (Eds.), *Psychiatric disorders in America* (pp. 258–290). New York: Macmillan.

Russell, A. T. (1994). The clinical presentation of childhood schizophrenia. *Schizophrenia Bulletin, 20*, 599–617.

Spencer, E. K., & Campbell, M. (1994). Children with schizophrenia: Phenomenology and pharmacology. *Schizophrenia Bulletin, 20*, 713–725.

State, R. C., Altshuler, L. L., & Frye, M. A. (2002). Mania and attention deficit hyperactivity disorder in a prepubertal child: Diagnostic and treatment challenges. *American Journal of Psychiatry, 159*(6), 918–925.

Stone, M. H. (1993). Long term outcome in personality disorders. *British Journal of Psychiatry, 162*, 299–313.

Tarrier, N., Lewis, S., Haddock, G., Bentall, R., Drake, R., Kinderman, P., Kingdon, D., Siddle, R., Everitt, J., Leadley, K., Benn, A., Grazebrook, K., Haley, C., Akhtar, S., Davies, L., Palmer, S., & Dunn, G. (2004). Cognitive-behavioural therapy in first-episode and early schizophrenia: 18-month follow-up of a randomised controlled trial. *British Journal of Psychiatry, 184*, 231–239.

Taylor, E. H. (1998). Advances in the diagnosis and treatment of children with serious mental illness. *Child Welfare, 77*, 311–332.

The Harvard Health Letter. (2007, May 11). *Bipolar Disorder in Children, 23*(11), 1–3.

The Harvard Mental Health Letter. (1997, December). *Copy Editor, 14*, 8.

Tolbert, H. A. (1996). Psychosis in children and adolescents: A review. *Journal of Clinical Psychiatry, 57*(3), 4–8.

Tsuang, M. T., Woolson, R. F., & Fleming, M. S. (1979). Long term outcome of major psychoses. *Archives of General Psychiatry, 36*, 1295–1301.

Turner, P., & Salzer, M. S. (2006). Consumer perspectives on quality of care in the treatment of schizophrenia. *Mental Health & Mental Health Service Research, 33*, 674–681.

Werry, J. S. (1992). Child and adolescent (early-onset) schizophrenia: A review in light of DSM-III-R. *Journal of Autism and Developmental Disorders, 22*, 601–624.

Woody, G. E., McLellan, T., Luborsky, L., et al. (1985). Sociopathy and psychotherapy outcome. *Archives of General Psychiatry, 42*, 1081–1086.

Wozniak, J., Biederman, J., Kiely, K., Ablon, J. S., Faraone, S. V., Mundy, E., et al. (1995). Mania-like symptoms suggestive of childhood-onset bipolar disorder in clinically referred children. *Journal of the American Academy of Child and Adolescent Psychiatry, 34*, 867–877.

Zanarini, M. C. (2000). Childhood experiences associated with the development of borderline personality disorder. *Psychiatric Clinics of North America, 23*(1), 89–101.

Zhang, M., Wang, M., Li, J., & Phillips, M. R. (1994). Randomised-control trial of family intervention for 78 first-episode male schizophrenic patients: an 18-month study in Suzhou Jiangsu. *British Journal of Psychiatry Supplement, 24*, 96–102.

Further reading

Gilbert, C. M. (1988). Children in women's shelters: A group intervention using art. *Journal of Child and Adolescent Psychiatric Nursing, 10*, 7–13.

Jacobsen, L. K., & Rapoport, J. L. (1998). Research update: Childhood schizophrenia: Implications of clinical and neurobiological research. *Journal of Child Psychology and Psychiatry, 39*, 101–113.

16 Evidence-Based Practice with Serious and Terminal Illness, Disabilities and Bereavement in Children and Adolescents

16.1. INTRODUCTION

Four serious health-related issues will be discussed in this chapter: Serious and terminal illness, disabilities, and prolonged bereavement. Significant personal growth often takes place when people cope with life threatening illnesses and bereavement. Kubler-Ross (1969/1997) believes that terminal illness frequently leads to life-changing growth. Greenstein and Breitbart (2000) write that "[e]xistentialist thinkers, such as Frankl, view suffering as a potential springboard, both for having a need for meaning and for finding it" (p. 486), while Frankl (1978) writes, "Even facing an ineluctable fate, for example, an incurable disease, there is still granted to man a chance to fulfill even the deepest possible meaning. What matters, then, is that the stand he takes in his predicament ... the attitude we choose in suffering" (p. 24).

Finn (1999) believes that spirituality becomes an important aspect of terminal illness because it leads to "an unfolding consciousness about the meaning of human existence. Life crises influence this unfolding by stimulating questions about the meaning of existence" (p. 487).

16.2. COPING WITH DISABILITIES

The U.S. Census Bureau (2000) indicates that the overall number of children served by special school programs for disabled children and adolescents grew from 3.72 million in 1977 to 5.68 million in 2000, an increase of 53%. The percent change per 100 000 between 1980 and 2000 in disabled children served were as follows: Children with health impairments: 169%; children with learning disabilities: 148%, and developmental delay: 390%; children with physical handicaps: 108%, children with emotional problems: 58%; children with traumatic brain injuries: 137% and children with autism: 215%.

Finn (1999) reports that "there are an estimated 1.7 million people with disabilities who are homebound and an additional 12.5 million who are temporarily homebound. There also are many caretakers of disabled youth who are essentially homebound as a result of their responsibilities at home" (p. 220). Finn (1999, p. 220) goes on to say that a number of social and emotional problems develop from being "alienated" or "socially quarantined" from the larger society, including depression, loneliness, alienation, lack of social interaction, lack of information and lack of access to employment (Braithwaite, 1996; Coleman, 1997; Shworles, 1983). In a study of the impact of physical and emotional disabilities, Druss et al. (2000) write that:

> *Combined mental and general medical disabilities were associated with high levels of difficulty across a variety of functional domains: bed days, perceived stigma, employment status, disability payments, and reported discrimination. These findings may best be understood by the fact that co-morbid conditions, unlike either mental or general medical conditions alone, are most commonly associated with deficits spanning several domains of function. In turn, respondents with deficits across multiple domains have few areas of intact function available to make up for their existing deficits. The uniquely high levels of functional impairment associated with combined conditions speak to the potential importance of integrated programs that can simultaneously address an individual's medical and psychiatric needs. (p. 1489)*

Finn (1999) studied the content of messages sent by people with disabilities using the Internet as a form of group therapy. He found that most correspondents wanted to talk about their health and about specific issues of treatment and quality of care, but that overall, the correspondents acted as a support group helping others cope with emotional, medical, and social issues. These issues included "highly technical descriptions of medications, procedures, and equipment to subjective accounts of treatment experiences. There also was considerable discussion of interpersonal relationship issues such as marital relationships, dating, and sexuality" (p. 228). Finn (1999) reminds us that many disabled people are homebound and that the Internet becomes an important part of the communicating they do each day. This is particularly true for homebound people who may also have difficulty speaking or hearing.

The author worked with profoundly disabled teens and young adults in the early part of his career. Many of the accidents that resulted in disabilities were either athletic in nature or the result of very impulsive behavior, either during the use of substances or following an event which left the person depressed or in great stress. Working in a rehabilitation center in Minneapolis, the majority of our patients were young men who had, for example, driven a motorcycle into a tree while very drunk. Another had dived into an empty swimming pool after he and his girlfriend broke up. Yet another had fallen from a building he was working on after a night of drinking and getting chewed out by the job site foreman. Many of the patients were suicidal after the accidents and not a few committed suicide. This is not to say that all accidents resulting in disability are the fault of the victim, because that is not the case. What is true is that many of the disabled young, even with the best of help, are profoundly depressed and suicidal. The following case is an example. Apologies to the reader for the language in the next case, but for those of you who work with adolescents or are about to, this really is often the way they talk when they are upset.

16.3. CASE STUDY: EVIDENCE-BASED PRACTICE WITH A HOMEBOUND DISABLED ADOLESCENT

Ginnie is a 14-year-old young woman with quadriplegia from a recent trampoline accident. She is profoundly disabled with only a small amount of ability to use her hands and must be cared for at home by her family and by community caregivers. She is too disabled to attend school because of the amount of time and the cost to drive her to school, although the school is providing tutoring via the Internet and some limited in-home instruction. Ginnie was an active and athletic young woman who did very well in school and had many friends. A year after the accident she is despondent and talks frequently about suicide. The worker providing case management to Ginnie is worried that she may become actively suicidal. Like many suicidal disabled youth, she knows a number of ways to kill herself and has begun contacting other quads on the Internet to share their thoughts about suicide and the unique methods many of them have learned about.

The case manager, a trained MFT with 10 years of experience with disabled youth, has begun seeing Ginnie at home in therapy sessions. Ginnie is silent most of the time and often cries. When she *does* talk it is usually about how her friends have forgotten her and how a best friend stopped coming by after her catheter malfunctioned and urine spilled all over the floor. Ginnie believes that her life is over. She told the worker, "You tell me life is worth living but how would you like to be stuck in the house tied to machines, smelling your own shit all day long. It's disgusting. I'm disgusting. Look at me. My legs are like sticks. I used to be cute but now I'm just a thing. Stop telling me how wonderful life is. It stinks. That's what I think and you would too if you were me."

The worker has seen similar behavior in newly traumatized adolescents and she knows the potential for suicide is great. She has been unable to get a non-suicide contract from Ginnie and has had to share her concerns with her family and to inform them of the more common ways quads attempt suicide. The family has promised to watch Ginnie closely but fear for her life. A double trauma in so short a period of time would be devastating, they told the worker and believe that in time Ginnie will regain her zest for life if she can just get over her anguish about the accident.

The worker has gone to the literature on disabilities and suicide and found the following: There is painfully little in the literature on predicting or preventing suicide in adolescent clients with serious disabilities. The literature is fairly clear that most adolescent suicide victims have at least one emotional disorder, usually severe depression, such that treatment attrition is a significant problem with depressed adolescents. Too little is known about the best treatment for potential adolescent suicide victims, although cognitive therapy is mentioned with caution since there is not strong research evidence as yet of its efficacy with potential adolescent suicide victims (Barbe et al., 2004; Compton et al., 2004; Friedberg and McClure, 2002). Barbe et al. (2004) report that "up to 60% of adolescent suicide victims have a depressive disorder at the time of death" (p. 44). If cognitive therapy is used, it should be used with considerable care since the assertive nature of the approach can often be misinterpreted by clients as being insensitive and uncaring, conditions that one would not want to convey to a client as depressed and despondent as Ginnie.

With this limited base to go on, the worker decided to use a very gentle form of cognitive-behavioral therapy with Ginnie. She began by asking Ginnie if she had any unfinished business she wanted to discuss. The following is a short interchange from this initial session:

Ginnie (G): What do you mean unfinished?

Worker (W): People you'd like to talk about. Anything you'd like to say to me or anyone else.

G: I'd like to tell my ex-boyfriend to kiss my ass. Is that what you mean?

W: Yes.

G: Yeah, sure, like he's going to come see me while I tell him what a jerk he is.

W: Maybe not, but we can role play what you'd say.

G: Ha!You don't look like him at all.

W: But if he was here, what would you say to him?

G: I'd tell him what a fucking prick he is.

W: Say it to him like he's here. Talk to him not me.

G: OK. You fucking prick, if you weren't pushing me to be so great on the trampoline, I wouldn't be here in this bed, you fucking asshole. You kept saying to go higher and make more rotations, and look at what happened to me? And then you have the nerve to stop seeing me (begins to sob).

W: (Let's Ginnie cry for a while). So you have a lot to tell him.

G: Yeah, and those friends of mine, too. They were there. They were saying, 'you can do it, go girl.' And when I broke my neck, they took off. Did you know that? My good friends. They left me on the floor of the gym with a broken neck. I haven't seen any of them since. I'd like to kill everyone of them. It was the janitor who found me and called the ambulance. My doctor said that if I'd been seen earlier maybe they could have saved some of my functioning, but they don't know.

W: There's a lot to be mad about, Ginnie, but taking it out on yourself isn't the best way to get even.

G: What is? Maybe I could hire someone to break their necks?

W: Or maybe you could start getting on with life and living it to its fullest. Maybe it's time to go to school and get out of the house. Maybe it's time to start making new friends.

G: Go to school, looking like this? Everyone will laugh at me.

W: There are schools specializing in kids with disabilities. No one laughs at anyone at those schools.

G: Schools for gimps and cripples, huh?

W: No. Serious schools for kids like you. Smart, funny, serious kids who had accidents like you had and now are getting on with their lives. I'd like to take you to a school I think you'd enjoy but I have to get your word that you won't do anything self-destructive. It's really important, Ginnie, that you give me your word you won't try and hurt yourself.

G: Ha! What a joke. Since you talked to my family they watch me like a hawk. It's like being in jail.

W: Time to get out of jail and smell the roses, huh?

G: Yeah, better than smelling my own shit.

After several more sessions, the worker and Ginnie and her parents went to see the new school. It is a residential school and Ginnie, in true adolescent style, said she hated it, that everyone was a gimp, and how could she go to a place like that? But later she spoke to the worker.

G: You think I'd like being there?

W: What do you think?

G: I sort of liked the guy who showed us around. He was pretty cute, and he's like my age and a former jock. I could get along with him.

W: Anything else?

G: The rooms aren't so bad, but having a roommate. I don't know. The food wasn't bad. Better than the dog crap I eat at home.

W: So?

G: I don't know, Barb. I'm pretty pissed off about everything that happened. I don't see much of a future. The people online who have blogs say they're in pain all the time and they get urinary tract infections, and they can't work, and living in boarding homes for gimps, they get treated bad.

W: What about the people who do well?

G: Yeah, there are those people. I've been online with a guy who's a quad and he's going to high school and doing well. He has a scholarship to some Ivy League school. He's like a genius or something. He says it's the shits to be a quad but he got over feeling sorry for himself and he's doing OK. He doesn't bullshit me at all. He's a computer whiz and he sends me all kinds of things to cheer me up. Cartoons and stuff like that.

W: So, why not think about it. It's close enough for your family to visit.

G: Yeah, I will. I'll think about it, Barb, and don't worry, I'm too chicken to do anything to myself. Puck, puck, puck.

After waffling for several months and continuing on in treatment, Ginnie agreed to attend the residential school where she is now a sophomore. She has done well academically and has made friends, but she continues to have bouts of depression and receives individual and group therapy and a mild anti-depressive. The worker sees her frequently and sometimes Ginnie is in despair. "I didn't do anything to deserve this, Barb," she told the worker. "I'm just a kid and I'll be in this bed and a wheel chair all my life." The worker sits and listens. She knows that were it herself in Ginnie's position, she'd probably feel the same way.

On their last visit, Ginnie said to the worker: "You made me think a lot when we talked about the best way to get back at people by being happy and successful. I found out from a friend that nobody talks to my ex and my ex-friends and that they think they're dirtballs for leaving me after the accident. They aren't worth ruining my life over, are they. That's what I think."

16.4. SERIOUS AND FATAL ILLNESS

Howarth (1972) reports that in a comparison of children with leukemia, cystic fibrosis and a non-fatal illness, children with leukemia and cystic fibrosis had a 40% higher incidence of psychiatric disorders than the non-fatal group. Although a causal relationship between family disturbance and the child's behavior was not demonstrated, there were clearly some families in whom the stress of a fatally ill child opened up widespread cracks in their functioning. The parents in particular need support, and any improvement in the family atmosphere will probably also alleviate indirectly the sick child's emotional disturbance. Almost without exception, the parents interviewed were eager to talk and ventilate their feelings. Many were very isolated, not just from friends and relations, but even from husband or wife, often for fear of causing the other distress by talking about their ill child. They need to be given time to talk and express their concerns.

Hardwig (2000) reports that terminally ill patients are often unable to deal with unfinished business in their lives because they feel abandoned by friends, family, their bodies, and by God. "Many [dying patients] find that the beliefs and values they have lived by no longer seem valid or do not sustain them. These are the ingredients of a spiritual crisis, the stuff of spiritual suffering" (Hardwig, 2000, p. 29). Hardwig (2000) believes that the medical care system complicates the client's ability to finish unfinished business because it often makes many treatment decisions without actually consulting the terminally ill patient, and that the use of medication often limits the patient's ability to think clearly. Loved ones may interfere with the patient's need to find closure on important family issues that may complicate and prolong bereavement. And since families often find it impossible to allow a loved one to die naturally, they may deny the patient's wish to die and prolong life by allowing the use of intrusive life supports and treatments.

While Caffrey (2000) believes there is a role for psychotherapy with terminal illness, he thinks that the reduction of anxiety and depression in dying patients (palliative care) is narrow-minded. In considering palliative care versus help with unfinished meaning-of-life issues, McClain et al. (2003) found that low levels of spirituality in terminally ill patients were highly related to "end-of-life despair, providing a unique contribution to the prediction of hopelessness, desire for hastened death, and suicidal ideation even after controlling for the effect of depressive symptoms and other relevant variables" (p. 1606). The authors report that high levels of spirituality in dying patients leads to hopefulness that results in a more cooperative relation with the treatment team, improved resolution of long-standing emotional problems, and the desire to live longer. As Kubler-Ross (1969/1997) wrote, "We can help them die by trying to help them live" (Caffrey, 2000, p. 519).

Lloyd-Williams (2001) found depression in 25% of the terminally ill patients he has screened, and cautions that depression seriously affects the success of medical treatment in prolonging life and helping the patient finish important unfinished business. Lloyd-Williams (2001, p.35) suggests the following treatment strategies with terminally ill patients to treat depression: (1) establish good rapport; (2) diagnose and treat emotional problems; (3) treat underlying organic problems which may be contributing to the depression; (4) differentiate normal sadness and grief from serious depression; (5) provide supportive therapy and reduce the patients' level of isolation from others; (6) provide family treatment and support if called for; and (7) use anti-depressives in selective cases.

Blundo (2001) believes that clinicians must make a substantial shift in their work with terminally ill patients in crisis. This shift requires that we engage clients in a highly collaborative dialogue that begins without any preconceived ideas of underlying pathology. Greenstein and Breitbart (2000) report that collaborative relationships with terminally ill patients often result in "patients reordering their priorities, spending more time with family, and experiencing personal growth through the very fact of having had to cope with their traumatic loss or illness" (p. 486).

Commenting on the environment in which patients who are terminally ill reside, Richman (2000) notes the need for an empathic and caring approach to terminal illness, and reports that a study of empathy found that 40% of the caregivers of patients whose physicians were described by patients as non-empathetic had symptoms of depression, while 27% of the caregivers whom patients described as empathic reported depression. Patients with non-empathic physicians "were more likely to consider euthanasia or doctor-assisted suicide" (p. 485).

In a finding that could have implications for the terminally ill, Finn (1999) studied the content of messages sent by people with disabilities using the Internet. He found that most people using the Internet wanted to discuss their health and to find out about specific issues of treatment and quality of care. Correspondents functioned as a support group by helping one another cope with emotional, medical, and social concerns which included, "highly technical descriptions of medications, procedures, and equipment to subjective accounts of treatment experiences. There also was considerable discussion of interpersonal relationship issues such as marital relationships, dating, and sexuality" (p. 228). Since many terminally ill people are homebound, the Internet becomes a significant part of the communicating they do each day. This is particularly true of terminally ill people who may have difficulty speaking or hearing.

16.5. A CASE STUDY: EVIDENCE-BASED PRACTICE WITH A TERMINALLY ILL ADOLESCENT

This case study first appeared in modified form in a book the author did on evidence-based practice (Glicken, 2005, pp. 203–207). The author wishes to that Sage Publications for permission to reprint this material.

Jacob Peterson is a 16-year-old high school student who has been diagnosed with advanced testicular cancer. Jacob had been experiencing discomfort and pain for over a year, but failed to seek medical help until he began noticing blood in his urine. The cancer metastasized quickly and has moved into a number of organs in his body. The doctor gives him less than a year to live. He has had surgery to remove both testicles and is on chemotherapy. Neither procedure seems to be helping. Jacob is depressed and ill from the chemotherapy treatments. He is seriously thinking of asking one of his schoolmates to buy some poison and help him commit suicide. His personal physician has recommended that Jacob seek help for the depression, but Jacob has been too depressed and weak to even consider it. A hospital social worker dropped by his room during one of his reactions to chemo when he was too ill to return home. The social worker sat and listened to Jacob talk about how angry he was that something like this could happen to him at such a young age. Jacob told her, "I used to be a happy kid with a girlfriend and a chance to play college baseball and look at me now. I'm bald and bloated and no one even comes to see me in the hospital anymore."

Talking to the social worker seemed strangely comforting, and when the social worker suggested that they continue talking the next day, uncharacteristically, Jacob agreed. Jacob hates the feminizing way helping professionals make him feel, and described what it felt like going to a school counselor when he first learned about his cancer and the terminal diagnosis. "I felt like he didn't care. He was just saying words that were supposed to be soothing but just pissed me off about how this would be a meaningful experience and I had a chance to make up with people I'd had arguments with, and shit like that. It really pissed me off so bad I almost slugged him. There's nothing meaningful about dying at 16, and anyone who thinks there is, is completely fucked."

The social worker seemed much more understanding than the counselor. As Jacob continued seeing the worker on a bi-weekly basis, he shared his life disappointments with her. She listened and observed that he was being very hard on himself. She felt that Jacob had done amazing things in his life. Jacob was not so sure he agreed and wondered if the worker was just trying to placate him as he moved toward death. The worker assured him that she did not believe placating ever worked, but it certainly would not work with a highly intelligent young man like Jacob. As Jacob thought about their conversations, he began to realize that he had been successful in many small and large ways, but that an inner voice, the voice of his father, kept insisting that he had been a failure. Gradually, the inner voice changed and Jacob felt that he was beginning to see what the worker meant. He also felt better physically, although his health was declining and death was imminent.

Jacob decided that he would return to school even if he did not make it through the semester. He felt he would be a much more considerate student and friend than he had been before his illness. He also decided to talk to everyone with whom he had stopped talking because of real or imagined conflicts. This included his father, his former girlfriend and several friends he had actually gotten into physical fights with when they had all had too much to drink. As Jacob began to talk to old friends and members of his family, he felt elated at being able to resolve old hurts before he died. The people he spoke to felt the same way and said that they had missed Jacob and were happy to have him back in their lives.

Jacob made it through the semester and, with a good deal of help from his doctors, through the next semester. By the time death was only days away, Jacob had developed a support network that consisted of estranged friends, family members, fellow students he only knew vaguely, and the terminally ill young and older people he had met in the hospital during his treatment. Before he passed away, Jacob told the worker,

> *"You saved my life. I was full of a lot of crap inside before we started talking, and now I know this sounds dumb because, hell, I'm going to die soon, but I feel happy. I think I've made a difference in people's lives the past year. I think I lived longer because I was able to get rid of a lot of the crap I had inside. You always treated me like an adult and you made me see that I wasn't a loser like I thought when all this happened. Feeling so good about myself helped me live longer. The doc said I'd die six months ago but here I am. I think it helped to make up with people. Like my doctor said, every day I live is a gift from God."*

In describing her work with Jacob, the worker said, like many dying patients, Jacob was very angry. He had his mind set on suicide because of the pain he was in and because he felt so helpless. Like most adolescents, death was not something he had ever considered. He had always thought he had control over his life and now he had no control at all. Helping him see his strengths, respecting his anger, encouraging his need to finish unfinished business, and watching his transformation from an angry and resentful teenager to a loving and kind person has been a very special experience for me. I see it so often that when people search for endings which include resolving old conflicts, they live longer, happier, and more pain-free lives. While death is not pleasant, I think people like Jacob die peacefully.

"One of the main helping approaches I used with Jacob was behavioral charting. We found several articles in the literature about people who had dealt with serious disabilities by charting their progress each day through their physical rehabilitation and then during their jobs and personal lives. We devised goal attainment scales with realistic expectations. Jacob liked the idea that he could assist his treatment by maintaining good health habits and that diet and exercise might have a very positive impact on prolonging his life. He created an elaborate chart, with some help from his school friends, one of whom is very good at math and science, which measured a number of different variables such as calorie and fat intake, sleep, how long it took to dress and shower, fatigue at certain hours of the day, and the times when he needed to rest. He could see that while his condition was terminal, he actually felt better and functioned better than he had at the beginning of the charting.

"The anticipation of meeting goals had a very positive impact on him physically and emotionally. He gained weight, he enjoyed the taste of food where before he hardly noticed what he ate, and his grades in school improved considerably. The charting also helped him understand how the illness was affecting him. He knew that mornings were his best time and arranged his school schedule to attend classes in the morning. He found that he sometimes became depressed at night and decided that being with friends and family helped lessen his depression. The end result was not only a happier and more fulfilled person, but someone who actually lived a year longer than his physicians had expected.

I see real value in helping terminally ill people, and I am certain his loved ones, while very saddened by his death, had a much more gentle and positive bereavement than they would have had without treatment. There are significant benefits to helping people deal with their terminal illness. We should not deny them the opportunity to grow and expand any more than we would with clients with other types of problems. In Jacob's view, he grew more in the last year of life than he had in the previous 16.

16.6. JACOB'S BEHAVIORAL CHART

The following goals represent a partial list of more than 40 goals Jacob developed in his behavioral chart.

1. Brought his weight back to his pre-diagnosed state. He achieved 80% of the goal, but the chemotherapy treatments made him nauseous and it was sometimes difficult for him to eat regularly.
2. Walked at least a mile a day when not hospitalized. He surpassed this goal by averaging 2 miles a day.
3. Improved his GPA in school from a C-average to at least a B average. He surpassed this goal with his last set of classes when he achieved a B+ average.
4. Improved sleeping from an average of 2 h a night to at least 6 h. Because the pain often kept him awake, he slept an average of 5 h a night, but napped in the afternoon for another hour.
5. Had dinner or attended a social or family event at least two times a week. He surpassed this goal by increasing social activities from less than once a week to five times a week.
6. Used biofeedback and other behavioral techniques to reduce pain and dependence on painkillers. At the start of the charting, Jacob was averaging eight Vicadin a day. When he entered the hospital the final time before he died, he was taking only two for very intense pain.
7. Used positive feedback and supportive statements with friends, family, students and treatment staff. Jacob went from no supportive or positive statements (most were neutral or negative) to more than 40 positive statements a day. Examples included words like "thanks," "that was really helpful," "well done," "I really appreciate what you did for me," and so on. Neutral statements were silence, and negative statements included such typical statements Jacob used to make as, "Stop being such an incompetent jerk," "When are you going to learn to do things right?" and, "How can anyone so stupid be a nurse?"
8. Finishing unfinished business. Jacob made a long list of people he wanted to see to apologize for past hurts and misunderstandings or just to reconnect with them because he had missed their company. Jacob had been very reclusive before working with the hospital social workers, but saw everyone on his list at least once and sometimes more before he died. He added names to the list when it became apparent he would finish it fairly easily.

9. Tried to involve himself in his family's religious practices. This was a less successful activity, but he attended Sunday services most Sundays and while they did not move him much, he liked meeting friends and neighbors and joining them for meals after services were completed.

16.7. BEREAVEMENT

Balk (1999) writes that bereavement is the loss of a significant person in one's life. This loss can result in long-lasting physical and emotional problems, including fear and anger, sleeping disturbances, substance abuse, cognitive difficulties and uncharacteristic risk-taking that may also significantly affect relationships with others. Jacobs and Prigerson (2000) warn that bereavement sometimes develops into a complicated or prolonged grief lasting more than a year. The symptoms of complicated grief include intrusive thoughts about the deceased, numbness, disbelief that a loved one has passed away, feeling confused, and a diminished sense of security. Prolonged grief may be unresponsive to interpersonal therapy or to the use of antidepressants.

Black and Urbanowicz (1985, 1987) surveyed parents regarding the length of grief reactions by children after the death of loved ones and found that grieving children have higher levels of emotional difficulties than non-grieving children for up to 2 years, and up to 40% of grieving children have emotional difficulties 1 year after bereavement. Weller et al. (1991) found that over a third of the pre-adolescent children studied had a major depressive disorder 1 year after bereavement. Rutter (1966) reported that very young children grieving the death of a loved one had five times the psychiatric disorders when compared to the general population. When an older sibling dies who previously assumed some of the parental responsibilities in the home, the child's reaction may be similar in severity to the death of a parent. Regarding prolonged bereavement, Black (1998) reports that a small number of children may experience more severe forms of grieving, particularly if they had something to do with the death of a parent or have experienced several traumatic bereavements in a short period of time. Adolescents who express suicidal ideas may also be at risk of a more serious and prolonged bereavement.

However, Harrington and Harrison (1999) point out that much of the research on bereavement with children and adolescents lacks objective methodologies, and as such, the conclusion that children often experience prolonged bereavement may not be valid. In fact, in their review of published research on childhood bereavement, they conclude that "[e]xisting data suggest that childhood bereavement is not a major risk factor for mental and behavioral disorder in either childhood or adult life. Indeed, some studies indicate that most children cope surprisingly well with this severe form of trauma" (p. 232). The relative immaturity of children may protect them from complications of bereavement because children seem to be much less prone to depression than adolescents or adults (Angold et al., 1998). The authors concede however that some children and their families will require help, particularly when children have prior emotional problems or when there are substantial problems within the family that make resolution of grief difficult.

Stroebe (2001) points out a number of problems with the grief work usually done to treat prolonged bereavement by suggesting that there is limited empirical evidence that resolving grief is a more effective process than letting it resolve naturally. Stroebe (2001) says that resolving prolonged bereavement is complicated by very different ways of resolving grief as prescribed by cultures, religions, genders, and socio-economic groups, and writes, "There is no convincing evidence that other cultural prescriptions are less conducive to adaptation than those of our own" (p. 654). Stroebe is also concerned that traditional treatments for grief work seem to be primarily concerned about complicated grief and lack precise definitions useful for research studies such that the researcher must ask, "What is being worked through? In what way?" (p. 655).

In trying to resolve these issues, Stroebe (2001) suggests that the following issues need to be studied in more detail: (1) What are the coping skills that allow some people to cope with loss while others do not? (2) What are the differences between normal and prolonged grief? (3) What are the primary reasons that some people resolve their grief in natural ways while others experience complicated and prolonged bereavements? (4) Is an existential approach to grief work in which meaning of life issues are dealt with any more effective than focusing on removal of grief-related symptoms? (5) Do those who resolve their grief naturally and in a normal period of time experience their grief later and, if so, is it a more severe grief than those who experience prolonged grief?

16.8. BEST EVIDENCE FOR GRIEF WORK

Black and Urbanowicz (1987) report that in a controlled trial of family therapy with children who had lost a parent, the incidence of emotional difficulty dropped from 40% at 1 year to 20% after six sessions of family therapy which focused on shared mourning and open discussion about the dead parent.

Piper et al. (2002) studied the relationship between the expression of positive affect in group therapy and favorable treatment outcomes for complicated (long lasting) grief. The authors found a strong positive correlation between these two variables in a number of therapy groups studied. The authors believe that positive affect (smiles, nods in agreement, sympathetic looks) conveys optimism in the person and has a positive effect on others in the group. The authors also found that positive affect correlates well with a cooperative attitude and a desire by clients to do the work necessary to resolve the complicated and traumatic grief they were experiencing. This was true regardless of the type of treatment that was offered, and no difference was seen in the effectiveness of cognitive behavioral approaches or interpersonal approaches. Client affect rather than the approach used was the overriding factor in successful resolution of prolonged grief, according to the authors.

Kendall (1994) found cognitive-behavioral therapy to be effective with children suffering from separation anxiety after the death of a loved one. The author reports that treated children had reduced fears, less anxiety, better social skills, and lower scores on depression scales. These gains continued in follow up a year after the end of treatment. The author is uncertain if this same finding would be applicable to adults suffering from prolonged grief.

Jacobs and Prigerson (2000) report that self-help groups have been an effective adjunct treatment to professional therapy by "offering the inculcation of hope, the development of understanding, social supports, a source of normalization or universalization, and a setting to learn and practice new coping skills" (p. 487). Raphael (1977) studied a 3-month psychodynamically-oriented intervention for high-risk, acutely traumatized widows during the first stages of grief. The author defined high risk as the lack of support by a social network, the suddenness or unexpected nature of the death, high levels of anger and guilt, ambivalent feelings about the marital relationship, and the presence of other life crises related to or predating the death of a spouse. The predating life crises were often financial, work-related, and involved children, substance abuse in the spouse of widow, or marital infidelity. When compared to the control group, the treatment group had better general health, was less anxious and depressed, and had fewer somatic symptoms. Marmar et al. (1988) compared brief psychodynamic therapy to a self-help group and found that both groups experienced diminished stress and improved social functioning. However, improvement in grief-related symptoms began at the end of treatment and continued on thereafter, making the researchers wonder if the improvement was caused by treatment or whether it was a delayed response to grief which would have taken place in time, with or without treatment.

Sireling et al. (1988) compared "guided mourning" with a control group instructed to avoid cues that might bring about memories of their grief. The treated group had a reduction in distress and physical problems related to their grief which was maintained for up to 9 months in follow-up studies. Kleber and Brom (1987) successfully used exposure and relaxation treatment, hypnosis, and brief psychodynamic therapy in clients experiencing prolonged grief of more than 5 years, and noted sustained improvement of symptoms in follow-up studies. The authors noted that low income clients benefited more from behavioral approaches than from psychodynamic therapy.

Because of their concern that traumatic grief should be considered a separate diagnostic category because of its unique set of symptoms, Jacobs and Prigerson (2000) call for the development of a specific therapy for the treatment of grief. By specific therapy they suggest one that "focuses on separation distress and relevant elements of traumatic distress and that addresses several tasks (such as educating about the nature of these types of distress), helps individuals to cope with the distress, and mitigates the distress using a variety of strategies" (p. 491).

To help provide diagnostic guidance for the assessment of prolonged grief, Jacobs and Prigerson (2000, p. 496) suggest the following symptoms lasting more than 2 months and having significant negative impact on social functioning: (1) frequent attempts not to remember the deceased; (2) feelings of hopelessness, meaningless, and futility; (3) a sense of emotional detachment and numbness; (4) feelings of shock; (5) difficulty accepting the death of a loved one; (6) difficulty imagining their lives without the presence of the deceased; (7) a lost sense of security; (8) assuming the physical and emotional symptoms of the deceased person, including negative behaviors; and (9) considerable signs of anger and bitterness toward the deceased.

16.9. CASE STUDY: EVIDENCE-BASED PRACTICE WITH AN ADOLESCENT'S PROLONGED GRIEF

Ellen Stern is a 15-year-old 10th grader whose father passed away suddenly following a major heart attack several years ago. She has a brother 14, and a sister 10. Her father Frank was obsessed with good health and worked out daily, often at the expense of spending time with his family. Frank began experiencing chest pains in the middle of the night. As is the case with some heart victims in extreme denial, he went to the gym at 4:00 a.m. and began vigorously working out until he passed out and was pronounced dead at the scene. Ellen's mother was left with a large number of debts, no insurance, and no health benefits, since Frank was self-employed and was trying to save money. She and the children get a social security survivors pension, but it is not enough to cover basic costs and she has had to apply for welfare to cover medical expenses.

Her father passed away over 2 years ago, but Ellen has traumatic grief as indicated by severe depression, high levels of anxiety, very angry and intrusive thoughts about her father and the condition he left the them in, and obsessive thoughts about what she wished she had said to him before he died – uncomplimentary and angry remarks which would convey her depth of despair and anger over the current situation in the family. She feels guilty about these intrusive thoughts about her father but her mother's anguish at the death and the financial problems they are left with have changed their lives for the worse. From being a happy teenager with thoughts of attending a good college, Ellen now has to work after school to help the family out and care for a depressed mother and two siblings who are also having symptoms of prolonged grief. Her schoolwork has suffered, and 2 years after the death of her father her physician referred Ellen to a therapist when she continued to complain of the symptoms of prolonged grief long after her father's death.

Ellen's therapist met with her and they immediately began a discussion of what was keeping Ellen from resolving her feelings of grief. Ellen was stymied, so the therapist suggested that she make a list of everything that came to mind and that she also do a literature search into the typical causes of prolonged grief and the best evidence of how to treat it so that they might continue the discussion at the next session. Ellen was initially angry that she was asked to do work that the therapist should be doing for her, and complained to her referring physician, who encouraged Ellen to give it a little more time. She half-heartedly did what the therapist had asked of her and came only slightly prepared for further discussion at the next meeting.

When asked why she was not better prepared, Ellen became angry and confrontational. "You haven't even said you're sorry about my loss," she said, and angrily confronted the therapist for doing what her mother was currently doing to her: Leaving major decisions up to Ellen. The therapist said she appreciated the feedback and *did* feel badly about Ellen's loss. Still, she wondered why Ellen was unprepared and explained that only by working together could they resolve Ellen's painful and extended grief. Ellen promised to do more work in preparation for the next session. With the help of her precocious and computer literate 14-year-old brother, she was able to find Internet articles that seemed to very clearly explain why her grief was not going away and what she might do about it.

The next session with the therapist was very business-like and purposeful. Ellen was excited about what she had read, described it to her therapist, and together they planned the following strategy to treat Ellen's symptoms of prolonged grief: (1) Ellen needed to discuss all of the reasons for her anger at her father. The therapist urged her to write them down and to bring the list with her the next time they met. Before she could resolve her anger, she had to be clear about why she was so angry. (2) If there was anything she could directly do about her anger, she would do it. Examples were trying to develop a financial strategy to help with college and ways of shifting some of the responsibilities of caring for the family to her mother and her siblings. (3) She would begin involvement in a self-help group for adolescents with prolonged grief begun by a remarkable woman who had also gone through a complicated grief after the death of her 15-year-old son in a car crash. (4) Ellen would be seen by a psychiatrist to evaluate the use of anti-depressive medications and to supervise the medical treatment of her depression. (5) She would start a daily regimen of exercise and diet available at her high school. (6) Her spiritual and religious ties had been broken after her father's death. She missed both and planned to reestablish them. (8) Her mother had distanced herself from her husband's family. While she had been close to them when her father was alive, her mother felt irrationally angry and blamed them for her father's obsessive worry about his physical condition. Frank's father began having heart attacks in his mid-40s. Her mother felt they had done too little to moderate Frank's anxiety about his health and subtly encouraged his over indulgence in exercise, which may have stressed his heart and contributed to his death. Ellen did not feel this way and decided that it was important for her to reestablish her contact with the family because she missed them. (9) She would continue on in individual treatment for at least 12 sessions.

Ellen's prolonged grief began to moderate itself after 2 months of treatment. By the third month, she was back to her old self, although she still attended the self-help group and saw the therapist once a month to monitor the depression. She no longer takes anti-depressants and has maintained her exercise regimen and diet. She sees her father's family regularly. She has been able to reestablishing her religious ties and recently had the *Bat Mitzvah* (Jewish confirmation ceremony for young women) that she had studied for but was unable to complete because of her grief over her father's death. She told her therapist, "I know it's something my dad wanted for me, and I feel good being back in synagogue with my old friends. Lots of times I go to services with my grandparents, and while my mom is still mad at God for my dad's death, it gives me a lot of pleasure to be with other Jews and worship. I guess I feel very close to my dad when I attend services, and I like the feeling of being together with other people who have lost a loved one and to say *Kaddish* (the prayer remembering lost loved ones) together. I never thought I'd be religious but it's given me a strength I never thought I had, or would ever need, and it's been a good thing because death happens in everyone's life and dealing with my dad's death has made me stronger."

In commenting on Ellen's grief, the therapist said:

> *"Ellen has a lot to be depressed about. I don't know that I would even call her depression prolonged. It seems to me that people experience grief in their own unique ways and Ellen's quick recovery, once she began therapy, is a good example of how therapy can be so helpful. Giving people assignments to help in their own recovery is energizing, and encouraging their own involvement in treatment can be very empowering. Ellen needed a little push and then she was better. She'll have moments of sorrow and despair. When you love someone and they pass on before their time, you expect that to happen. But on every measure of social functioning, Ellen is doing a great deal better. From the limited amount of sound evidence about the treatment of grief, one can't help but think that even at a professional level, we are still a death-denying society. One last thought. Grief and depression are two separate issues. Grieving people often feel depressed, but you have to treat the grief as a separate issue. Many people find it difficult to talk about death, but you can't help people cope with the death of a loved one without talking about that experience and the impact it's had. And you have to talk to people about their own notions of death because that's what drives their grief. Ellen has reconnected with her faith and it's been a strong reason for her improvement. The experiences she has during religious services and the ability to publicly remember her father by reciting an ancient prayer in Hebrew cause her to feel close to her father and the connection she now feels has helped her recover from what might have altered her life for a very long time to come."*

16.10. SUMMARY

This chapter discusses EBP with serious and terminal illness, disabilities and bereavement. Much of the chapter focuses on finding meaning in the crisis of illness and death. Several case studies are offered which demonstrate the use of EBP in the treatment of terminal illness and bereavement. The concept of prolonged or complicated grief is discussed, and the differences between normal grief and prolonged grief are noted. Suggestions are made regarding the treatment of prolonged grief using best evidence and a personal story of the resolution of grief is included.

16.11. INTEGRATING QUESTIONS

1. In some cultures and societies, prolonged grief is considered normal. Why is there an expectation in our society that we resolve our grief quickly or we fear that the grief will be debilitating?
2. The suggestion that we let people die without a struggle which may include treatments that leave people confused, unable to communicate, or to resolve unfinished business, is troubling. Is not it to our benefit that we struggle so hard to keep people with terminal illnesses alive for as long as possible?
3. Do you think grieving would be easier for most of us if terminally ill patients were allowed to die in their homes surrounded by their loved ones rather than in sterile and often uncaring hospitals?
4. The death of a parent, even a parent who is very elderly and infirmed, often creates a serious emotional response in children. Why do you think this occurs?
5. People who never grieve at the death of loved ones are often thought to be unfeeling or emotionally disengaged. Do you think that at some point in life this lack of grief catches up with people and shows itself in a number of emotional problems?

References

Angold, A., Costello, E. J., & Worthman, C. M. (1998). Puberty and depression: The roles of age, pubertal status and pubertal timing. *Psychological Medicine, 28*(5), 1–61.

Balk, D. E. (1999). Bereavement and spiritual change. *Death Studies, 23*(6), 485–493.

Barbe, R. P., Bridge, J., Birmaher, B., Kolko, D., & Brent, D. A. (2004). Suicidality and its relationship to treatment outcome in depressed adolescents. *Suicide & Life-Threatening Behavior, 34*, 44–55.

Black, D. (1998, March 21). Bereavement in childhood. *British Medical Journal, 316*(7135), 931–933.

Black, D., & Urbanowicz, M. A. (1985). Bereaved children-family intervention. In J. E. & Stevenson (Ed.), *Recent research in developmental psychopathology* (pp. 179–187). Oxford: Pergammon.

Black, D., & Urbanowicz, M. A. (1987). Family intervention with bereaved children. *Journal of Child Psychology and Psychiatry, 28*, 467–476.

Blundo, R. (2001). Learning strengths-based practice: Challenging our personal and professional frames. *Families in Society, 82*(3), 296–304.

Braithwaite, D. O. (1996). Exploring different perspectives on the communication of persons with disabilities. In E. B. & Ray (Ed.), *Communication and disenfranchisement: Social health issues and implications* (pp. 449–464). Hillsdale, NJ: Lawrence Erlbaum.

Caffrey, T. A. (2000). The whisper of death: Psychotherapy with a dying Vietnam veteran. *American Journal of Psychotherapy, 54*(4), 519–530.

Coleman, L. M. (1997). Stigma: An enigma demystified. In L. J. & David (Ed.), *The disability studies reader* (pp. 216–231). New York: Routledge.

Compton, S. N., March, J. S., Brent, D., Albano, M., & Weersing, R. (2004). Cognitive-behavioral psychotherapy for anxiety and depressive disorders in children and adolescents: An evidence-based medicine review. *Journal of the American Academy of Child and Adolescent Psychiatry, 43*, 930–959.

Druss, B. G., Marcus, S. C., Rosenheck, R. A., Olfson, M., et al. (2000). Understanding disability in mental and general medical conditions. *American Journal of Psychiatry, 157*(9), 1485–1491.

Finn, J. (1999). An exploration of helping processes in an online self-help group focusing on issues of disability. *Health & Social Work, 24*(3), 220–231.

Friedberg, R. D., & McClure, J. M. (2002). *Clinical practice of cognitive therapy with children and adolescents: The nuts and bolts*. New York: Guilford.

Frankl, V. E. (1978). *Psychotherapy and existentialism: Selected papers on logotherapy*. New York: Touchstone Books.

Glicken, M. D. (2005). *Learning from resilient people: Lessons we can apply to counseling and psychotherapy*. Thousand Oaks, CA: Sage Publications.

Greenstein, M., & Breitbart, W. (2000). Cancer and the experience of meaning: A group psychotherapy program for people with cancer. *American Journal of Psychotherapy, 54*(4), 486–500.

Hardwig, J. (2000). Spiritual issues at the end of life: a call for discussion. *The Hastings Center Report, 30*(2), 28–30.

Harrington, R., & Harrison, L. (1999, May). Unproven assumptions about the impact of bereavement on children. *Journal of the Royal Society of Medicine*, 92.

Howarth, R. V. (1972, November). The psychiatry of terminal illness in children. *Proceedings of the Royal Society of Medicine, 65*(11), 1039–1040.

Jacobs, S., & Prigerson, H. (2000). Psychotherapy of traumatic grief: A review of evidence for psychotherapeutic treatments. *Death Studies, 24*(6), 479–496.

Kendall, P. C. (1994). Treating anxietydisorders in children:Results of a randomized clinical study. *Journal of Consulting and Clinical Psychology, 62*, 100–110.

Kleber, R. J., & Brom, D. (1987). Psychotherapy and pathological grief: Controlled outcome study. *Israeli Journal of Psychiatry and Related Sciences, 24*, 99–109.

Kubler-Ross, E. (1969/1997). *On death and dying*. New York: Touchstone.

Lloyd-Williams, M. (2001). Screening for depression in palliative care patients: A review. *European Journal of Cancer Care, 10*(1), 31–36.

Marmar, C. R., Horowitz, M. J., Weiss, D. S., Wilner, N. R., & Kaltreider, N. B. (1988). A controlled trial of brief psychotherapy and mutual help group treatment of conjugal bereavement. *American Journal of Psychiatry, 145*, 203–209.

McClain, C. S., Rosenfeld, B., & Breitbart, W. (2003). Effect of spiritual well-being on end-of-life despair in terminally-ill cancer patients. *Lancet, 361*(9369), 1603–1608.

Piper, W. E., Ogrodniczuk, J. S., Joyce, A. S., & McCallum, M. R. (2002). Relationships among affect, work, and outcome in group therapy for patients with complicated grief. *American Journal of Psychotherapy, 56*(3), 347–362.

Raphael, B. (1977). Preventive intervention with the recently bereaved. *Archives of General Psychiatry, 34*, 1450–1454.

Richman, J. (2000). Introduction: Psychotherapy with terminally ill patients. *American Journal of Psychotherapy, 54*(4), 482–486.

Rutter, M. (1966). *Children of sick parents*. Oxford: Oxford University Press.

Sireling, L., Cohen, D., & Marks, I. (1988). Guided mourning for morbid grief: A replication. *Behavior Therapy, 19*, 121–132.

Shworles, T. R. (1983). The person with disability and the benefits of the microcomputer revolution: To have or to have not. *Rehabilitation Literature, 44*(11–12), 322–330.
Stroebe, M. S. (2001). Bereavement research and theory: Retrospective and prospective. *American Behavioral Scientist, 44*(5), 854–865.
U.S. Bureau of the Census. (2000). *Statistical Abstract of the United States*, p. 175.
Weller, R. A., Weller, E. B., Fristad, M. A., & Bowes, J. M. (1991). Depression in recently bereaved prepubertal children. *The American Journal of Psychiatry, 148*, 1536–1540.

Part Four
Violence and Anti-Social Behavior

17 Evidence-Based Practice with Spoiled Children and Cyber-Bullies

This chapter deals with two serious behavioral problems for which there are no specific diagnostic categories but which we all know cause the community a great deal of pain: spoiled children and cyber-bullies. Many of these children come from affluent but sometimes uncaring homes where parenting has become a type of friendship, a buddy system in which discipline and modeling of moral behavior have taken a back seat to giving in to whims, however negative the consequences. This behavior often results in children who treat others with contempt and place their own needs far higher than those of others, including their parents who often protect them and facilitate this behavior. In the case of cyber-bullies, the Internet has given rise to harmful and cruel rumors about peers that damage the lives of children and adolescents.

To be sure, these are not new problems in our society. We have always had badly parented children whose lives are shaped by parents who have little sense of what parenting means. These parents seem to be unaware that moral values and positive behavior have to be modeled and not just spoken. What *is* new are the numbers of children who feel no allegiance to the community, believe the world revolves around them, and know that someone will protect them and come to their rescue if they ever have a problem. These are the children of the "sibling society" which Robert Bly talks about – the children who rely on others to care for them and who, in their eternal state of adolescence, never grow up. They often live with their parents well into their parents' old age, feel little commitment to care for their parents, have little concept of money and the labor required to make it, and when asked about their behavior, always have an excuse and seldom take responsibility for themselves.

In Japan these children are known as "parasite singles" (Orenstein, 2001) because they live with their parents well into their 30s and often until their parents pass away. While some of these children help with household chores or pay rent, most do not and many even receive allowances from parents. Most are unmarried and never plan to marry or have love relationships. Orenstein (2001) describes the parasitic young women she met in Japan and wonders how many American young men and women have similar attitudes:

> *More than half of Japanese women are still single by 30 – compared with about 37% of American women – and nearly all of them live at home with Mom and Dad. Labeled "Parasite Singles," they pay no rent, do no housework and come and go freely. Although they earn, on average, just $27 000 a year,*

they are Japan's leading consumers, since their entire income is disposable. Despite Japan's continuing recession, they have created a boom in haute couture accessories by Louis Vuitton, Bulgari, Fendi and Prada, as well as in cell phones, minicars and other luxury goods. They travel more widely than their higher-earning male peers, dress more fashionably and are more sophisticated about food and culture. (p. 1)

The following is an essay written by the author for a book on writing (Glicken, 2008, pp. 188–189) that spells out the societal consequences of spoiling children and concerns about the future of American youth if this trend continues.

In his book, The Sibling Society (1996), the American poet Robert Bly suggests that a new generation of Americans has lost its ability to function as responsible citizens. Rather than being trained for adulthood and the responsibilities of adulthood, children are now being trained for eternal adolescence. As adolescents, they lack responsibility to anyone, including the families that raise them. Characteristics of members of the sibling society are lack of a work ethic, an inability to treat others with care and consideration, a feeling of entitlement, and an inability to accept, or discharge, their responsibilities to society.

Guided by the need for pleasure and by an endless belief that they are entitled to be irresponsible, members of the sibling society provide convenient excuses when its citizens fail. There is an excuse for every failure and Bly argues that over time, the responsible few will be forced to take care of the irresponsible many. Often the responsible few are immigrants and their first-generation children, or the children of healthy parents who provide their children with a work ethic. The sibling society lives off the hard work and the social concern of this growing minority. Where once college students fought against the war in Viet Nam and racial injustice, the sibling society riots when beer privileges are taken away from them on high-profile campuses.

Bly believes that the sibling society invents excuses for failure that affect our legal system. The issue is no longer guilt or innocence, or whether the trial was fair, but a series of excuses that justify, explain, absolve, and ultimately encourage its citizens to act out again.

Bly argues that the continuation of the sibling society will create adults incapable of dealing with the responsibilities of a democracy. Citizens of the sibling society will be so disassociated from the necessities to think of the community, to exercise restraint in daily living, or to act for the greater good, that Americans will permit the nation to slip into an autocracy because adult members of the sibling society are unwilling to vote, to know issues, to understand the democratic process, to be activists, or to speak out when there are injustices.

Bly believes that welfare and unemployment will mark the sibling society because its members lack motivation to care for themselves and feel certain that others will take care of them in any eventuality.

Bly sees the American parent as a partner in the sibling society. Instead of providing values and moral lessons that assist the society in dealing with new social and economic problems, Bly believes that American parents want a partnership with their children. Such a partnership blunts the lines between parent and child so that children find it difficult to accept moral messages, when given, because the messenger is their buddy, their companion, their playmate, and not their parent.

As evidence of the existence of a sibling society, expectations in universities have dwindled. American business can no longer find enough American-born workers to fill its requirements and depend, increasingly, on immigrant labor. And while we suffer from intense xenophobia (the fear of immigrants) in America, the reality is that hard-working immigrants propel the economy and permit us to live in a high degree of affluence. Much as Rome depended on slave labor, the sibling society depends on its immigrants to do the many tasks it is unwilling to do for itself.

Bly believes that the American mass media and the liberal philosophies of the helping professions are largely responsible for the creation of the sibling society. As the power of the American media affects other societies, he believes that the sibling society will become a worldwide reality, and that national agendas will be determined by a sense of entitlement and narcissism. The end result, according to Bly, bodes badly for the future of our planet.

17.1. SPOILED CHILDREN

Schmitt (2006) indicates that a spoiled child is undisciplined, manipulative, and unpleasant to be with much of the time and behaves in many of the following ways by the time he or she is 2 or 3 years old: Does not follow rules or cooperate with suggestions; does not respond to "no," "stop," or other commands; protests everything; does not know the difference between his needs and his wishes; insists on having his own way; makes unfair or excessive demands on others; does not respect other people's rights; tries to control people; has a low tolerance for frustration; frequently whines or throws tantrums and continually complains about being bored. Often the main cause of children being spoiled is lenient and permissive parents who try to rescue children from normal frustrations. These parents, or the caretakers who raise them, have a difficult time allowing children to learn proper attention-seeking behaviors and tend to respond in a protective and oversolicitous way even when the child should be able to cope with small frustrations by himself.

Without changes in child-rearing, spoiled children often experience rejection by other children and adults by the time they reach school age. Other children dislike them because they are overly controlling and self-centered, and adults tend to dislike them because they are rude and make excessive demands. Because of problems with relationships with others, spoiled children are often unhappy children whose school work often declines and who experience increased incidences of drug abuse and other risk-taking behaviors. A case study at the end of this section on spoiled children describes the symptoms and treatment of a spoiled pre-schooler.

17.2. PREVENTION

Schmitt (2006) suggests the following ways to prevent spoiling a child and with a spoiled child, ways of unspoiling him or her: rule setting that is age-appropriate; cooperation and even involvement as the child ages (4–5 years of age) in democratic discussions of rules and their importance; not allowing temper tantrums to sway your limit setting and the rules you have developed; teaching children patience and ways of dealing with boredom; not protecting children from normal life challenges; not overpraising, and teaching children to respect the rights of others. Obviously there is a fine line between spoiling a child and developing a healthy child, but the line becomes clearly drawn when the child responds badly. That should tell parents and other caretakers that the child-rearing strategies are not working and that a bit of evaluation will help understand which child-rearing approach is at fault and should be changed. Obviously this requires a good deal of cooperation between partners and caretakers. It is not unusual for parents who are not getting along to be indecisive in their child rearing approaches or to have one partner rescind the discipline of another. When this happens the child will almost always side with the parent who is most lenient and the process of spoiling and confusing the child has begun in earnest. The following case study illustrates the behavior of spoiled children and some possible treatment strategies.

17.3. CASE STUDY: EVIDENCE-BASED PRACTICE WITH A SPOILED CHILD

Alice is the 5-year-old daughter and only child of Larry and Margaret, a successful professional couple in their late 30s. The couple contacted the therapist because Alice is entering first grade and the early childhood issues they had with her of her insisting on occupying all of their time, being demanding, and not being considerate of their needs, have not only continued but seem worse than ever. Alice is doing well academically in school; however her teachers report that she demands a great deal of the teachers' attention and when she does not get it, sulks and complains bitterly that they do not like her. The other children tend to keep a distance from Alice because she can be bossy and controlling.

The parents have begun to use the tough love tactics of withdrawing attention when she misbehaves at home with little success. They admit to feel guilty when they discipline Alice, who often cries and tries to come out of her room where she has been sent for an infraction, claiming she has done nothing wrong and that her parents are just being mean. When the family has company, Alice takes center stage and wants even more attention. When she does not get it she claims that she is ill. On many occasions the parents admit that dinners out with friends often result in Alice wanting to go home, largely, they think, because she gets angry when people are talking about other things and ignoring her. The phantom illnesses she claims to have always go away within minutes of arriving home.

The therapist interviewed Alice and wrote, "Alice is a very pretty, bright child of five. She's attending kindergarten and likes it but thinks that the teacher is mean to her. She explains that the teacher likes the other kids better and never pays attention to Alice. When that happens, Alice gets a stomachache and has to go see the nurse or her mother is called to take her home. Alice asks her mother to report the teacher to the principal and to complain that the teacher is always mean to Alice even though Alice reads better than anyone else. She also complains that she doesn't get any presents when her mom goes shopping – Alice expects her mom and dad to bring her presents whenever they return to the house after shopping. Alice also feels that her parents are too strict, and that when they try to discipline her she believes it means that they don't love her anymore. When asked how she feels about the other kids in her class, she says they talk too much and always need the teacher's attention, and they say mean things to her. One of the girls in her class called her a "spoiled brat," which Alice thinks is the worst thing you can ever say about a kid. Alice says she's not spoiled, she's just special, and she requires more attention than the other kids because special kids will be able to do a lot for the world when they grow up. When asked what she would do for the world, Alice said that she'd make sure that other people loved her and played with her and said nice things to her. No one would be mean or say bad things about her."

A home visit revealed that Alice has so many toys and clothes that her room barely held them all. Alice informed the therapist that she could not use Alice's bathroom, but maybe she could use her parents'. She told the therapist where she could sit, and during the 1-h visit with the parents present, never once let her parents talk without interrupting them or trying to show how well she read or played with a toy. Obviously embarrassed, the parents tried to quiet her but were unable to do anything about her constant interruptions. The therapist suggested the meeting continue in her office with just the parents present. They readily agreed.

Later when they were in the office, the parents told the therapist they were mortified by Alice's behavior and apologized. They wondered how things had gotten to this point and if there was any hope that Alice would develop in a more normal way. They realized that they had been far too lenient and thought that praising her continually, whether she deserved praise or not, had resulted in Alice becoming very self-centered.

The therapist listened and agreed that there was a need to intervene with Alice, and that the parents were the ones who must have control over what happened to

Alice. It would, she told them, require a very consistent approach against which Alice would rebel, and to expect a great deal of resistance. It was not that the parents were not willing to discipline her, the therapist told the parents, it was more a failure on their part to follow through. They were correct in wanting to change the behavior but the trouble came when they failed to stick with a discipline. Unless they were willing to do so, Alice would continue with the behavior they were concerned about and it would very likely become worse over time. As it became a more serious problem Alice would experience rejection by the other children and the adults in her life. The therapist also referred them to a parent effectiveness group, gave them several articles to read with research evidence that spoiled children do badly as teen-agers and adults, and that the time to correct the problem was while the child was still young. The therapist also encouraged them to do some extensive reading about children like Alice. She was hesitant to use the term "spoiled" because of its pejorative connotation, and instead spoke of children who needed a great deal of attention and seemed overly demanding. She agreed to see the parents weekly to help with any problems they might encounter.

In the next session with the therapist they said they had consistently disciplined Alice and that she had had temper tantrums each time. They ignored the tantrums, and very quickly Alice learned that tantrums would not work. She then stopped eating. The parents were concerned that she would become ill but in time they discovered that Alice was sneaking food from the refrigerator after her parents went to bed. As Alice's options began to decrease, she became sullen and would not speak to her parents. She kept a continual monolog going throughout the day and evening about how mean her parents were and how much she wished she had different parents. After two difficult months the complaining stopped and the parents began, with the therapist's guidance, to establish expectations for Alice's behavior. After 6 months she was generally compliant, with only occasional outbursts of self-pity.

The worker made another home visit after six months and Alice seemed almost happy to see her and told the worker she could use her bathroom anytime she wanted to. She also showed the worker her newly cleaned up room. The toys and clothes that seemed excessive had been given to "kids who need them more than I do."

Alice's parents spoke to the therapist a year after treatment began. They said that the process of undoing the harm they had done was excruciating. Alice was a bright child who came up with an endless list of strategies to make them pull back on the discipline. Thankfully, the parent effectiveness training (PET) group they went to was supportive and the therapist had helped them understand the personal reasons each had been so inconsistent with Alice. Not surprisingly there were problems in the marriage that were resolved in treatment, problems in which Alice was used as a way for each partner to get back at the other. Each parent tended to rescind the discipline of the other parent and each parent found him or herself being critical of the spouse in front of Alice. This process led to Alice feeling that whatever she did, her parents were too self-involved with their marital problems to do anything about it. Alice also worried that the marriage would end and her behavior was, in many ways, a display of anxiety and a need to control that from happening.

The parents felt the articles suggested by the worker had helped a lot and knowing that many other parents had similar problems was very helpful. Finally, they began to realize several months into treatment that the parents of Alice's friends were also badly spoiling their children, and that when Alice was around them, the old behavior came back. They distanced themselves from these parents, a difficult decision since many of them were also friends of theirs with many of the same marital problems they had in their marriage. Margaret said,

> *I could see, after a few months of therapy, that we'd chosen our friends because they reinforced the bad behavior we were experiencing in our marriage, especially the sort of bitchy ways we were treating each other. Being around them was comfortable because we all acted the same way. It took a lot of soul searching for us to find new friends who were on the same track as we were, but in the PET group we made some new friends and they're healthy friends who make us feel very loving toward one another. Who would have thought that helping Alice would end up helping us as well?*

17.4. CYBER-BULLYING AND RELATIONAL AGGRESSION IN CHILDREN AND ADOLESCENTS

Thanks to Meghan Anaya, an exceptional MSW student in my graduate research class at Arizona State University, for permission to use the following information about cyber-bullying and relational aggression.

Cyber-bullying is the use of communication technologies such as e-mail, cell phone and pager text messages, instant messaging, defamatory personal Websites, and defamatory online personal polling Websites to support deliberate, repeated, and hostile behavior by an individual or group that is intended to harm others (Belsey, 2004). Cyber-bullying can also include three-way calling, blogs, chat rooms, cell phone cameras in locker rooms, and unflattering use of computer photo editing programs (Garinger, 2006). In short, cyber-bullying is harassment via means of electronic communication.

Cyber-bullying is a type of relational aggression expressed through the hurtful manipulation of peer relationships and friendships which inflicts harm on others through social exclusion and malicious rumor spreading (Anderson and Sturm, 2007; Crick and Grotpeter, 1995). Also known as indirect or social aggression, relational aggression is used as a social strategy which is part of a developmental process that peaks in late childhood and preadolescence (Archer and Coyne, 2005). This type of non-physical aggression is unique to the human species and exists in every age group of participants and in many different social contexts (Archer and Coyne, 2005). The purpose of relational aggression is to create and maintain power through social exclusion and by decreasing the social standing of another member of the group. Because of their concern for social standing and social relationships, the non-physical nature of relational aggression as a social strategy has been found to be more prominent among females and is becoming more prevalent in school-age girls (Keith and Martin, 2005). The term "mean girls" is sometimes used to describe pre-adolescent and adolescent girls who use cyber-bullying tactics with others.

There are several explanations for the existence of cyber-bullying. Mason (2008) suggests that the Internet and other electronic communication sources offer the anonymity which face-to-face confrontation lacks (Anderson and Sturm, 2007; Li, 2005; Mason, 2008; Ybarra and Mitchell, 2004a, 2004b). The lack of cues such as body language and voice tone in victims allows cyber-bullies to experience lowered feelings of remorse (Mason, 2008). Another aspect of anonymity in cyber-bullying is the activation of a social identity that can differ from a child's individual identity and allows the child to use a persona that hides his or her real identity (Mason, 2008). Mason (2008) believes that the ability to create new Internet identities for the purpose of harassing others is aided by poor parental monitoring and poor relationships between parent and child.

Compared to traditional, physical bullying, cyber-bullying has several unique advantages: anonymity and 24 h accessibility of technology (Anderson and Sturm, 2007) which allows the bully to harass a victim at home or at school and feel relatively safe from being caught (Anderson and Sturm, 2007). Because of stricter school rules against Internet and cell phone usage, cyber-bullying occurs more frequently at home than at school (Garinger, 2006; Smith et al., 2008). Cyber-bullying is also made possible by a parental gap in understanding technology, problems in taking down hateful Web sites because of free-speech laws, and attitudes among victims that nothing can be done to stop cyber-bullying (Keith and Martin, 2005; Li, 2005; Smith et al., 2008).

Relational aggression begins early in childhood and begins to increase between ages 8 and 11, with girls more likely to use this form of aggression than boys (Archer and Coyne, 2005). In 2006, Fight Crime, an organization comprised of a team of more than 3000 police chiefs, sheriffs, prosecutors, other law enforcement officers, and violence survivors who are dedicated to protecting children from crime and violence, released a report of national statistics that approximately 13 million children ages 6–17 are victims of cyber-bullying (Kharfen, 2006). Of these 13 million, more than 2 million told no one (Kharfen, 2006). Of those who did tell someone, about half of the children ages 6–11 told their parents, while only 30% of older teens told their parents (Kharfen, 2006).

Common themes in cyber harassment include physical appearance, sexual promiscuity, poverty, grades, diseases, and disabilities (Anderson and Sturm, 2007). These types of harassment issues can cause severe psychological distress in victims, including increased feelings of stress, tension, low self-esteem, and depression (Anderson and Sturm, 2007). Mason (2008) found that victims of cyber-bullying reported serious emotional problems, including suicidal ideations, eating disorders, chronic illness, and poor self-esteem causing adjustment difficulties later in life (Garinger, 2006). Signs in children of being harassed include spending a great deal of time on the computer, problems with sleeping, depression or crying without reason, extreme mood swings, feeling unwell, withdrawing from friends and family, and falling behind in school work (Keith and Martin, 2005). Cyber-bullies experience many of the same problems affecting bullies in general, including antisocial behaviors later in life and higher rates of crime (Mason, 2008). Children who participate in bullying but have also been victimized are more likely to experience substance use, depression, and low school commitment (Ybarra and Mitchell, 2004a, 2004b).

In trying to better understand cyber-bullying, Li (2005) studied 177 seventh grade students with low to moderate socioeconomic status in an urban school setting and found that 60% of the victims were female, 70% of the aggressors were Caucasian, 50% of the aggressors had above average grades, and aggressors reported that they used computers more often than students who had not cyber-bullied others. Li (2005) found that only 34% of victims told adults that they were being cyber-bullied and of all the students sampled, 70% believed that adults did not try to stop cyber-bullying when they knew of it.

In a study examining whether or not relational aggression should be included in the DSM-V under disruptive behavior disorders, Keenan et al. (2008) researched the reliability and validity of relational aggression in boys and girls aged 9–17 when reported by parents and youth as informants and found adequate reliability and validity. They also examined the overlap between relational aggression, oppositional defiant disorder (ODD) and conduct disorder (CD) and found that relational aggression was only moderately correlated with symptoms of ODD and CD. The researchers concluded that there was not enough information to warrant a diagnostic placement in the DSM-V based on informant criteria (Keenan et al., 2008). Perhaps this suggests that relational aggression is a widely practiced phenomenon among American youth encompassing children and adolescents whose aggression would not be as prevalent were it physical in nature. The opportunity to harass others, if anonymous, may indicate that youth are much more hostile and envious of their classmates than we would like to believe.

Sandstrom (2007) examined the link between maternal disciplinary strategies and relational aggression in 82 fourth grade students. The participants completed peer nominations of overt and relational aggression, and mothers completed a questionnaire regarding the disciplinary strategies they used. Sandstrom (2007) found a positive association between authoritarian disciplinary styles and relational aggression as well as a positive association between maternal permissiveness and relational aggression among girls. Ybarra (2004) studied characteristics of the aggressor, including depressive symptoms and caregiver–child relationships in 1501 youth ages 10–17 using a telephone survey and a nine-item questionnaire based upon criteria of a depression diagnosis from the DSM-IV. Requirement for participation included having used the Internet at least six times in the previous 6 months. The study found a strong positive correlation between Internet harassment and depressive symptoms, suggesting that those who participate in cyber-bullying may be more likely to be depressed and express their negative feelings in the form of Internet harassment. Ybarra and Mitchell (2004a, 2004b) found that 44% of online harassers reported a poor emotional bond with a parent and that poor caregiver-child relationships increased the likelihood of cyber-bullying.

As a way of preventing cyber-bullying, Anderson and Sturm (2007) suggest that parents use preventative strategies such as blocking unwanted friends on instant messaging and monitoring any behavioral changes in their child which may be related to victimization, including changes in academic performance, sleep patterns, eating habits, nervous behaviors, and choice of friends. Garinger (2006) recommends that parents attend parent-training programs as a way of learning developmentally appropriate parenting skills and methods to help children who may display antisocial behaviors. Mason (2008) believes that school professionals should be encouraged to implement anti-bullying programs to promote positive social relationships, such as the Olweus Bullying Prevention Program (Mason, 2008). This includes teaching "Netiquette" or Internet etiquette and other appropriate ways to act online (Mason, 2008). Overall, the most important strategies to implement in order to reduce cyber-bullying include educating children and parents about cyber-bullying, parental monitoring of technology used by children, and encouraging students to tell a trusted adult when cyber-bullying is occurring (Anderson and Sturm, 2007; Garinger, 2006).

17.5. CASE STUDY: MEAN GIRLS GET CAUGHT

We often think that cyber-bullies are not really bullies but the term "mean girls" is one used to describe cyber-bullying by children and adolescents who are often popular and good students. The following case study illustrates that bullying behavior is much more prevalent than we might assume.

Jennifer is a 14-year-old high school freshman who is a good student and involved in a number of activities. She was referred by the school for counseling when she and three other girls were discovered to be cyber-bullying a classmate and former friend. The girls sent out anonymous e-mails to many students in their class portraying their former friend as a "slut" who slept around and who had sex with guys she did not know after school in the boys' bathroom. To make things as graphic as possible, they produced a video supposedly showing their former friend in the midst of a sex act. The girl they cyber-bullied was so distraught by the e-mails that she had to change schools and was being treated for depression when the identities of the three girls were discovered.

In an initial interview with Jennifer's parents, Jim and Darlene, they attacked the school for accusing their daughter of sending out the e-mails and said there was no proof their daughter had been involved, even though 10 people who knew what the girls had done and one of the girls who cyber-bullied with Jennifer implicated her. Jennifer's mother told the worker that Jennifer was a nice girl who would never do such a thing. However, a further investigation confirmed that Jennifer had shoplifted when she was in 6th grade, had been picked up by the police for driving without a license and being under the influence of a substance, and had been accused once before of cyber-bullying when a former boyfriend was the subject of a website suggesting that he slept with prostitutes and had sex with one of his male teachers. The parents said that all of these accusations were untrue and the therapist could believe whatever he wanted, but Jennifer was a normal 14-year-old who went to church on Sunday and did well in school. The father threatened to sue the therapist if she tried to work with Darlene, but later apologized and said that perhaps all of them could use some help to "clear this up."

Jennifer told the worker that she cyber-bullied frequently and that everyone in her class did it and many of the girls just did it as a form of retaliation and no one took it seriously. She claimed the last girl she cyber-bullied really was a slut and this thing about being depressed and having to go to another school was just a big act. Everyone shoplifted, she told the worker, and the only thing different about her was that she had been caught. "Get a life," she told the worker. "This is like a different time and nobody acts like a Girl Scout anymore." She figured most of the girls in her class were sleeping around by age 12 and most were using drugs, and anyway, "What's the big deal? I do well in school and I'm a cheerleader for heaven's sake. Doesn't that count for something?"

The worker and Jennifer met for eight sessions, with Jennifer blowing off the things she had done and criticizing the school for making her come to treatment. On the ninth session she admitted she was quite unhappy and knew that what she had done was wrong. She told the worker her parents were so oblivious to her and spent so little time with her she wondered if they even knew she existed or cared about her. Her mother spent her day gossiping with friends and her father was almost never home because of work. She wondered if she was really their daughter and could not imagine that they actually planned on having her. She began to cry and told the worker she knew that her former friend was very hurt by the cyber-bullying because she knew that she had been in counseling before any of this happened because of depression. The three girls chose her because she was so vulnerable. "How could we do such a mean thing?" she asked the worker, and was told that this was why therapy might be so helpful. That and helping her become happier with her life.

After the ninth session, Jennifer settled in to treatment and became cooperative and motivated to change. She read the articles on cyber-bullying the worker suggested and found some on her own. She told the worker, "They are pretty much about me. I can see myself in almost everything the articles say about girls who cyber-bully." The worker thought it might be a good idea to include her parents in the next few sessions. The parents were hostile in the beginning, but when Jennifer began to cry and confronted them about how she felt about their parenting, they became silent and a deep look of hurt came over the father's face. "You're right, Jennifer" he said. "Your mom and I have been ignoring you because we've been ignoring each other." Jennifer's mother began to cry and shook her head. "How could our family be so messed up?" she asked. "We used to be a happy family, now look at us."

The family continued in treatment for five sessions. Jennifer began self-disclosing her general feeling of deep resentment of others she felt had happy family lives, admitted her two friends were emotional wrecks who, like her, were deeply envious and said that she craved a happy family life. So did the parents who agreed they needed marital counseling in addition to the work they were doing in family treatment. The family met 6 months later and agreed that everything was much better now, both in the family and in their marriage. Jennifer was doing better as well and had joined a self-help group for teenagers who had been involved in cyber-bullying. "God, what a disgusting thing to do to people," she told the worker. "Some of the kids in the groups were victims and it's messed up their lives badly. One of the three girls I did the stuff with against my former friend got caught again. She's a mess and they've expelled her from school. She never went for therapy and made a big joke out of me going. Look who's laughing now?"

In summarizing her work, the therapist said the following:

> *I've begun to work with a number of girls like Jennifer. They come from good homes and middle class families of the sort we used to think were the moral backbone of our community. In reality the parents ignore their children and assume a passive parenting style whose message to children is that they don't really care what the children do as long as they leave them out of it and don't get caught doing anything that will embarrass the parents. Many of the parents have serious marital problems and some resent ever having had a child. It's a statement about our society that many of these children are so deeply unhappy with their lives that they lash out at others who are vulnerable just because it gives them a small sense of satisfaction and superiority. I don't think traditional diagnostic categories capture the lives of these unhappy children. Sure you could say they have conduct disorders, but they often do well in school and haven't a history of difficulty or early signs of ODD. This seems to happen in middle school and into high school. If I could compare it to anything, it would be gang behavior, in which children form cliques with like-minded friends and feel the power of group membership as a form of protective shield against their unhappy lives.*
>
> *I don't think traditional pathology-oriented therapy works with cyber-bullies. From my reading, I'd suggest the use of the strengths approach because in time these kids talk about their unhappiness and my experience is that when you mobilize families they do well in treatment. That isn't often true of children with CD. Also, they seldom have the deep-seated pathology caused by a malfunctioning family life that you see with conduct disorders at this age. Although the literature on cyber-bullying lags the more traditional literature on CD and ODD, I did find a beginning literature including recent article by Keenan et al. (2008) and Keith and Martin (2005) that were helpful. I think cyber-bullying is so pervasive that it has to be seen as a statement about the condition of our society. I believe the DSM-V needs to include it as a diagnostic category just to show how unhappy many of our children are and how badly functioning family life is for too many American kids.*

As more research becomes available I think a better approach might be developed to prevent relational aggression and cyber-bullying, but for now, strong parental involvement in the lives of children, understanding who their friends are, awareness of the power of the Internet to hurt others, and the limits parents need to place on computer usage at home are all behaviors parents need to consider as children grow up in this new world of cyber communicating.

17.6. SUMMARY

This chapter discussed spoiled children and cyber-bullies, a new form of bullying that uses the Internet to harass others. The chapter notes that in both cases, parents often do a limited job of preparing their children for life and either opt out of parenting by ignoring their children or give in to every whim without a sense of proper moral behavior. Parents also tend to not encourage their children's ability to exist in a society in which people must earn the right to be thought highly of through hard work and persistence. Many of the children who bully and use the Internet to mask their identities are children who feel detached from the harm cyber-bullying causes, and do not think of it as much more than a social contrivance which most people do. Many have themselves been victims. Both issues need prompt attention from parents, school personnel and therapists because spoiled children and cyber-bullies perform badly as adults without changes in parenting and treatment from knowledgeable professionals.

17.7. QUESTIONS FROM THE CHAPTER

1. How would parents know that their children are cyber-bullying when it is done on someone else's computer? Do not we expect too much of parents who, after all, have a full plate just dealing with their own life issues?
2. What is the big deal about using the Internet to gossip or put down classmates and ex-friends? We have always done this by passing notes around or gossiping about kids we do not like. Anyway, kids always know who is doing it and just do it back, so what is the harm?
3. I do not get how you can spoil a child. Most of the problems discussed in this book are caused by parents who put down children or abuse them. Is not spoiling children something they get over, but which helps them have a positive self-concept?
4. We put a lot of pressure on parents to do the right thing but parents are human too and they do the best they can. Rather than criticizing them, as the author does in this chapter, why not be a little more supportive and recognize that without parents we would not have anyone to raise kids and, for the most part, they do a good job.
5. Is not having computers in the home an invitation to cyber-bullying? Should not we only allow kids to use their parents' computers and it should not they be set up by professionals to block e-mail and any other ways of communicating online or, if cell phones are used, by text messaging?

References

Anderson, T., & Sturm, B. (2007). Cyber bullying: From playground to computer. *Young Adult Library Services*, 24–27.

Archer, J., & Coyne, S. M. (2005). An integrated review of indirect, relational, and social aggression. *Personality and Social Psychology Review, 9*(3), 212–230.

Belsey, B. (2004). *What is cyber-bullying?* Retrieved on April 8, 2008 from www.bullying.org

Bly, R. (1996). *The sibling society*. Boston: Wesley-Addison Longman.

Crick, N. R., & Grotpeter, J. K. (1995). Relational aggression, gender, and social-psychological adjustment. *Child Development, 66*(3), 710–722.

Garinger, H. M. (2006). Girls who bully: What professionals need to ask. *Guidance and Counseling, 21*(4), 1–10.

Glicken, M. D. (2008). *A guide to writing for the human service professionals*. New York: Rowman and Littlefield.

Keenan, K., Coyne, C., & Lahey, B. B. (2008). Should relational aggression be included in the DSM-V. *Journal of the American Academy of Child and Adolescent Psychiatry, 47*(1), 86–93.

Keith, S., & Martin, M. E. (2005). Cyber-bullying: Creating a culture of respect in a cyber world. *Reclaiming Children and Youth, 13*(4), 224–228.

Kharfen, M. (2006, August 17). *1 of 3 teens and 1 of 6 preteens are victims of cyber-bullying: Teenager recounts harrowing tale of online death threats*. Retrieved April 12, 2008, from http://www.fightcrime.org/releases.php?id=231

Li, Q. (2005). New bottle but old wine: A research of cyber-bullying in schools. *Computers in Human Behavior, 23*, 1777–1791.

Mason, K. L. (2008). Cyber-bullying: A preliminary assessment for school personnel. *Psychology in the Schools, 45*(4), 323–348.

Orenstein, P. (2001, July). Parasites in Prêt-à-Porter. *New YorkTimes Magazine*. http://query.nytimes.com/gst/fullpage.html?res=9B01E1DE1030F932A35754C0A9679C8B63&sec=&spon=&pagewanted=all

Sandstrom, M. J. (2007). A link between mothers' disciplinary strategies and children's relational aggression. *British Journal of Developmental Psychology, 25*, 399–407.

Schmitt, B. D. (2006). *Your child's health: Spoilded Children*. New York: Bantom Books.

Smith, P. K., Mahdavi, J., Carvalho, M., Fisher, S., Russell, S., & Tippett, N. (2008). Cyber-bullying: its nature and impact in secondary school pupils. *Journal of Child Psychology and Psychiatry, 49*(4), 376–385.

Ybarra, M. L. (2004). Linkages between depressive symptomatology and internet harassment among young regular internet users. *Cyber Psychology and Behavior, 7*(2), 247–257.

Ybarra, M. L., & Mitchell, K. J. (2004a). Online aggressors/targets, aggressors, and targets: a comparison of youth associated characteristics. *Journal of Child Psychology and Psychiatry, 45*(7), 1308–1316.

Ybarra, M. L., & Mitchell, K. J. (2004b). Youth engaging in online harassment: associations with caregiver-child relationships, internet use, and personal characteristics. *Journal of Adolescence, 27*, 319–336.

18 Evidence-Based Practice with Children and Adolescents Coping with Abuse and Neglect

18.1. INTRODUCTION

Lambie (2005) reports that approximately 5 million cases of suspected child abuse were reported to Child Protective Services nationally in 2000. By 2003, 2400 *children* were found to be victims of abuse everyday. Nationally, each week, CPS agencies receive more than 50 000 reports of suspected child abuse but estimates indicate that for every report of abuse, there are an additional five abused and neglected children who go unreported (Prevent Child Abuse America, 2003). According to Lambie, over 18 000 children a year suffer permanent injuries as a result of child abuse.

Miller (1999, p. 32) indicates that common symptoms of children who have been abused include: High levels of anxiety and hyper-vigilance causing the child's nervous system to constantly be on alert; irritability, denial, and intrusive thoughts that sometimes create panic attacks; nightmares with themes of violence that are similar to their abuse; impaired concentration and memory lapses; withdrawal and isolation; acting-out behavior; repetitive play; self-blame; a foreshortened future where abused children believe that they will only live a short length of time; regression, periods of amnesia, and somatizing the trauma into physical illnesses including headaches, dizziness, heart palpitations, breathing problems, and stomach aches.

Similar problems have been noted in adult survivors of child abuse, but additional common symptoms include substance abuse; difficulty in maintaining intimate relationships; prostitution; severe psychosomatic disorders; abusive behavior; violent crime; depression; bi-polar disorder; psychosis; anxiety and panic disorders; and a host of problems that suggest the terrible consequences of child abuse.

In the classroom, abused children are 25% more likely to repeat a grade, and 75% of all high school dropouts have a history of abuse or neglect (Sechrist, 2000). Long-term harm caused by child abuse may include possible brain damage; developmental delays; learning disorders; problems forming interpersonal relationships and social difficulties; aggressive behavior; depression; low academic achievement; substance abuse; teen pregnancy; sexual revictimization; and criminal behavior (Lambie, 2005). Lambie goes to note,

> *The more immediate effects include feeling helpless, hopeless, and ashamed. Victims may feel unworthy of having friends and fearful that their "family secret" will be revealed; therefore, they may isolate themselves and withdraw. Such students may have increasingly pessimistic feelings about themselves, leading to decreased self-worth, self-blame, guilt and shame, as well as negative feelings about their own bodies (Russell, 1999). In some cases, these destructive feelings about "self" can manifest in self-mutilation. Other abused students may develop perfectionist tendencies and focus on overachievement as a form of escapism by concentrating on areas that may provide them with some sense of control (e.g., school success) (Horton and Cruise, 2001). This type of perfectionism may be accompanied by anxiety and inflexibility (p. 256).*

Pollak (2002) found that *abused children* are highly sensitive to signs of anger in facial expressions. As a result, they tend to see maladaptive intentions in others when none may exist, and they may act on their misperceptions in a variety of incorrect ways including anger, withdrawal, fear, and flight.

In an analysis of national child abuse reports, Sedlak (1997) reports that the average abused child was 7.2 years old, ranging from a mean of "5.5 years of age for physical abuse to 9.2 years of age for sexual abuse" (p. 153). Fifty-four percent of the victims were male children who had been physically abused. Male children also accounted for 23% of sexual abuse cases (p. 153), suggesting a much higher rate for male victims of sexual abuse than had previously been thought. In the National Family Violence Survey conducted by Straus and Gelles (1990), it was estimated that 110 out of every 1000 children in the general population experience severe violence by their parents and that 23 in 1000 experienced very severe or life threatening violence. Severe violence was defined as kicking, biting, punching, hitting, beating up, threatening with a weapon, or using a knife or gun (Sedlak, p. 178). Very severe violence resulted in serious bodily damage to a child. Since lower income families are much more likely to have abuse reported by an outside party than are more affluent families, it was estimated by Straus and Gelles (1990) that inclusion of potential abuse by more affluent families could raise the actual amount of abuse by 50%.

In her study of the factors that influence the multiple forms of child abuse and neglect, Sedlack (1997) reports that family income is a strong factor. When compared to children whose families had incomes of $30 000 a year or more, children from families with incomes below $15 000 per year were found to have:

1. Twenty-one times greater risk of physical abuse.
2. More than 24 times the risk of sexual abuse.
3. Between 20 and 162 times the risk of physical neglect (depending on the children's other characteristics).
4. More than 13 times greater risk of emotional maltreatment.
5. Sixteen times greater risk of multiple maltreatment, and
6. Between 78 and 97 times greater risk of educational neglect (in Geffner, 1997, p. 171).

When the home situation becomes extremely dysfunctional and abusive, children may run away. A study by Finkelhor et al. (2000) indicated that about 133 000 children run away from home each year and while away, stay in insecure and unfamiliar places. The same study reports that almost 60 000 children were "thrown out" of their homes. Almost 140 000 abused and neglected children were reported missing to the police while 163 000 children were abducted by one parent in an attempt to permanently conceal the whereabouts of the child from the other parent. These additional data suggest that the impact of abuse and neglect often leads to children being abandoned or running away to other unsafe environment where they can experience additional harm (NCJ-180753).

Children who are subjected to domestic violence, even when they are not the victims, have a higher than normal potential of abusing others. Dodge et al. (1990) believe that physical abuse in early childhood is a risk marker for the development of aggressive behavior patterns. The authors report a threefold increase in the risk to be abusive in children who have witnessed abuse in their families and a significant increase in the way in which these children incorrectly view the hostile intent of others.

As we know, however, many children who experience abuse are able to cope with it in admirable and even heroic ways and have made life adjustments demonstrating behavior that is well within normal limits. In a highly controversial article, Rind et al. (1997) suggest that the impact of child sexual abuse may be much less than we think and write:

> *Our goal in the current study was to examine whether, in the population of persons with a history of CSA, this experience causes pervasive, intense psychological harm for both genders. Most previous literature reviews have favored this viewpoint. However, their conclusions have generally been based on clinical and legal samples, which are not representative of the general population. To address this viewpoint, we examined studies that used national probability samples, because these samples provide the best available estimate of population characteristics. Our review does not support the prevailing viewpoint. The self-reported effects data imply that only a small proportion of persons with CSA experiences are permanently harmed and that a substantially greater proportion of females than males perceive harm from these experiences. Results from psychological adjustment measures imply that, although CSA is related to poorer adjustment in the general population, the magnitude of this relation is small. Further, data on confounding variables imply that this small relation cannot safely be assumed to reflect causal effects of the CSA (p. 253).*

Among a number of researchers who tested the above conclusions, Duncan (2000) studied the finding that college students who had been sexually abused as children did as well as non-abused students. She found that abused college students were much more likely to suffer from symptoms of PTSD and to drop out of college prematurely, often after one semester. In a highly critical article suggesting that the Rind et al. research promoted pedophilia since it argued against the long-term harm of sexual abuse, Dallam (2002) writes

> *A number of researchers have demonstrated that the Rind et al.'s (1998) data either fails to support their case, was presented in a misleading or biased way, or equally supports alternative explanations. A review of the authors' previous writings reveals that Rind and Bauserman formed many of their opinions about the relative harmlessness of sexual relationships between adults and children years prior to performing any meaningful research into the issue. In addition, the authors' views on sex between adults and children have more in common with the ideology of advocates of "intergenerational" sexual relationships, than the reasoned opinions of most other scientists who have studied this issue. After reviewing the available evidence, Rind et al. is perhaps best described as an advocacy paper that inappropriately uses science in an attempt to legitimize its findings (p. 128).*

18.2. JUDGING RISK FACTORS OF CHILD ABUSE

The problem of determining the risk factors of abuse is a daunting one for many child protective service workers. Shlonsky and Wagner (2005) argue that before child abuse and neglect can be contained from very high current levels, a much better risk assessment approach must be used. The current system of identifying children and families at risk requires the worker to make the assessment quickly because of potential danger to the child and to sift through a great deal of complex information resulting in "Clinical decisions involving the assignment of risk [that] are marked by cognitive biases and thinking errors, resulting in decisions that tend to have limited predictive validity" (p. 409). The authors believe that one way to resolve the problem of determining risk of child abuse is to substitute clinical judgment based on intuition and experience for formal risk assessment instruments that are "compiled by "experts" who may draw upon previous research findings, clinical experience, or a combination of both' (p. 409) something that is not often done at present. The authors believe that models of assessment based on empirical research are far superior to clinical judgment and write, "Put simply, carefully validated actuarial models outperform clinical judgment at estimating future behavior" (p. 409). Commenting further on the need for an evidence-based model of risk assessment the authors write

> *The primary mission of every CPS agency is to manage risk to children (i.e., the risk of maltreatment), essentially meaning that cases need to be managed in a way that reduces harm to children. Effective agency case management, therefore, requires a reliable and valid estimate of future child maltreatment in order to inform key decisions that involve risk to children (Rycus and Hughes, 2003). Actuarial risk assessments do not yield infallible estimates of future harm but there is evidence that they provide the best available mechanism for estimating the probability of future maltreatment at a critical point – the close*

of the protective service investigation (Baird and Wagner, 2000; Baird et al., 1999)

In determining when child abuse and neglect exist, child protective agency workers frequently use the following federal and state mandated guidelines (Feller, 1992; DePanfillis and Salus, 1992; Brokenburr, 1994):

1. **The age of the child:** State laws provide upper age limits of children protected by reporting laws, however, it is important to recognize that abuse and neglect can have more harmful effects on younger children. If a parent has slapped an infant and believes that slapping and shaking a child is an appropriate discipline, the infant could be in danger where an older child might not be.
2. **The location of the injury:** Physical injuries to the face and head are more likely to cause severe or permanent damage than on other parts of the body. Accidental injuries will commonly leave bruises on the shins, knees, elbows and forehead. The bruises will not have any uniform pattern if they are accidentally caused, for example, by a fall from a bicycle. Injuries inflicted on purpose will often have some patterns to them and may, for example, appear on both buttocks, both sides of the neck, and both hands or both ears.
3. **The use of an object:** Objects such as coat hangers, sandals, straps, belts, kitchen utensils, electric cords, pipes or fists are more likely to cause serious injuries than an open-handed spanking. Often, the instrument used can be recognized by the distinctive shape of the injuries they inflict. Electrical cords will often leave a long loop shaped bruise. Teeth marks are easily recognized in bite injuries.
4. **When corporal punishment becomes physical abuse:** Parents will often try to excuse the marks on their child by saying that the child deserved punishment for their misbehavior. However, an injury to a child cannot be condoned or ignored. The worker may understand the provocation that triggered the abuse and this will be helpful in working with the parents. Sometimes the punishment doesn't leave marks but it is still abusive. An example might be when a child is locked in a closet or chained in the yard.
5. **Examples of physical neglect:** Neglect can be defined as a failure to provide a proper level of care including food, clothing, shelter, hygiene, medical attention and supervision. One form of neglect can be medical. If a child has an ear infection and the parents are not using the medical options available to them, then the worker might need a court order to ensure that the child gets immediate care. Shelter that is unheated in the winter or bug ridden would be a reason for the worker to intervene. Malnutrition and failure to thrive are clear grounds for intervention. Inadequate clothing for the season or clothing that isn't washed would also require intervention. When money is used for drugs or alcohol by the parents and the children are deprived of basic needs such as food, shelter, clothing or medical care, this would be considered neglect in most states.
6. **Educational neglect:** Poor school attendance is another form of parental neglect that would be considered a reason for child protective services intervention. The child may be missing school because of poor health or a parent may require an older child to stay home and care for younger siblings. Often, children may not be attending school because of chaos, domestic violence, child abuse or other forms of crisis and in the home.

7. **Insufficient supervision:** There are many aspects to consider when determining that a lack of parental supervision constitutes neglect. The ages of the children, the time of day or night they may be left unsupervised, and the length of time they were alone are all important factors. Whether the parents left a phone number and food for the children are also considerations. Abandonment is an extreme form of neglect. "Throwaways" are a term used for children whose parents "kick" them out of the home or move away leaving the children to fend for themselves.
8. **Moral neglect:** Children who are allowed or encouraged to steal or prostitute themselves suffer from moral neglect. Sometimes parents will use children to make pornography. Runaways have often been victims of moral neglect as well as physical neglect and abuse.
9. **Emotional abuse and neglect:** Emotional abuse is parental behavior that causes psychological harm to the child. Abusive threats to lock the child up, have them arrested by the police, or send them away, thoroughly frighten and immobilize children and are examples of emotional abuse. When a parent or caretaker fails to provide adequate love and caring or intellectual stimulation, the child may often suffer from emotional neglect. Children with emotional abuse problems may exhibit developmental lags, withdrawal, or attachment problems that make it difficult for them to bond with others. They may also appear apathetic and have difficulty developing intimate relationships.
10. **Sexual abuse:** When a parent or any caretaker responsible for a child commits or allows any sexual act to be committed on a child, it is considered sexual abuse. Sexual abuse occurs most often within a family. The sexual activity between a family member and child is called incest with the most common form of incest being father–daughter sexual abuse. Another form of sexual abuse is sexual contact between the child and a non-relative known to the child. This form of sexual abuse is considered "sexual assault." Sexual assault also includes sexual activity initiated by a stranger. Sexual assault and incest are extremely traumatic to the child because force or threats are often used. Incest is also very damaging to the victim because the person responsible is usually in a position that would normally engender trust and should have protected rather than exploited the child. There is no question of degree or definition in the case of sexual abuse. Any sexual activity between a child and an adult or someone significantly further along in their physical and emotional development is considered sexual abuse.

18.3. EVIDENCE-BASED PRACTICE WITH ABUSED CHILDREN

Most helping professionals believe that child abuse ultimately results in serious emotional problems in childhood and adulthood unless treated early in the abuse cycle. But there is still a great deal to learn about treating the various forms of child abuse. In a book review of *Treatment of Child Abuse*, edited by Robert M. Reece (2000) Lukefahr (2001), writes:

> *Although there is a very strong effort throughout to base findings and recommendations on the available evidence, these chapters highlight the reality that this young, evolving specialty remains largely descriptive. A common theme of several authors is the prominent role of cognitive-behavioral therapy*

> *for child abuse victims, but therapists may be disappointed in the lack of specific protocols for implementing CBT (Lukefahr, 2001, p. 36).*

Kaplan et al. (1999) report that the effectiveness of treatment for children who have been physically and sexually abused "has generally not been empirically evaluated. In a review of treatment research for physically abused children, Oates and Bross (1995) cite only 13 empirical studies between 1983 and 1992 meeting even minimal research standards" (p. 1218). Delson and Kokish (2002) report the following conclusions about the effectiveness of conventional therapy with abused children:

> *Conventional wisdom recommends early treatment for child victims of sexual abuse and professional literature is rich with articles describing treatment methodology and anecdotal case reports. But controlled studies of treatment outcomes are rare. Here's one of the few. Eighty-four sexually abused children ages 5–15 were assessed at intake, along with a group of community controls. (Oates et al., 1995) When reassessed 18 months later, 65% of the abused children had received therapy – 35% had not.*
>
> *The abused group was more dysfunctional at intake than the control group. As time went by the abused children made greater strides towards normalcy than the controls. At the end of eighteen months, the abused group was still more dysfunctional, but had closed the gap considerably. The greatest improvement was in depression. Self-esteem did not improve and actually deteriorated over time in many of the victims, regardless of treatment. The use of "avoidance" as a coping strategy by mothers correlated positively with deterioration in children's self esteem.*
>
> *The best predictor of improvement was adequate maternal and family functioning. It may be that supportive social services and counseling for care givers would prove more effective than direct counseling for victims, at least in terms of short term adjustment (Delson and Kokish, 2002, p. 1).*

Finkelhor and Berliner (1995) reviewed 29 studies regarding the effectiveness of treating sexually abused children. The researchers report that the studies they reviewed showed "that sexually abused children improve over time with or without treatment" (p. 1409) and that the current research is so methodologically flawed "that the effectiveness of sexual abuse treatment has yet to be proven" (p. 1415). Seligman (1994) cautioned against therapy for the sexually abused and believed that there is no evidence to support current thinking that molested children need to relive the experience and experience a catharsis in order to improve (Bushman et al., 1999; Seligman, 1994). In fact Seligman suggested that reliving the event may cause harm since it strengthen the memory of the event in the child's mind and negatively impacts the child's ability to heal naturally (pp. 234–235). In a review of the findings of the effectiveness of treatment for sexually abused children, Oellerich (2000) concludes that a large mental health industry has developed since the 1970s when the impact of child sexual abuse began to be seriously discussed which provides little by way of research to support its existence and instead, functions by way of popular belief that sexually abused children need help and that all help, regardless of any evidence, is better than no help at all.

Oellerich (2000) believes that it is time to stop assuming that sexually abused children routinely need help or that referral for treatment is always necessary. He recommends that therapy should only be used when there is demonstrable harm done to the child and that children and parents should be advised that our knowledge of treatment for sexually abused children is at a very early stage which requires us to inform children and parents of the validity of our interventions and that with our lack of knowledge may come unwanted and even harmful results. Validity of our interventions should include full disclosure of treatment used and whether it has been empirically validated, is experimental, or has been deemed unhelpful.

This, of course leaves unanswered when referral *is* necessary. Oellerich says that treatment should be initiated when there has been coercion, threat or demonstrable harm. He leaves unanswered what constitutes demonstrable harm but it seems obvious that children who are suffering from depression, anxiety or symptoms of PTSD following a molestation should be referred for effective help. Similarly, eating and sleep disorders, which continue on for an unusual length of time should be referred. Regression to early stages of childhood and overtly age inappropriate sexual behavior are reasons to refer as are lethal anger against other children and deterioration in school functioning. While I disagree with the conclusion that sexual abuse of children does little long-term hard (I think it often causes harm in adult sexual relations and issues of intimacy) I do think giving the child time to heal before assuming emotional difficulty is wise before we refer for help. And I agree that treatment is in its infancy and before we initiate treatment we should be very aware of what works, when it works, and with whom it works.

In further evaluations of treatment approaches with potential to help abused and neglected children and their families, Chaffin and Friedrich (2004) examined 24 mental health interventions for children who were victims of intra-familial physical or sexual abuse and their families. Only one treatment, trauma-focused cognitive–behavioral therapy (TF-CBT; Cohen and Mannarino, 1997; Deblinger et al., 1996) was given a rating of well-supported and efficacious. One treatment, attachment therapy (the Evergreen Model), was found to have significant potential for harm. A second effort, funded by the Kauffman Foundation, found three treatment models with potential to help children and their families: Trauma-Focused Cognitive Behavioral Therapy (TF-CBT; Cohen and Mannarino, 1997; Deblinger et al., 1996), Abuse-Focused Cognitive–Behavioral Therapy (AF-CBT; Kolko, 1996), and Parent–Child Interaction Therapy (PCIT; Chaffin and Friedrich, 2004; Hembree-Kigin and McNeil, 1995; Urquiza and McNeil, 1996).

Chaffin and Friedrich (2004) argue that even though research on treatment effectiveness of work with abused children "is not a scientifically mature field, there is currently a small, but not insignificant number of models that have proven efficacious in these types of trials" (p. 1099), the evidence they offer seems very limited. Most of studies they cite are either methodologically flawed by the researchers own evaluations or there lacks uniformity in what the study is trying to measure. In a summary of some "promising" findings regarding the treatment of abuse and neglect, Chaffin and Friedrich (2004) provide the following:

1. **Preventing future abuse:** Perinatal home-visits for preventing future physical abuse and neglect among new parents have had disappointing results. The Nurse Family Partnership model (Olds et al., 1998) is the best-supported model currently being practiced, although methodological problems exist in the research efforts.
2. **Preventing future sexual abuse:** Sexual abuse prevention programs usually try to educate young children (potential victims) to avoid sexual abuse or to disclose abuse if it occurs. Chaffin and Friedrich (2004) report that "none of these victimization programs have been evaluated in randomized trials for actual abuse prevention outcomes. Quasi-experimental studies have yielded mixed findings of some possible benefit, but also the concerning finding that children receiving these programs may be more likely to be injured" (p. 1107).
3. **Preventing future neglect:** Although neglect comprises the majority of child welfare system cases, there are few studies of intervention. Chaffin and Friedrich (2004) found Project 12-Ways/SafeCare model to be one of the more widely studied and supported approaches (Gershater-Molko et al., 2002; Lutzker and Rice, 1987; Lutzker et al., 2001). The model uses behavioral methods, focusing on various problems within families related to neglect. Chaffin and Friedrich (2004) caution that although the findings are promising, methodological problems exist and further research is necessary to confirm its use in treating and reducing neglect.
4. **Treating children and families where abuse exists:** Chaffin and Friedrich (2004) report that two models show promise in treating physically abusive parents: Parent–Child Interaction Therapy (PCIT), a live-coached behavioral parent training intervention (Chambless and Ollendick, 2001). Chaffin and Friedrich (2004) report that PCIT can significantly reduce rates of future physically abusive behavior among abusive parents. Multisystemic Therapy (MST) (Brunk et al., 1987) was also found to be effective in treating abused children and their abusive families.
5. **Treating sexually abused children:** Chaffin and Friedrich (2004) write that "Trauma-focused cognitive–behavioral therapy, using the principles of gradual exposure and cognitive restructuring has been evaluated in a series of randomized trials (Cohen & Mannarino, 1997; Deblinger et al., 1996) and has consistently been found superior to competing approaches" (p. 1109). The researchers believe that because of the positive research findings that it is a clear choice for this population.

18.4. EBP WITH AN ABUSED CHILD: A CASE STUDY UTILIZING THE STRENGTHS PERSPECTIVE

Although the strength's perspective has yet to demonstrate a strong research literature, the approach offers promise in the treatment of children who have suffered abuse and neglect. Anderson (1997) has written with wisdom about the use of the strengths perspective with abused children. Before we begin the case, it might be helpful to note some of her suggestions and observations in working with abused children. They are:

1. Regarding the treatment plan Anderson (1997) writes:

   ... it is essential to formulate specific and clear guidelines for treatment that center on survival abilities because gathering this information helps children to take pride in their accomplishments. Rebuilding self-esteem and pride is extremely important for children who have been sexually abused because the trauma permeates their identity and may leave them lacking in feelings of self-worth. (Anderson, 1997, p. 593)

2. To understand the meaning of a maltreated child's behavior, Anderson (1997) suggests, "The psychological scars will never disappear completely; however, focusing on the child's strengths and resiliency can help limit the power of sexual abuse over the child" (p. 597). Anderson (1997) notes that many maltreated children use wishful thinking or daydreaming to emotionally distance themselves from the abuse. Rather than seeing these coping mechanisms as dysfunctional, Anderson suggests that we recognize all of the child's survival strategies as a way of understanding the way in which maltreated children cope. The child's coping strategies should be seen as strengths and not as impediments or dysfunctions.
3. Anderson (1997) explains why pathology models are not likely to work with abused children.

   A pathology focus encourages practitioners to perceive clients as having some disorder or deficit that creates negative expectations about their potential to address the stressors in their lives (Barnard, 1994; Saleebey, 1997). Identifying and building on the positive aspects of the self that helped the child survive trauma open up creative ways to work with children who have been sexually abused. (Anderson, 1997, p. 597)

4. Having a positive mindset about our treatment and the child's ability to change helps the therapeutic process. Anderson (1997) offers hope in our work with abused children and writes

   ... somehow as children they not only endure the sexual abuse but find ways to go on with their lives. They have the burden of not revealing that anything has happened to them. This prevents them from seeking assistance, and they are left to develop strategies for surviving the trauma on their own. Their capacity for self-repair takes tremendous energy, preventing them from accomplishing important developmental tasks. Because their survival abilities are overshadowed by the trauma, these strengths may be overlooked during treatment if the practitioner limits the definition of resiliency to the exhibition of competency (Anderson, 1997, p. 595).

18.5. LYNN

Lynn is a 9-year-old child who has been physically and sexually abused by her mother, Jolene, since Lynn was 4. Jolene has been diagnosed with schizophrenia and is currently in a state hospital where she is being treated to achieve competence to stand trial for abusing Lynn. Lynn has had some clear signs that she is not coping well with either the abuse or her mother's absence. She has been experiencing depression and anxiety since her mother was hospitalized and reports occasional enuresis and bulimia. The worker sees both Lynn and her mother, separately, since it is vital that Lynn maintain even indirect contact with her mother and that the two maintain a relationship although they will be separated for some time to come. Children have loyalty to parents, even abusing parents, and Lynn wants to maintain contact with her mother. The purpose of the treatment Lynn is receiving is to help her understand her mother's behavior, disassociate it from anything Lynn has done, and to help Lynn develop positive feelings about herself. The symptoms of depression, anxiety, bedwetting and bulimia will also be treated.

Lynn believes that she is responsible for her mother's abusive behavior and thinks that there is something evil about her. These are messages given to Lynn by her mother who believed that Lynn was possessed by evil forces. The worker has allowed Lynn to express these feelings while noting her many positive achievements, even in the midst of abuse that would be more than most children could endure. The worker brought a note from Lynn's mother saying how much she loves Lynn, how sorry she is for what she did, and that it had nothing to do with Lynn, but was something that had to do with her illness. She thinks Lynn is a very special child, and prays for her everyday, and asks God His forgiveness for her bad behavior. Lynn is very moved by her mother's notes and returns from treatment feeling loved and cherished. "I forgive my mom," she told the worker, "and I pray every night that my mom will get well and we'll be together."

Lynn lives with her grandmother who is a stable and positive support. Her grandmother is religious and Lynn has begun to find solace in the religious experiences she shares with her grandmother. The church she attends has been supportive and caring and many of the children she meets at services have been abused or neglected and are living with relatives or foster parents who attend the church. She has chosen her friends wisely and has developed a small support network of friends who have been abused and neglected and know, without needing to have it explained, that a certain level of sadness never quite leaves an abused child. Some days are difficult for Lynn, but with the kindness of her grandmother and friends, she does well in school and has discovered a gift for music. Her depression and anxiety are lifting but she still has days when she feels blue.

In describing her therapy, Lynn said, "I like seeing Mrs. Redman. She's always nice to me and treats me like an adult. Sometimes when I'm really upset and can't talk much, she's patient and we can sit together and she lets me cry. She makes me feel that I can do anything in life. I like that she's helping my mother and understands that it's her mental illness that makes her act so bad. My mom is a wonderful person when she's not sick and even Mrs. Redman tells me so. When I see Mrs. Redman, she always tells me about the good things I can do. When I get really sad, she tells me that many children haven't done as well as I have and there must be something pretty special about me. I don't know if that's true because sometimes I feel awful inside, but it sure makes me feel better. The people I have at church and at school help a lot too, and Mrs. Redman always says that nice people are attracted to each other. I hope my mom is OK, and I hope she can see me a lot. She's still my mom and it doesn't matter what she did. You only have one mom in your life, and if God meant for her to have this sickness, it must be for a reason. Maybe it helps me care more about other people. I hope so."

18.6. DISCUSSION

Like many abused children, Lynn is loyal to her mother. She understands the harm her mother did to her but also recognizes the impact of her mother's mental illness. This understanding attitude is one that will very likely have a positive impact on Lynn as she matures. The treatment she is receiving is supportive, positive, and caring. Lynn feels that her worker is a sensitive person and that her treatment helps her feel better about herself. She is honest about the feelings of sadness she experiences and has been wise in her choice of friends. Her grandmother and the religious experiences they share together have been strengths that have helped Lynn cope with the abuse and the loss of her mother. Rather than focusing on the harm done to her by her mother, her grandmother and the therapist have focused on Lynn's many positive attributes. By doing this, Lynn is beginning to internalize a positive self-view that helps offset the many times when she has negative thoughts about herself. She feels sad and the worker allows her to feel that way without suggesting that it is a dysfunctional behavior she allows Lynn to process her feelings even if it involves long silences. Helping Lynn feel she's in control of her treatment is a way of helping her feel that she's in control of her life. In many important ways, the therapist is modeling for Lynn what a kind and supportive mother would be like and Lynn has begun to understand that being nurtured and loved are important qualities in any relationship. This understanding helps Lynn separate her fantasies about her mother from the realities of coping with a mother who may have a limited ability to nurture or to love.

I asked the worker why she chose the strengths perspective and how it worked in practice with Lynn. She told me, "I went to the literature when I began working with abused children and I was surprised to learn how little had been written about effective treatment. I found many suggestions but few that were research tested so I chose the strengths model because it seemed the least likely to cause harm. I know that sounds wishy-washy, but it's true. Consistent with the literature on the use of the strengths perspective (Glicken, 2004; Saleebey 2000, 1996, 1994, 1992) I focused on the positives in Lynn's life. I tried not to use pejorative words that implied pathology like depressed, or anxious, or fearful. Instead, when Lynn talked about her emotions she used words like blue, or down, or nervous, everyday words we all use. I let her talk and I didn't dwell on any of her unhappiness. I listened respectfully, involved her in the issues we would discuss, valued what she said, never tried to steer the conversation in a direction, and focused instead on Lynn recognizing the amazing degree of resilience and mental health she exhibited in face of some terribly abusive behavior. Thanks to the work of Anderson (1997), I focused on helping Lynn build self-esteem.

"As a social worker I'm mainly interested in social functioning. To determine whether she was doing better as a result of treatment I checked with the school, her grandmother, and the pastor of her church. Her grades had improved from a 'C' average to a 'B' average since the beginning of treatment 6 months ago. Lynn's grandmother confirmed she hadn't wet her bed in almost 4 months and that she was eating normally. The pastor said that Lynn was a wonderful child whose warmth and compassion for others were felt by everyone in the small congregation. I counted the number of times Lynn used words to describe her behavior that implied emotional distress, words like sad, or nervous, or scared. The number of words with negative connotations fell from over 50 a session to perhaps 1 or 2 after 6 months. Conversely, the number of positive words such as proud, happy, like, doing well, good grades, good friend rose from none the first session to over 50 by the end of 6 months. I realize that some of this could be explained by Lynn trying to please me by emphasizing positives in her life that aren't really there, but she assures me she isn't doing this, and I tend to believe her.

"I like the strengths perspective for abused children and I wish there was more in the literature to suggest what works. For the time being, I'm going to continue using the strengths approach and try and do my own evaluation of how effective it is with a variety of children by age, race/ethnicity, and gender. I had you in class for research, Dr. Glicken, and when you told us to evaluate our work I thought I could always tell when clients were better just by how they responded in a session. I don't believe that anymore and find it strangely satisfying, for a non-researcher, to continually check myself on how well I'm doing. Satisfying and, I have to admit, reinforcing. Instead of believing I do well with clients I now feel pretty certain that I am and that's pretty reinforcing."

18.7. SUMMARY

This chapter discusses the staggering numbers of abused children in United States, the causes of abuse, and best evidence for the assessment and treatment of abused children. The chapter notes that even abused resilient children who do well on many behaviorally oriented measures sometimes suffer negative emotional consequences including depression and low self esteem. Concern was raised for the limited amount of knowledge at present on effective treatment approaches for abused and neglected children. A case study describes treatment with a severely abused child.

18.8. QUESTIONS FROM THE CHAPTER

1. It is hard to imagine why we do not have a better understanding of how to best help abused and neglected children. Suggest some reasons why we still have such little concrete evidence about helping children after so many years of providing services to abused and neglected children in America.
2. We have a staggering amount of child abuse and neglect in the United States. What are the reasons for the large amount of abuse, in your opinion?
3. The Rind, Tromovitch, and Bauserman article stating that child molestation is not traumatic for most victims is controversial to say the least. What is your reaction to the conclusions of the authors?
4. In many states, less than 10% of all reported cases of child abuse are investigated. Do you think this suggests wide spread incompetence on the part of child protective services in America or might there be other reasons?
5. If you leave your 2-year-old alone in the car while you run into the store for a quick shopping trip, do you think this would constitute child endangerment and if so, what would the correct community response be?

References

Anderson, K. M. (1997, November). Uncovering survival abilities in children who have been sexually abused. *Families in Society: The Journal of Contemporary Human Services, 78*(6), 592–599.

Baird. , & Wagner, D. (2000). The relative validity of actuarial and consensus-based risk assessment systems. *Children and Youth Services Review, 22*(11–12), 839–871.

Baird, C., Wagner, D., Healy, T., & Johnson, K. (1999). Risk assessment in child protective services: Consensus and actuarial model reliability. *Child Welfare, 78*(6), 723–748.

Barnard, C. (1994). Resiliency: A shift in our perception?. *American Journal of Family Therapy, 22*, 135–144.

Brokenburr, D. (1994). The author acknowledges the contribution of Ms. Doyle Brokenburr in the development of parts of this chapter.

Brunk, M., Henggeler, S. W., & Whelan, J. P. (1987). Comparison of multisystemic therapy and parent training in the brief treatment of child abuse and neglect. *Journal of Consulting and Clinical Psychology, 55*, 171–178.

Bushman, B. J., Baumeister, R. F., & Stack, A. D. (1999). Catharsis, aggression, and persuasive influence: Self-fulfilling or self-defeating prophecies?. *Journal of Personality and Social Psychology, 76*, 367–376.

Chaffin, M., & Friedrich, B. (2004). Evidence based treatment in child abuse and neglect. *Children and Youth Services Review, 26*, 1097–1113.

Chambless, D. L., & Ollendick, T. H. (2001). Empirically supported psychological interventions: Controversies and practices. *Annual Review of Psychology, 52*, 685–716.

Cohen, J. A., & Mannarino, A. P. (1997). A treatment study of sexually abused preschool children: Outcome during a one year follow-up. *Journal of the Academy of Child and Adolescent Psychiatry, 36*, 1228–1235.

Dallam, S. J. (2002). Science or Propaganda? An examination of Rind, Tromovitch and Bauserman (1998). *Journal of Child Sexual Abuse, 9*(3–4), 109–134.

Deblinger, E., Lippmann, J., & Steer, R. (1996). Sexually abused children suffering post-traumatic stress symptoms: Initial treatment outcome findings. *Child Maltreatment, 1*, 310–321.

Delson, N., & Kokish, R. (2002). *Treating sexually abused children: Disturbing information about effectiveness.* Article found on the Internet November 25, 2002. http://www.delko.net/CSA%20kid%20treatment.htm.

DePanfillis, D., & Salus, M. (1992). *Child protective services: A guide for caseworkers.* National Center for Child Abuse and Neglect. McLean, Virginia: The Circle, Inc..

Dodge, K. A., Bates, J. E., & Peteit, G. S. (1990). Mechanisms in the cycle of violence. *Science, 28*.

Duncan, R. D. (2000). Childhood maltreatment and college drop-out rates: Implications for child abuse researchers. *Journal of Interpersonal Violence, 15*, 987–995.

Feller, J. (1992). *Working with the courts in child protection.* McLean, Virginia: National Center on Child Abuse and Neglect. The Circle, Inc..

Finkelhor, D., & Berliner, L. (1995). Research on the treatment of sexually abused children: A review and recommendations. *Journal of the American Academy of Child and Adolescent Psychiatry, 34*, 1408–1423.

Finkelhor, D., Hotaling, G.T., & Sedlack, A. (2000). Missing, abducted, runaway and throwaway children in America. First report: Numbers and characteristics, National Incident Report, 1988. Reported in 1999 National Report Series: Juvenile Justice Crime Bulletin, May 2000, NCJ-180753.

Gershater-Molko, R. M., Lutzker, J. R., & Wesch, D. (2002). Using recidivism data to evaluate project SafeCare: An ecobehavioral approach to teach "bonding", safety, and health care skills. *Child Maltreatment, 7*, 277–285.

Glicken, M. D. (2004). *Using the strengths perspective in social work practice.* Boston, MA: Allyn and Bacon/Longman.

Hembree-Kigin, T., & McNeil, C. B. (1995). *Parent–child interaction therapy.* New York: Plenum.

Horton, C. B., & Cruise, T. K. (2001). *Child abuse and neglect: The school's response.* New York: The Guilford Press.

Kaplan, S. J., Pelcovitz, D., & Labruna, V. (1999). Child and adolescent abuse and neglect research: A review of the past 10 years. Part I: physical and emotional abuse and neglect. *Journal of the American Academy of Child and Adolescent Psychiatry, 38*(10), 1214–1222.

Kolko, D. J. (1996). Individual cognitive behavioral therapy and family therapy for physically abused children and their offending parents: A comparison of clinical outcomes. *Child Maltreatment, 1*, 322–342.

Lambie, G. W. (2005). Child abuse and neglect: A practical guide for professional school counselors. *Professional School Counseling, 8*(3), 249–259.

Lukefahr, J. L. (2001). Treatment of child abuse (book review). *Journal of the American Academy of Child and Adolescent Psychiatry, 40*(3), 383.

Lutzker, J. R., & Rice, J. M. (1987). Using recidivism data to evaluate Project 12-Ways: An ecobehavioral approach to the treatment and prevention of child abuse and neglect. *Journal of Family Violence, 2*, 283–290.

Lutzker, J. R., Tymchuk, A. J., & Bigelow, K. M. (2001). Applied research in child maltreatment: Practicalities and pitfalls. *Children's Services: Social Policy, Research, and Practice, 4*, 141–156.

Miller, L. (1999). Juvenile crime statistics 1998. Victim Advocate. U.S. Department of Juvenile Justice. Washington, DC: U.S. Government Printing Office.

Oates, R. K., & Bross, D. C. (1995). What have we learned about treating child physical abuse? A literature review of the last decade. *Journal of Child Abuse & Neglect, 19*, 463–473.

Oellerich, T. D. (2000). Rind, Tromovitch, and Bauserman: Politically Incorrect – Scientifically Correct. *Sexuality & Culture, 4*(2), 67–81.

Olds, D. L., Henderson, C. R., Cole, R., Eckenrode, J., Kitzman, H., Luckey, D., et al. (1998). Long-term effects of nurse home visitation on children's criminal and antisocial behavior: 15-year follow-up of a randomized controlled trial. *Journal of the American Medical Association, 280*, 1238–1244.

Pollak, S. D. (2002, June 25). Early experience is associated with the development of categorical representations for facial expressions of emotion. *Proceedings of the National Academy of Sciences, 99*(13), 9072–9076.

Prevent Child Abuse America. (2003). *What everyone can do to prevent child abuse: 2003 child abuse prevention community resource packet*. Chicago: Author.

Rind, B., Tromovitch, P., & Bauserman, R. (1997). A meta-analytic review of findings from national samples on psychological correlates of child sexual abuse. *Journal of Sex Research, 34*(3), 237–255.

Russell, D. E. (1999). *The secret trauma: Incest in the lives of girls and women* (Rev. ed.). New York: Basic Books.

Rycus, B., & Hughes, R.C. (2003). Issues in risk assessment in child protective services: A policy white paper, North American Resource Center for Child Welfare Center for Child Welfare Policy, Columbus, Ohio.

Saleebey, D. (1992). *The strengths perspective in social work practice*. White Plains, NY: Longman.

Saleebey, D. (1994). Culture, theory, and narrative: The intersection of meanings in practice. *Social Work, 39*, 352–359.

Saleebey, D. (1996). The strengths perspective in social work practice: Extensions and cautions. *Social Work, 41*(3), 296–305.

Saleebey, D. (1997). The strengths approach to practice. In D. & Saleebey (Ed.), *The strengths perspective in social work practice* (pp. 49–57). New York: Longman.

Saleebey, D. (2000). Power in the people; strength and hope. *Advances in Social Work, 1*(2), 127–136.

Sechrist, W. (2000). Health educators and child maltreatment: A curious silence. *Journal of School Health, 70*(6), 241–243.

Sedlack, A. (1997). Risk factors for the occurance of child abuse and neglect. *Journal of Agression Maltreatment and Trauma, 1*(1), 149–181.

Seligman, M. E. P. (1994). *What you can change and what you can't*. New York: Alfred A. Knopf.

Shlonsky, A., & Wagner, D. (2005, April). The next step: Integrating actuarial risk assessment and clinical judgment into an *evidence-based practice* framework in CPS case management. *Children & Youth Services Review, 27*(4), 409–427.

Straus, M. A., & Gelles, R. J. (1990). *Physical violence in American families: Risk factors and adaptations to violence in families*. New Brunswick, NJ: Transaction Publishers.

Urquiza, A. J., & McNeil, C. B. (1996). Parent–child interaction therapy: An intensive dyadic intervention for physically abusive families. *Child Maltreatment, 1*, 132–141.

Further reading

Abrams, M. S. (2001). Resilience in ambiguous loss. *American Journal of Psychotherapy* (2), 283–291.

Arend, R., Gove, F., & Sroufe, L. (1979). Continuity of individual adaptation from infancy to kindergarten: A predictive study of ego-resiliency and curiosity in preschoolers. *Child Development, 50*, 950–959.

Baldwin, A., Baldwin, C., Kasser, T., Zax, M., Sameroff, A., & Seifer, R. (1993). Contextual risk and resiliency during adolescence. *Development and Psychopathology, 5*, 741–761.

Byrd, R. (1994). Assessing resilience in victims of childhood maltreatment. Doctoral diss. Pepperdine University. Dissertation Abstracts, 5503.

Cohler, B. (1987). Adversity, resilience, and the study of lives. In E. J. Anthony, B. J. & Cohler (Eds.), *The invulnerable child* (pp. 363–424). New York: Guilford.

Egeland, E., Carlson, E., & Sroufe, L. (1993). Resilience as process. *Development and Psychopathology, 5*, 517–528.

Furey, J. A. (1993). Unknown soldiers: Women veterans and PTSD. *Professional Counselor, 7*(6), 33–34.

Garmezy, N., Masten, A., & Tellegen, A. (1964). The study of stress and competence in children: A building block for developmental psychopathology. *Child Development, 55*, 97–111.

Henry, D. L. (1999, September). Resilience in maltreated children: Implications for special needs adoptions. *Child Welfare, 78*(5), 519–540.

Kauffman, C., Grunebaum, H., Cohler, B., & Gamer, E. (1979). Superkids: Competent children of psychotic mothers. *American Journal of Psychiatry, 136*, 1398–1402.

Luthar, S. (1993). Annotation: Methodology and conceptual issues in research on childhood resilience. *Journal of Child Psychology and Psychiatry, 34*, 441–453.

Mandleco, B. L., & Peery, J. C. (2000, July–August). An organizational framework for conceptualizing resilience in children. *Journal of Child & Adolescent Psychiatric Nursing, 13*(3), 99–112.

Masten, A. (1989). Resilience in development: Implications of the study of successful adaptation for developmental psychopathology. In D. & Cicchetti (Ed.), *The emergence of a discipline: Rochester symposium on developmental psychopathology* (pp. 261–294). Hillsdale, NJ: Lawrence Erlman Publishers.

Masten, A. S. (2001). Ordinary magic: Resilience processes in development. *American Psychologist, 56*, 227–238.

Masten, A. A., & Powell, J. L. (2003). A resilience framework for research, policy, and practice. In S. S. & Luthar (Ed.), *Resilience and vulnerabilities: Adaptation in the context of childhood adversities* (pp. 1–25). New York: Cambridge University Press.

Okun, A., Parker, J., & Levendosky, A. (1994). Distinct and interactive contributions of physical abuse, socioeconomic disadvantage, and negative live events to children's social, cognitive, affective adjustment. *Development and Psychopathology, 6*, 77–98.

Radke-Yarrow, M., & Brown, E. (1993). Resilience and vulnerability in children of multiple-risk families. *Development and Psychopathology, 5*, 581–592.

Tiet, Q. Q., Bird, H., & Davies, M. R. (1998, November). Adverse Life Events and Resilience. *Journal of the American Academy of Child and Adolescent Psychiatry, 37*(11), 1191–1200.

Walsh, F. (1998). *Strengthening family resilience*. New York: The Guilford Press.
Werner, E. (1989). High-risk children in young adulthood: A longitudinal study from birth to 32 years. *American Orthopsychiatric Association, 59*, 72–81.
Werner, E. (1993). Risk, resilience, and recovery. Perspectives from the Kauai longitudinal study. *Development and Psychopathology, 5*, 503–515.

19 Evidence-Based Practice and Sexual Violence by Children and Adolescents

19.1. INTRODUCTION

The author wishes to thank Pearson Education, Inc. for permission to use material from a book he wrote on violence by children under the age of 12 (Glicken, 2004, pp. 80–97)

Few of us think of young children as predatory sexual offenders but as we will note in this chapter, a considerable amount of the adolescent and adult sexual offending, particularly child molestation, often begins well before the onset of puberty. In studies that will be discussed in this chapter, the average age of the onset of sexual molestation may occur before the age of ten. And since most of the children who begin their sexual offending that young molest their own younger siblings or close family friends, the sexual offending is very likely to continue on at an ever more dangerous level as the child ages. The victims of molestation, in far too many cases, become the offenders as they age, and a cycle that should never have started, had we been more vigilant, continues on until the molested child becomes the molester and is caught. How much suffering might have been prevented had we been more aware of the early onset of sexual deviances and done something proactive to prevent it from happening? Hopefully this chapter will aid in that process.

19.2. LEGAL DEFINITIONS OF SEXUAL VIOLENCE

The following definitions of sexually violent acts are a compilation of terms used by a number of reporting groups, including the National Crime Victimization Survey (NCVS), The Uniform Crime Reports (UCR), and The National Incident-Based Reporting System (NIBRS). The definitions are taken from The Bureau of Justice Report entitled, "Sex Offenses and Offenders" (Lawrence Greenfeld, February 1997, NCJ-163392, pp. 31–33).

Forcible Rape: The carnal knowledge of a person forcibly and/or against his or her will, or in which the victim is incapable of giving consent because of age, mental status, or physical incapacity. Assaults and attempts to commit rape by force or threat of force are also included;

however, statutory rape without force and other sex offenses are excluded.

Statutory Rape: The carnal knowledge of a person without force or threat of force in which the person is below the statutory age of consent.

Forcible Sodomy: Oral or anal sexual intercourse with another person, forcibly and against his or her will, or in which the person is unable to consent because of age, mental or physical incapacity.

Sexual Assault With An Object: Assault in which the offender uses an instrument or object to unlawfully penetrate the genitalia or anal opening against a victim's will.

Forcible Fondling: Touching the private parts of another person against his or her will for the purpose of sexual gratification.

Incest: Non-forcible intercourse between persons who are related to one another and would not legally be permitted to marry.

Lewd Acts With Children: Fondling, indecent liberties, immoral practices, molestation and other indecent behaviors with children.

19.3. EVIDENCE OF SEXUAL VIOLENCE BY CHILDREN AND ADOLESCENTS

Knopp (as cited in Araji, 1997), using the 1980 Uniform Crime Reports, notes that 208 children under the age of 12 were arrested for rape. More recent surveys of sexually acting out children reveal much higher rates of sexually abusive behavior by preadolescent children. English and Ray (as cited in Araji, 1997) reported that the Washington Department of Social and Health Services had 641 active cases of children under the age of 12 who had raped, molested, or were involved in such non-contact sexual acts as exposing, masturbating in public, or peeping. Ryan et al. (1996) report that in a sample of 616 adolescents seen for evaluation or treatment for committing a sexual offense, 25.9% had been sexually abusive prior to their 12th birthday.

In self-reports by almost 500 juveniles being evaluated by the police for possible involvement in sexual offenses, Zolondek et al. (2001) found that over 60% reported involvement in child molestation, over 30% in pornography, and 10–30% in exhibitionism, fetishism, frottage, voyeurism, obscene phone calls and phone sex. Juveniles reported involvement, on the average, in 9-46 incidents of sexual offenses. The average age of onset for the sexual offenses was between 10 and 12 years of age. Of the boys who reported never having been accused of molesting children, 41.5% reported that they had molested a younger child. The authors suggest that between 15% and 20% of all sexual offenses are committed by youth younger than 18, and as many as 50% of all child molestations may be committed by youth younger than 18 (Davis & Leitenberg, 1987; Furby et al., 1989).

Commenting on the very early age of onset of various sexual behaviors in their sample (9.7 to 12.4 years of age), Zolondek et al. (2001) note that the average age of onset of sexual acting out is considerably younger than had been reported by other researchers, including Abel et al. (1985) and Weinrott (1996). Previous studies, they report, relied on retrospective reports by adult offenders who may have been giving socially desirable responses or whose memories may have been poor. The authors believe that adolescents begin their sexual offending prior to puberty, and that this finding is cause for concern, particularly since many of the offenders in their sample had been molesting younger siblings or close family friends. The authors call for early identification of youthful sexual offenders and point out that by the time a young offender is caught, he or she may have committed several offenses with several victims. They urge clinicians and researchers to go back to the offender's preadolescent years. They caution that very early deviant sexual behavior is a strong predictor of later predatory sexual behavior.

Caputo et al., 1999 report that juvenile sex offenses constitute a large number of all sex offenses. Groth et al., 1982 note that juveniles have been identified as the perpetrators in more than 25% of all child sexual abuse cases. Davis and Leitenberg (1987) report that juveniles committed 20% of the forcible rapes reported to the FBI in 1981. Caputo et al., 1999 note that while it is assumed that juvenile sexual offenses are merely exploratory and will not be repeated in adulthood, Groth et al. (1982) found that about a half of all adult sexual offenders report committing their first sexual offense as teenagers. Groth et al. (1982) further note that the patterns of the sexual offenses in terms of the age and characteristics of the victim, the amount of force used, and other aspects of the assault appear to have first developed in adolescence and continue into adulthood.

Saunders et al., 1992 found that 44% of respondents who were raped as children reported that the offender was younger than 21 years old. Berliner (1998) indicates that studies of adult sexual offenders have found that half of the offenders had begun having deviant sexual thoughts in adolescence or during preadolescents. Berliner also believes that juvenile sex offenders have very similar characteristics to adult sex offenders. "They may engage in serious sexual crimes, have multiple victims, exhibit deviant sexual preferences, have comparable cognitive distortions, and lack victim empathy" (Berliner, 1998, p. 645). Because the characteristics of juvenile sexual offenders are similar to those of adult offenders, Berliner believes that treatment programs for juveniles are similar to those of adults, without any strong evidence that an adult treatment model is necessarily the correct model for young offenders.

Snyder and Sigmund (1995) report that the number of juvenile offenders arrested for sexual crimes has increased steadily over the past decade. Barbaree et al., 1993 indicate that current studies estimate that juveniles are responsible for 15–20% of all rapes and 30–60% of all child sexual assault cases committed in the United States each year. Araji (1997) says that reports of sexual aggression in children as young as three and four are not uncommon, with the most common age of the onset of sexual aggression appearing to be between six and nine. Girls are more likely to be early onset sexual aggressors than older adolescents who have been sexually abused. The sexual acting out of early onset female offenders is just as aggressive as that of young male sexual offenders. Victims of preadolescent sexual abusers have an average age of between four and seven, are most often female, and are usually siblings, friends, or acquaintances (Araji, 1997). Araji (1997) further notes that victimized children who have been sexually abused have been very frequently sexually abused, and, according to Pithers et al. (1998b), have higher rates of abuse and neglect victimization experiences than those found among their adolescent counterparts (English and Ray, as cited in Araji, 1997). The preadolescent victims of sexual abuse have also been found to have frequent academic and learning difficulties and impaired peer relationships (Friedrich and Luecke, as cited in Araji, 1997; Pithers and Gray, as cited in Araji, 1997). Pithers et al. (1998a) found that the families of children with sexual behavior problems tended to live with high levels of poverty and with the frequent existence of child sexual abuse and domestic violence.

English and Ray (as cited in Araji, 1997) compared preadolescent sexual offenders with adolescent offenders. Both groups had a high number of family risk factors related to repeat offending. The families of preadolescent sexual offenders had more family problems than the adolescent offenders. The younger children had much higher levels of social isolation and current life stresses than the adolescent offenders. Lane and Lobanov-Rostovsky (1997) found that girls represent 5–8% of the juvenile sex offenders and often sexually offended while involved in childcare. Mathews et al., 1997 compared 67 girls and 70 boys with sexual offense histories. While both male and female offenders were alike in many ways, and both groups tended to molest young children of the opposite sex, girls had many more severe experiences as victims of childhood sexual abuse than boys.

In discussing juvenile dating experiences, James et al., 2000 reported that half of all early adolescent children report some degree of violence in dating situations including scratching, hitting, pushing, grabbing, or shoving their dates. About 25% of the children exhibited this behavior an average of four to nine times per date. Thirty-three percent of the children in dating situations threw something that hit their dating partners, kicked them, and slapped them. Twenty percent of the children twisted their partners' arms, slammed or held their dating partners against a wall, bent their fingers, bit them, choked them, dumped them from a car, burned them, beat them up, or hit them with something harder than a fist (James et al., 2000). Cascardi et al., 1994 found that 32% of the males and 52% of the females in their study of high school students had used aggression against a dating partner, while O'Keefe (1997) found that 39% of the males and 43% of the females had been physically aggressive with a dating partner at least once. Foshee (1996) reports that females were more likely to be perpetrators of dating violence. Jezl et al., 1996 found that 59% of their adolescent sample had experienced physical violence at least once in a dating relationship, 96% had experienced some form of psychological maltreatment, and 15% had been forced to engage in sexual activity. Significantly, more males than females reported being victims of physical abuse. Gray and Foshee (1997) found that about 66% of the adolescents who reported violence in dating relationships stated that it had begun with mutual consent and then escalated.

Veneziano et al., 2000 studied the sexual behavior of adolescent sexual offenders. They believe that youthful offenders relive their own sexual molestations by the choice of victims and the circumstance in which they were molested. The authors were able to prove the following hypotheses guiding their study:

Hypothesis 1: Adolescent sexual offenders victimize children of an age close to the age that they had been when they were sexually abused. That is, if they had been victimized at age six, they would be more likely to victimize a 6-year-old.

Hypothesis 2: Adolescent male sexual offenders who had been sexually abused by a male would be more likely to victimize a male.

Hypothesis 3: Adolescent sexual offenders victimize children related to them in the same way that they were related to their perpetrator. That is, if a relative had victimized them, they would victimize a relative. If a non-relative had victimized them, they would victimize a non-relative.

Hypothesis 4: Adolescent sexual offenders engage in the same abusive behaviors with their victims as the abusive behaviors that had been forced on them. That is, if they had been fondled, they would fondle their victims. (Veneziano et al., 2000, p. 365)

19.4. CHILD VICTIMS OF SEXUAL ASSAULT

In their sample of 500 juveniles undergoing evaluation for sexual offenses, Zolondek et al. (2001) found that when youth in the sample molested children, most of the children tended to be younger siblings or known non-family members. Juveniles in the sample used coercion and deception rather than force in the molestations and tended to select victims they knew and who were easily available. Ryan et al. (1996) found in their sample of adolescent child molesters that the victims were blood relatives in 38.8% of the cases, while Johnson (1988) found that 46% of the children molested by juveniles were family members. Many of the juveniles in this sample had engaged in child molestation that had gone undetected. A large number of youth in the sample had not been arrested for child molestation but for other sexual deviancies. The authors report that 42% of those in the sample arrested for sexual offenses other than molestation admitted that they had molested children before they were arrested. The authors strongly recommend that all juveniles arrested for sexual offenses should be evaluated for possible molestation of children.

What makes victimization such a tragic situation is that prior childhood sexual molestation of sexual offenders has been a frequent finding in both the adult and juvenile literature (Ford and Linney, 1995; Langevin et al., 1989; Pierce & Pierce,

1987). We have knowledge from child abuse reports that almost 40% of all adolescent sexual offenders have been sexually abused in childhood (Ryan et al., 1996). A study of very young perpetrators indicates that at least 49% have been sexually abused (Johnson, 1988), while other studies have found even higher rates (50% to 80%) of prior sexual abuse (Friedrich & Luecke, 1988; Ryan et al., 1987). It is important to keep in mind that this data were known to us before the juvenile began sexually abusing children. It is highly likely that another significant population of juvenile offenders were molested as children but failed or refused to confirm their molestation (or perhaps, had no memory of the molestation), raising the number of youthful sexual molesters who themselves have been abused to even greater numbers.

Victimization of children by sexual perpetrators not only results in a large range of symptoms, but also results in a high probability that the molested child might become a molester. As Glicken notes (2004), children who are molested develop symptoms in childhood that worsen in adolescence and often become unmanageable in adulthood. Symptoms of childhood molestation include depression, suicidal thoughts, eating disorders, substance abuse, the inability to establish and maintain relationships, sleep disorders, anxiety problems with panic attacks, failure at school and at work, sexual deviancies, sexual acting out including child molestation, rape and prostitution, inability to form attachments with significant others and a range of somatic concerns.

19.5. EBP WITH YOUTHFUL SEXUAL OFFENDERS

Lab et al., 1993 compared recidivism rates for juveniles in a specialized sex offender treatment program with recidivism rates for juveniles in non-specialized programs for sex offenders. The researchers found that recidivism rates for both groups were low and that specialized treatment programs did no better than non-specialized programs for juvenile sex offenders. The authors concluded, "These results suggest that the growth of interventions has proceeded without adequate knowledge of how to identify at-risk youth, the causes of the behavior, and the most appropriate treatment for juvenile sex offending" (p. 543). However, Kimball and Guarino-Ghezzi (1996) found that juveniles receiving specialized sex offender treatment were more likely to accept responsibility for their behavior, to indicate remorse for what they had done, and to provide evidence that would suggest the ability to resist relapse. Follow up to treatment suggested that involvement in a specialized program for adolescent sex offenders resulted in lower rates of re-offending.

Lea et al., 1999 note that attitudes toward sex offenders and sex crimes vary among members of the different professional groups assigned to work with offenders. Akerstrom (1986) believes that prison staff may see sex offenders as outcasts in the prison system and may relate to them in ways that inhibit treatment. Hogue (1993) studied the attitudes of various staff working with sex offenders and found that probation officers and psychologists had more positive attitudes toward offenders than prison officers and police officers. Not surprisingly, Hogue (1993) also found that sex offenders had more positive attitudes toward other sex offenders than did any of the professionals, suggesting that supervised peer groups might be an effective way to offer treatment. Hogue (1995) also found that police and prison officers who were selected for special training to work with sex offenders came away from the training with much more positive attitudes than were held before the training. This finding may apply to helping professionals who work with sex offenders but have no specialized training.

Hilton et al. (1998) report on their experiences with high school students using half-day workshops to help reduce the numbers of date rapes and other forms of violence related to intimate and non-intimate relationships. Unfortunately, the authors found that self-report rates of sexual violence were as high for their sample attending a half-day workshop on sexual violence as they were for students who had no anti-date violence training. This was found to be so even though most students attending the workshop did not endorse sexual violence. The authors suggest that the workshops might have been more effective if only high-risk students had attended. Perhaps, the authors suggest, the material would have had more impact had it become part of the regular classroom curriculum and more opportunities for experiential work had been given. Lonsway et al. (1998) report that college students gave better answers to hypothetical scenarios of sexual conflict and positive changes in attitudes after a semester-long date-rape education course. Hilton et al. (1998) believe that there is value in repeating emotional information such as the discussion of date-rape. Resistance to discussing sexually violent behavior that may describe the behavior of many of the participants takes time to overcome. Hilton et al. (1998) warn that date-rape education courses should not be viewed as "innocuous" since they may actually make things worse. Programs to reduce sexual violence need to be carefully thought through, should use the available research as a guide, and must develop empirically sound forms of evaluation to determine whether they work.

A number of treatment approaches have been used with perpetrators of sexual violence, including those molesting children and perpetrators of rape of intimates and of strangers. The literature suggests that the primary approaches used in various treatment settings include the following traditional and less traditional approaches: Insight-Oriented Individual Psychotherapy, Group Psychotherapy, Family Therapy, Psycho-Educational Skills Training, Behavioral Treatments, Chemical Castration, Sexual Addiction Twelve Step Recovery Programs, Relapse Prevention, Parents United, and several model approaches that combine each of the above. Several of the therapies used with sexual offenders are provided here.

19.5.1. Chemical Castration

This highly controversial treatment is used primarily with intransigent adult offenders to decrease sexual obsessiveness by significantly lowering libido, erotic fantasies, erections, and ejaculations. Not a single study read suggests that it should be used with children. One commonly used drug is Depo-Provera, a testosterone-suppressing agent. Side effects of the drug include weight gain, lethargy, cold sweats, nightmares, hot flashes, hypertension and elevated blood pressure, high blood sugars, and shortness of breath. Berlin (1982) reports an 85% effectiveness rate in eliminating deviant sexual behaviors, "as long as the medication was taken on a regular basis. It is not a cure and relapse often follows discontinuation of medication and is not recommenced as an exclusive treatment" (reported in Brown & Brown, 1997, p. 347). Furthermore, the motivation to rape is often less sexual than it is hostility toward women. Consequently, perpetrators may continue to rape even though they lack any sexual or physical desire.

19.5.2. Psycho-Educational Skills Training

Because sexual offenders as a group tend to be uninformed about human sexuality (Groth, 1978), and often have difficulty expressing their feelings, skills training groups focus on "... multiple aspects of assertiveness skills, including making eye contact, duration of reply, latency of response, loudness of speech and quality of affect." (Becker et al., 1978, in Brown & Brown, 1997, p. 345). Rosen and Fracher (1983) also recommend teaching offenders tension reduction and anger management in those offenders who may experience anxiety and anger before the assault. Groth (1983) believes that the majority of offenders has very little awareness of the short- and long-term impact of sexual assault on their victims and suggests the use of empathy training to help offenders understand the impact of the offender's behavior on the victim.

19.5.3. Behavioral Treatments

These interventions include covert sensitization, electrical aversion, odor aversion, chemical aversion, and suppression and satiation techniques. *Covert sensitization* is a procedure in which the therapist describes a deviant sexual scene followed by an aversive scene. The aversive scene may include going to jail, blood, odors, community responses, and other aversive stimuli the therapist has determined to be effective in a screening interview. Scenes last about 10 minutes and two scenes are presented at each session (Mayer, 1988). This same concept can be used with the addition of unpleasant odors or electric shock with the aversive scene. In Satiation Procedures, the offender is told to masturbate to non-deviant fantasies and then ejaculate. The client is then asked to continue masturbating to deviant fantasies for 45 minutes. Throughout, the client is asked to verbalize his fantasies, which are recorded and monitored for client compliance. Satiation procedures attempt to destroy the erotic nature of deviant urges by boring the client with his own fantasies (Johnson et al., 1992).

More traditional treatment approaches use insight, moral revulsion, concern for the victim, the consequences of continued sexual abuse, group treatment to reinforce the messages given during individual treatment, and empathy training to help the youthful offender recognize the harm done by their behavior through contact with victims who have been sexually assaulted. Most of these approaches have limited effectiveness because they fail to replace deviant sexual attitudes and impulses with those that are more socially acceptable. Changing sexual behavior is difficult, particularly in youthful offenders whose sexual needs are considerable and whose fear of being caught may not as yet be very strong. When age and impulsivity are combined, the probability of behavioral change may not be high. Sexual assault may not be about sexual gratification as much as it may be about power, control, and humiliation. Nowhere is that more likely to exist than in prior victims of sexual abuse who relive their abuse as perpetrators rather than as victims.

Prendergast (1991) notes that children he has worked with in the 6th grade often lack knowledge of the fundamentals of sex and suggests that some sexual assault may be a function of lack of knowledge in meeting and relating to others. He suggests that in addition to the usual material presented in sex education courses, additional material should be included on the social aspects of dating and relationships that would include the following:

> *How to meet someone and initiate a social conversation; how to successfully ask for a date; meaningful small-talk; how to say "no" in an acceptable and appropriate manner; how to be laughed at and not take it personally (this includes being the center of attention in a group, making an error or acting silly and laughing at yourself with the group); and all other aspects of a normal adult social life that may be suggested by the class (Prendergast, 1991, p. 177).*

The National Task Force on Juvenile Sexual Offending suggests the following approach to the treatment of youthful sex offenders (NAPN, 1993):

1. Following a full assessment of the juvenile's risk factors and needs, individualized and developmentally sensitive interventions are required.
2. Individualized treatment plans should be designed and periodically reassessed and revised. Plans should specify treatment needs, treatment objectives, and required interventions.
3. Treatment should be provided in the least restrictive environment necessary for community protection. Treatment efforts also should involve the least intrusive methods that can be expected to accomplish treatment objectives.
4. Written progress reports should be issued to the agency that has mandated treatment and should be discussed with the juvenile and parents. Progress "must be based on specific measurable objectives, observable changes, and demonstrated ability to apply changes in current situations" (NAPN, 1993, p. 53).
5. Although adequate outcome data are lacking, NAPN (1993) suggests that satisfactory treatment will require a minimum of 12 to 24 months.

The primary goals in the treatment of youthful sex offenders, according to Cellini (1995), are community safety, control over abusive behaviors, increasing pro-social interactions, preventing further victimization, stopping the development of additional sexual problems, and helping youth develop appropriate relationships (Becker & Hunter, 1997). To accomplish these goals, highly structured individual and group interventions are recommended (Morenz & Becker, 1995). Treatment approaches include individual, group, and family interventions. Treatment content usually includes sex education, changes in thinking, victim awareness training, values clarification, impulse control, social skills training, reduction of deviant sexual arousal, and relapse prevention (Becker & Hunter, 1997).

Research by Izzo and Ross (1990) regarding the effectiveness of interventions with juveniles who commit various types of offenses, not just sex offenses, suggests that programs using cognitive therapy are twice as effective as those using other approaches. Lipsey and Wilson (1998) found that treatments focusing on interpersonal skills using behavioral approaches had the best results. Unfortunately, programs treating youthful sexual offenders experience high treatment attrition (Becker, 1990; Hunter and Figueredo, 1999). Hanson and Bussière, 1998 found that failing to complete treatment correlated highly with a great deal of recidivism. Apparently, there is little evidence that segregating sexual offenders from other offenders in treatment leads to better results, according to Morenz and Becker (1995).

In an extensive meta-analysis of the treatment effectiveness of juvenile sexual offender treatment programs, Winokur et al., 2006 concluded that there is a small to moderate reduction in recidivism rates of treated juvenile sexual offenders (JSO). They also note that "juveniles who complete a cognitive-behavioral treatment program are less likely to commit a sexual or nonsexual re-offense than are juveniles who do not receive treatment, receive an alternative treatment, or do not complete treatment" (p. 23). Of the many empirical studies of treatment effectiveness of JSOs, only a few were considered strong enough to use data and of those, all had some methodological weaknesses, according to the researchers. Nonetheless, they agree with (Hunter, 2000, p. 2) that there is a sufficient evidence base to "provide empirical support for the belief that the majority of juvenile sex offenders are amenable to treatment and achieve positive treatment outcomes."

In a cautionary note on making more of the findings of any meta-analysis, and particularly one done on such a difficult subject with such limited information, Winokur et al., 2006, p. 25) write that because studies of recidivism rates for treated juveniles who do not commit sexual crimes show better results than those for sexual offenders, even when cognitive therapy is used,

> *...[C]ognitive-behavioral treatment programs for JSO may not completely address all of the causes of sexual recidivism. For example, Hanson and Morton-Bourgon (2005) recently found that "variables commonly addressed in sex offender treatment programs (e.g., psychological distress, denial of sex crime, victim empathy, stated motivation for treatment) had little or no relationship with sexual or violent recidivism" (p. 1154).*

19.6. CASE STUDY: SEXUAL VIOLENCE AND CHILD MOLESTATION

Johnny is a 10-year-old boy living with his mother and three younger siblings. Johnny was sexually molested by his mother's boyfriend between ages six and eight. The boyfriend was very sadistic in his molestation and Johnny is an angry and deeply troubled boy. The molestation was never reported to the authorities and the mother discontinued the relationship with the boyfriend when it became clear to her what was happening. The boyfriend threatened to kill Johnny if he told his mother and Johnny all too readily believed him, although a later investigation revealed that Johnny was reported by his elementary school to child protective services who, through an all-too- frequent glitch in the system, failed to investigate the case. Johnny was coming to school with many signs of neglect and physical abuse, including bruises on his hands, arms, and face and clothes that were dirty and badly worn.

The mother felt that the best way to help Johnny was to give him extra attention. She was fearful of seeking treatment because she thought the worker would report the boyfriend to the authorities. Like Johnny, the mother was afraid that the boyfriend would harm her.

Johnny has begun to sexually molest younger children. He is sadistic in his molestation and often leaves bruises and cuts on his victims. He doesn't care if the victim is male or female and usually does damage to the child's genital areas by using pliers with young boys and bottles or broom sticks to penetrate young girls. Johnny feels a rage come over him before he molests a child. Sometimes he steals liquor from his mother to provide the courage to commit the molestation.

A teacher caught Johnny molesting a young boy in the restroom of his school. Johnny is a withdrawn child, and when he was caught and the police were called in, he became silent and emotionless. The crisis worker who saw him initially diagnosed Johnny as having post traumatic stress disorder. There was no indication from the school that Johnny had violent sexual tendencies. He was considered a mild, introverted child by his teachers, on the low end of intelligence, and generally compliant. Like many compliant children, his quiet behavior hid a great deal of rage. Johnny was remanded to juvenile court and awaits disposition by the court following a pre-sentence investigation.

19.7. DISCUSSION

Johnny was seen initially by a forensic psychologist for psychological testing and then by a clinical social worker to gather a precise social history. During the history-taking, it was determined that the mother's boyfriend had sexually and physically abused Johnny. Many of the sadistic things Johnny does to other children were first done to him by the boyfriend. The depth of Johnny's pathology was determined during the psychological examination when the psychologist wrote:

> *"Johnny is a ten-year-old Caucasian child who was sexually and physically molested by his mother's boyfriend from ages six to eight. He is a child with above average intelligence who was developing normally before the molestation by the mother's boyfriend. He is deeply withdrawn and has repressed feelings of rage at the boyfriend and at his mother for not protecting him. He is now taking that rage out on other children. He knows that what he is doing is wrong but feels that he can't control the impulse to hurt others. He is unable to talk about his feelings at a level that would suggest potential success in treatment and isn't certain that what he is doing is personally wrong, given what was done to him. He sees it as payback for not being protected. His prior molestation and his risk to others suggest that he should be placed in a closed facility with supervised treatment. The prognosis is very poor."*

The social work report noted the following: "Johnny's molestation by his mother's boyfriend was exacerbated by the mother's unwillingness to provide professional treatment for her child. Rather than seeking help, the mother compounded the boy's problems by overly sexualizing their relationship. Johnny slept with his mother after the boyfriend's departure and has memories of being touched and fondled by his mother, although the mother denies this. When Johnny molests other children, he has fantasies about being touched by his mother. Johnny needs supervised treatment in a protected facility where he cannot do harm to himself or to others. He has an underlying depression that makes suicide or violence to others very likely. He is confused about who he should hurt and often thinks that it might be best to hurt himself. The prognosis for improvement is very poor. This is a highly traumatized child who needs a protected and safe environment for a very long time to come."

Johnny was found guilty of molesting children and was placed in a guarded and locked facility for violent children. He is withdrawn, unsociable, compliant, and a non-participant in group therapy. He has learned the system of the facility and seems relieved that he is finally getting some needed protection. He volunteers for extra work and seems almost happy. He refuses to see his mother or any members of his family and has become a believer in the devil. He secretly worships with other believers in the facility and thinks he has found a philosophy of life that is satisfying. The staff of the facility has previously seen similar behavior in molested children and understands the harm that can be done by physical and sexual abuse. They also believe that age 10 is too early to give up on a child and think that some children, particularly those like Johnny who had some degree of normal development, have a chance to change their behavior as they mature. A good deal of the likelihood of change, they feel, has to do with continued help and the willingness of the staff to accept Johnny's current behavior as a sign of deep rage and resentment that may improve as he matures. The head therapist at the facility said this about Johnny and children who have been molested: "Lots of people talk about resilience and how wonderful the human spirit is. But when you see a child whose spirit is broken, you begin to understand the severe harm adults can do to children like Johnny. We are hopeful with Johnny but the odds are not good and traumas like the one Johnny suffered take a long time to heal, perhaps forever."

A young MSW student was assigned to work with Johnny offering, what her field placement director termed "supportive help." The student was taking a research course from the author and was being taught EBP. She decided to do a research proposal on the effectiveness of cognitive therapy with children below age 12 who had committed sexual crimes, and used what she found in the research literature to do "supportive work" with Johnny. To her surprise, Johnny was very receptive to looking at his thoughts and perceptions and could easily link many of them back to his own molestation. He could not see, however, how it could help control angry feelings that he took out on others.

The student set up homework assignments where Johnny was taught ways of logically coping with situations that made him angry, and where the impulse to sexually act out was great. Johnny excelled, using a number of examples in the locked facility of how he had learned to control his rage and not act out. Because of the change in his behavior, Johnny was sent to a half-way house in the community where he attended regular school and is doing well.

Before leaving the placement, the student evaluated her work: "I read all the reports about Johnny, and, of course I was pretty miffed that they would place me with such a limited client where no one thought anything good could happen. But they let me do my supportive work, and much to my amazement, Johnny loved what we were doing. He's a bright child and no one had recognized that he had good intelligence, which was often undermined by his internal rage. He liked mystery novels and he liked solving mysteries so I gave him the mystery to solve of why he was acting out sexually. And you know what? He knew exactly why. No beating around the bush with him. He also saw that his molester was taking his life away, and that made him doubly motivated to get better."

"Why did I help when others gave up on him? Maybe because I'm young, optimistic and full of hope. Maybe it's contagious and maybe the low opinion of the staff was a self-fulfilling prophecy for Johnny not getting better. When you get right down to it, I was offering him hope and everyone else was offering him hopelessness. Will he stay healthy and continue the positive changes he made with me during the nine months I worked with him? Boy, I sure hope so, but so much of what I encountered in the facility was this overlay of hopelessness and cynicism, that I wonder if the system does more harm for kids like Johnny than good. And what can you say about the fact that Johnny was never helped while he was being so severely abused? The only time the system worked was when Johnny's rage and need to retaliate for what was done to him caused him to act out against other kids. I wonder how many kids like Johnny never receive the help they need early on when it could so such good, but wait and wait and wait, and when they finally receive help, it's long after they've given up and everyone around them has done the same."

19.8. SUMMARY

Children who act out sexually may begin doing so well before we are prepared for the behavior. The studies in this chapter suggest that sexual acting out may begin well before the onset of puberty and that much of it is directed at younger siblings or friends of family members. These victims of sexual abuse by older siblings, in turn, often begin molesting children, and a vicious cycle begins to develop. There is a fairly imprecise and unreliable literature on the treatment of early childhood sexual acting out, much of it geared to older adults and consequently not of great value for children. The chapter also considered the victims of sexual abuse and noted the frequent and long-term problems brought about by sexual abuse throughout the victim's life.

19.9. QUESTIONS FROM THE CHAPTER

1. Do you believe that the average age that children begin molesting others is less than 10 years of age? Are children sexually active that early in life?
2. Chemical castration for sexually acting out children? Are you kidding? That is too awful a thing to do even to adult sexual predators. Do not you agree?
3. There seems to be a link between child sexual abuse and sexual acting out. Would not you think that being molested would sensitize people to how awful it is and make them less likely to molest others?
4. Girls seem to be sexual abusers. We have had some high profile stories of young teachers molesting adolescent boys. Do you think a woman molesting a boy is as harmful as a man molesting a girls? Why?
5. Most clinicians believe that adults who sexually abuse others are not very amenable to treatment. Would you say the same thing about children who molest other children? Why?

References

Abel, G. G., Mittleman, M. S., & Becker, J. V. (1985). Sex offenders: Results of assessment and recommendations in treatment in clinical criminology. In M. H. Ben-Aron, S. J. Hucker, C. D. & Webster (Eds.), *The assessment and treatment of criminal behaviour* (pp. 191–205). Toronto, Canada: M and M Graphics.

Akerstrom, M. (1986). Outcasts in prison: The cases of informers and sex offenders. *Deviant Behaviour*, 7, 1–12.

Araji, S. (1997). *Sexually Aggressive Children: Coming To Understand Them.* Thousand Oaks, CA: Sage Publications.

Barbaree, H. E., Hudson, S. M., & Seto, M. C. (1993). Sexual assault in society: the role of the juvenile offender. In H. E. Barbaree, W. I. Marshall, S. M. & Hudson (Eds.), *The Juvenile Sex Offender* (pp. 10–11). New York: Guilford Press.

Becker, J. V., & Hunter, J. A. (1997). Understanding and treating child and adolescent sexual offenders. In T. H. Ollendick, R. J. & Prinz (Eds.), *Advances in Clinical Child Psychology* (pp. 19). New York: Plenum Press.

Becker, J. V., et al. (1978). Evaluating social skills and social aggression. *Criminal Justice and Behavior, 514*, 357–367.

Becker, J. V. (1990). Evaluating social skills and social aggression. *Criminal Justiceand Behavior, 514*, 357–367.

Berlin, F. S. (1982). Sex Offenders: A biomedical perspective.. In J. Greer, I. & Stuart (Eds.), *The Sexual Aggressor: Current Perspectives on Treatment* (pp. 83–126). New York: Van Nostrand Reinhold.

Berliner, L. (1998, October). Juvenile sex offenders: Should they be treated differently? *Journal of Interpersonal Violence, 13*(5), 645–646.

Brown, J. L. & Brown, G. S. (1997). Characteristics of incest offenders: A review. *Journal of Aggression, Maltreatment and Trauma, 1*(1), Haworth Press.

Caputo, A. A., Frick, P., & Brodsky, S. L. (1999, September). Family violence and juvenile sex offending: The potential mediating role of psychopathic traits and negative attitudes toward women. *Criminal Justice & Behavior, 26*(3), 338–356.

Cascardi, M., Avery-Leaf, S., & O'Leary, K. (1994, August). Building a gender sensitive model to explain adolescent dating violence. Paper presented at the 102nd Annual Meeting of the American Psychological Association, Los Angeles, CA.

Cellini, H. R. (1995). Assessment and treatment of the adolescent sex offender. In B. K. Schwartz, H. R. & Cellini (Eds.), *The sex offender: Vol. 1. Corrections, treatment and legal practice* (pp. 6.1–6.12). Kingston, N.J: Civic Research Institute.

Davis, G. E., & Leitenberg, H. (1987). Adolescent sex offenders. *Psychological Bulletin, 101*, 417–427.

Foshee, V. (1996). Gender differences in adolescent dating abuse prevalence, types, and injuries. *Health Education Research, 11*(3), 275–286.

Friedrich, W. N., & Luecke, W. J. (1988). Young school-age sexually aggressive children. *Professional Psychology: Research and Practice, 2*, 155–164.

Ford, M. E., & Linney, J. A. (1995). Comparative analysis of juvenile sexual offenders, violent nonsexual offenders, and status offenders. *Journal of Interpersonal Violence, 10*, 56–69.

Furby, L., Weinrott, M., & Blackshaw, L. (1989). Sex offender recidivism: A review. *Psychological Bulletin, 105*, 3–30.

Glicken, M. D. (2004). *Violent young children.* Boston, MA: Allyn and Bacon.

Greenfeld, L.A. (1997, February). Sex offenses and offenders: An analysis of rape and sexual assault. US Department of Justice, Publication NCJ-163392.

Gray, H., & Foshee, V. (1997). Adolescent dating violence: Differences between one-sided and mutually violent profiles. *Journal of Interpersonal Violence, 12*(1), 126–141.

Groth, N. A., et al. (1978). Patterns of sexual assault against children and adolescents. In A. Burgess (Ed.), *Sexual Assault of Children and Adolescents* (pp. 3–24). Lexington, MA: D.C. Heath and Company.

Groth, N. A., Longo, R. E., & McFadin, J. B. (1982). Undetected recidivism among rapists and child molesters. *Crime and Delinquency, 128*, 450–458.

Hanson, R. K., & Morton-Bourgon, K. E. (2005). The characteristics of persistent sexual offenders: A meta-analysis of recidivism studies. *Journal of Consulting and Clinical Psychology, 73*, 1154–1163.

Hanson, R. K., & Bussière, M. T. (1998). Predicting relapse: A meta-analysis of sexual offender recidivism studies. *Journal of Consulting and Clinical Psychology, 66*, 348–362.

Hilton, N., Zoe, H., Rice, G. T., Krans, M. E., et al. (1998). Antiviolence education in high schools. *Journal of Interpersonal Violence, 13*(6), 726–742.

Hogue, T. E. (1993). Attitudes towards prisoners and sexual offenders. In N. K. Clark, G. M. & Stephenson (Eds.), *Sexual offenders: Context, assessment and treatment* (pp. 27–32). Leicester: BPS.

Hogue, T. E. (1995). Training multi-disciplinary teams to work with sex offenders: Effects of staff attitudes. *Psychology, Crime & Law, 1*, 227–235.

Jr.Hunter, J. A. (2000). Understanding sex offenders: Research findings and guidelines for effective management and treatment, *Juvenile Justice Fact Sheet*. Charlottesville, VA: Institute of Law, Psychiatry, & Public Policy, University of Virginia.

Hunter, J. A., & Figueredo, A. J. (1999). Factors associated with treatment compliance in a population of juvenile sexual offenders. *Sexual Abuse: A journal of Research and Treatment, 11*(1), 49–67.

Izzo, R. H., & Ross, R. R. (1990). Meta-analysis of rehabilitation programs for juvenile delinquents: A brief report. *Criminal Justice and Behavior, 17*(1), 134–142.

James, W. H., West, C., & Deters, K. E. (2000 Fall). Youth dating violence. *Adolescence, 35*(139), 455–465.

Jezl, D., Molidor, C., & White, T. (1996). Physical, sexual and psychological abuse in high school dating relationships: Prevalence rates and self-esteem issues. *Child and Adolescent Social Work Journal, 13*(1), 69–88.

Johnson, P., et al. (1992). The effects of masturbatory reconditioning with nonfamilial child molestors. *Behavior Research and Therapy, 30*, 559–561.

Johnson, T. C. (1988). Child perpetrators-children who molest other children: Preliminary findings. *Child Abuse and Neglect, 72*, 219–229.

Kimball, L. M., & Guarino-Ghezzi, S. (1996). Sex offender treatment: An assessment of sex offender treatment within the massachusetts department of youth services, *Juvenile Justice Series Report: No. 10*. Boston, MA: Northeastern University, Privatized Research Management Initiative.

Lab, S., Shields, G., & Schondel, C. (1993). Research note: An evaluation of juvenile sexual offender treatment. *Crime and Delinquency, 39*(4), 543–553.

Lane, S., & Lobanov-Rostovsky, C. (1997). Special populations: Children, families, the developmentally disabled and violent youth. In G. D. Ryan, S. L. & Lane (Eds.), *Juvenile sexual offending: Causes, consequences, and correction.* (pp. 322–359). San Francisco, CA: Jossey-Bass Publishers.

Langevin, R., Wright, P., & Handy, L. (1989). Characteristics of sex offenders who were sexually victimized as children. *Annals of Sex Research, 2*, 227–253.

Lea, S., Auburn, T., & Kibblewhite, K. (1999 Mar). Working with sex offenders: The perceptions and experiences of professional and paraprofessionals. International. *Journal of Offender Therapy & Comparative Criminology, 43*(1), 103–119.

Lipsey, M. W., & Wilson, D. B. (1998). Effective interventions for serious juvenile offenders: A synthesis of research.. In R. Loeber, D. P. & Farrington (Eds.), *Serious and violent juvenile offenders: Risk factors and successful interventions* (pp. 313–345). Thousand Oaks, CA: Sage Publications.

Lonsway, K. A., Klaw, E. L., Berg, D. R., Waldo, C. R., Kothari, C., Mazurek, C. J., & Hegeman, K. E. (1998). Beyond "no means no": Outcomes of an intensive program to train peer facilitators for campus acquaintance rape education. *Journal of Interpersonal Violence, 13*, 73–92.

Mayer, A. (1988). *Sex offenders: Approaches to understanding and management.* Holmes Beach, Florida: Learning Perspectives.

Mathews, R. Jr., Hunter, J. A., & Vuz, J. (1997). Juvenile female sexual offenders: Clinical characteristics and treatment issues. *Sexual Abuse: A Journal of Research and Treatment, 9*(3), 187–200.

Morenz, B., & Becker, J. V. (1995). The treatment of youthful offenders. *Applied and Preventative Psychology, 4*(4), 247–256.

Nationalationaladolescent Adolescent Perpetrator Network. (1993). The revised report from the national task force on juvenile violence sexual offending. *Jouvenile Justice and Family Court Journal, 44*(4), 1–120.

O'Keefe, M. (1997). Predictors of dating violence among high school students. *Journal of Interpersonal Violence, 12*, 546–568.

Pierce, L. H., & Pierce, R. L. (1987). Incestuous victimization by juvenile sex offenders. *Journal of Family Violence, 2*, 351–364.

Pithers, W. D., Gray, A., Busconi, A., & Houchens, P. (1998a). Caregivers of children with sexual behavior problems: Psychological and familial functioning. *Child Abuse and Neglect, 22*(2), 129–141.

Pithers, W. D., Gray, A., Busconi, A., & Houchens, P. (1998b). Children with sexual behavior problems: Identification of five distinct child types and related treatment considerations. *Child Maltreatment, 3*(4), 384–406.

Prendergast, W. E. (1991). *Treating sexual offenders on correctional institutions and outpatient clinics: A guide to clinical practice.* New York: The Haworth Press.

Rosen, R. C., & Fracher, J. C. (1983). Tension-reducing training in the treatment of compulsive sex offenders. In J. G. Greer, I. & Stuart (Eds.), *The Sexual Aggressors* (pp. 144–159). New York: Van Nostrand Reinhold.

Ryan, G., Miyoshi, T. J., Metzner, J. L., Krugman, R. D., & Fryer, G. E. (1996). Trends in a national sample of sexually abusive youths. *Journal of the American Academy of Child and Adolescent Psychiatry, 33*, 17–25.

Ryan, G., Lane, S., Davis, J., & Isaac, C. (1987). Juvenile sex offenders: Development and correction. *Child Abuse and Neglect, 11*, 385–395.

Saunders, B., Kilpatrick, D., Resnick, H., Hanson, R., & Lipovsky, J. (January 1992). *Epidemiological characteristics of child sexual abuse: Results from Wave II of the National Women's Study.* Presented at the San Diego Conference on Responding to Child Maltreatment, San Diego, CA.

Snyder, H. N., & Sigmund, M. (1995). *Juvenile offenders and victims: A focus on violence.* Pittsburgh, PA: National Center for Juvenile Justice.

Veneziano, C., Veneziano, L., & LeGrand, S. (2000 April). The relationship between adolescent sex offender behaviors and victim characteristics with prior victimization. *Journal of Interpersonal Violence, 15*(4), 363–374.

Weinrott, M. R. (1996). Juvenile sexual abuse: A critical review. Unpublished manuscript.

Winokur, M., Rozen, D., Batchelder & Valentine, D. (2006, June). Applied Research in Child Welfare Project, Social Work Research Center, School of Social Work, College of Applied Human Sciences, Colorado State University. Final Report. http://www.ssw.cahs.colostate.edu/centers_institutes/swrc/files/JSOTSystematicReview.pdf.

Zolondek, S. C., Abel, G. F., William, J., & Alan, D. (2001). The self-reported behaviors of juvenile sexual offenders. *Journal of Interpersonal Violence, 15*(1), 73–85.

Further reading

Becker, J. V., Kaplan, M. S., & Tenke, C. E. (1992). The relationship of abuse history, denial, and erectile response profiles of adolescent sexual perpetrators. *Behavior Therapy, 23*, 87–89.

Zolondek, S. C., Abel, G., Northey, W. F., & Jordan, A. D. (2000). The self-reported behaviors of juvenile sexual offenders. *Journal of Interpersonal Violence, 73–85*(16 no 1), 73–85.

20 Evidence-Based Practice and School Violence

20.1. INTRODUCTION

The author wishes to thank Pearson Education, Inc. for permission to reprint material from his book on violent young children (Glicken, 2004, pp. 35–45).

Although American schools claim that school violence has decreased, more recent data compared to data from the 1990s show that this often is not the case. Recent high profile shootings on schools and college campuses suggest that violence is still prevalent in or near American schools. While school violence usually makes us think of school shootings, in this chapter it has an expanded meaning, and includes bullying, intimidation, threats, theft, sexual harassment and violence near schools grounds. As we will see in the following discussion, school violence is a very serious problem in American schools. Further, the profiles which define children most likely to commit school violence may not adequately include the "invisible children," "Goth," or the "End-Times Children," who are often the recipients of bullying and intimidation by schoolmates and who harbor deep resentments which sometimes resolve themselves in school shootings and other acts of violent retribution.

20.2. THE AMOUNT OF SCHOOL VIOLENCE

The North Carolina Department of Juvenile Justice and Delinquency Prevention Center for the Prevention of School Violence (2007, pp. 2–3) compiled the following national statistics on school violence:

1. From July 1, 2004 through June 30, 2005, there were 48 school-associated deaths in elementary and secondary schools in the United States.
2. Incidents of crime are reported at 96% of high schools, 94% of middle schools, and 74% of primary schools.
3. In 2005, 6-1/2% of students surveyed reported that they had carried a weapon onto school property within the last 30 days, while 18% said they carried a weapon anywhere during the past month.
4. Six percent of students had not gone to school on one or more of the 30 days preceding the survey because they felt they would be unsafe at school or on their way to or from school.
5. The percentage of public schools experiencing one or more violent incidents increased between the 1999–2000 and 2003–2004 school years from 71% to 81%.
6. The youth who were surveyed graded adults for the following questions: For protecting kids and teens from gun violence, 30.5% graded a C, and 30.3% graded a B; for

keeping schools safe from violence and crime, 30.2% graded a C; and for getting rid of gangs, 32.7% graded a C.

7. In 2004, more than 78% of school resource officers surveyed reported they had taken a weapon from a student on school property in the past year.
8. In 2004, more than 35% of school resource officers surveyed reported that violent incidents on school buses had increased in their districts during the past two years.
9. In 2003–2004, 10% of teachers in central city schools were threatened with injury by students, compared with 6% of teachers in urban fringe schools and 5% of teachers in rural schools. Five percent of teachers in central city schools were attacked by students, compared with three percent of teachers in urban fringe schools, and 2% of teachers in rural schools.

Sprague and Walker (2000) report that more than 100 000 students bring weapons to school each day and more than 40 students are killed or wounded with these weapons annually. They note that many students experience bullying and other behaviors which have a negative impact on their school-related functioning. The authors report that over 6000 teachers are threatened each year and that over 200 teachers each year are assaulted by students on school grounds. Schools are often used by gangs to recruit new gang members, and gang activities often disrupt normal classroom functioning and give students a sense of danger (Committee for Children, 1997; National School Safety Center, 1996; Office of Juvenile Justice and Delinquency Prevention, 1995; Walker et al., 1995). Crowe (1991) notes that a National Institute of Education study revealed that 40% of the robberies and 36% of the assaults against urban youth took place on or near school grounds. Of the students who admit to bringing weapons to school, half say the weapons are for protection against other youth with weapons.

The W.M. Keck Foundation (2007) reports that:

> *Every year, three million young people in the United States fall victim to crimes at school. Almost two million of these incidents involve violence. Although most school violence takes the form of minor assaults, some episodes are far more serious. Some end in tragedy. For example, in two recent academic years, a total of 85 young people died violently in U.S. schools. Seventy-five percent of these incidents involved firearms (p. 1).*

The 1999 Youth Risk Behavior Survey (National Center for Injury Prevention and Control, 2001), summarized school-related violence by noting that:

- 35.7% of high school students reported being in a physical fight within the past 12 months, and 4% of students were injured in a physical fight seriously enough to require treatment by a doctor or nurse.
- 17.3% of high school students carried a weapon (e.g., gun, knife, or club) during the 30 days preceding the survey.
- 4.9% of high school students carried a gun during the 30 days preceding the survey.
- 14.2% of high school students had been in a physical fight on school property one or more times in the past 12 months.

- 7.7% of high school students were threatened or injured with a weapon on school property during the 12 months preceding the survey.
- 6.9% of high school students carried a weapon on school property during the 30 days preceding the survey.
- 5.2% of students had missed one or more days of school during the 30 days preceding the survey because they had felt too frightened to go to school. (NCIPC, 2001, p. 2)

In a study by Petersen et al. (1998), 202 teachers, building administrators, and district administrators in 15 school districts of varying sizes from 12 states, representing all geographical regions of the country, participated in a study of school violence. The authors report that most respondents had experienced some level of violence at least one or more times in the past two years. Sixty-three percent of the respondents said they had been verbally threatened or intimidated, 28% had been physically threatened or intimidated, 11% had been sexually threatened or intimidated, 68% had been verbally attacked, 9% had been physically attacked, and 55% indicated that their room, their personal property, or the school in which they worked had been seriously vandalized. Twenty-six percent of the respondents said violence was increasing or greatly increasing at the preschool level, and 53% said violence was increasing or greatly increasing at the elementary school level. Almost 65% of the respondents said violence was increasing at the middle school, junior high, and senior high school level.

Stevens (1995) reports that almost three million crimes are committed on or near a school campus each year, constituting 11% of all reported crimes in America (Sautter, 1995). Kauffman (1997) notes that 80–90% of all school-age children and youth, in reports to others, indicate that that they have been involved in acts of violence and aggression. Siegel and Senna (1994) report that a large proportion of these violent acts occur in school. Murray and Myers (1998) indicate that only 9% of the juvenile violent crimes committed in schools are reported to criminal justice authorities, compared to the 37% report rate for similar juvenile street crime. The authors believe that these data suggest that schools are avoiding involvement in the juvenile-justice system.

Fitzpatrick (1999) reports that even as violence has declined in the United States, violence among children and adolescents remains a very problematic area of concern. Although national homicide rates have been fairly stable during the last two decades, homicides by youth under the age of 25 have more than doubled in the last 20 years. Since the early 1980s, youth under the age of 18 were victims of violence at a rate of five to six times that of adults (Bureau of Justice Statistics, 1997). Much of this violence happens near schools and may have its origins in the interactions children have with other schoolmates. Of the children victimized by violence, males, particularly Black males, were victims of violence at twice the rate of White males. Children from households earning less than $15 000 a year were two to three times more likely to be victims of violence compared to their higher income counterparts (Bureau of Justice Statistics, 1997). Clearly, there are conditions of gender, income, and neighborhoods which increase the probability of school violence.

20.3. THE REASONS FOR INCREASED SCHOOL VIOLENCE

In a study by Petersen et al. (1998), the primary reasons for the increase in school violence, as suggested by the authors, were:

> *Lack of rules or family structure, 94%; lack of involvement or parental supervision, 94%; violence acted out by parents, 93%; parental drug use, 90%; student drug/alcohol use, 90%; violent movies, 85%; student poor self-concept/emotional disturbance, 85%; violence in television programs, 84%; nontraditional family/family structure, 83%; and gang activities, 80%. (Petersen et al., 1998, p. 348).*

Fitzpatrick (1999) believes that another reason for increased school violence is the unwillingness of large numbers of youth to walk away from fights. Youth at all age ranges, who believe that it is not possible to walk away from a fight, are at significant risk of violence, either during the confrontation or later through acts of revenge. Fitzpatrick suggests that often, once a child is challenged, he must fight or lose the respect of his peers. This reaction often leads non-violent children into violent acts and victimization. Fitzpatrick reports that boys in elementary and middle schools have a greater chance of being involved in violence than girls, but that girls tend to become involved in fighting and aggressive behavior later in their teenage years. Myles and Simpson (1998) believe there are three major reasons for increased school violence in America:

1. A significant increase in aggression and violence in America (Kauffman, 1997; Walker et al., 1995). Frequent exposure to acts of violence make violence socially acceptable and serves to desensitize children from its significance.
2. Increasing numbers of seriously disturbed, violent, and socially maladjusted children in the classroom increase school aggression and violence. This comes at a time when there are fewer resources available to refer children with potential for school violence.
3. There is a lack of teachers trained to work with violent children in the general classroom. Appropriate support systems to help teachers cope with violent children are lacking.

In his study of school violence, Fitzpatrick (1999) came to the interesting conclusion that a major predictor of school victimization was how safe students assessed their school environments to be. He found that students in elementary schools and middle schools who had more negative views of the safety of their school environments were also victimized more often. Fitzpatrick (1999) believes that children who perceive dangerous environments often find themselves in the midst of those very environments and, as a result, experience a higher degree of violence. This is particularly true for elementary age children who may know that certain children in the school are dangerous, but are unable to avoid them.

20.4. GANG INFLUENCES ON SCHOOL VIOLENCE

The influence of gangs on younger children is significant and is particularly problematic for schools. Young people join gangs for a variety of reasons which may include: A search for love; structure and discipline; a sense of belonging and commitment; the need for recognition and power; companionship, training, excitement, and activities; a sense of self-worth and status; a place of acceptance; the need for physical safety and protection; and being a part of a family tradition (Glicken and Sechrest, 2003).

Not all children who are at risk for gang affiliation actually join gangs. Some common characteristics among children living in poverty and adverse situations who seem to be stress-resistant and who avoid gang affiliation are: (a) the children are well-liked by peers and adults and have well-developed social and interpersonal skills; (b) they were reflective rather than impulsive about their behavior; (c) they have a high sense of self-esteem, self-efficacy, and personal responsibility; (d) they have an internal locus of control and believe they are able to influence their environment in a positive manner; (e) they demonstrate an ability to be flexible in their coping strategies; (f) they have well-developed problem-solving skills and intellectual abilities; (g) they have positive role models and have been exposed to more positive than negative experiences; (h) they have a sense of hope for the future and a belief in their own abilities; and (i) they have an ability to cope with the crises and problems that arise in their lives (Sechrest, 2001).

While reasons for gang membership continue to be studied in considerable detail, there is relatively little information on the process of transitioning from gang life. Hughes (1997) studied ex-gang members who successfully made the transition from gang life to other more socially acceptable activities. She reports four reasons for the transition from gang involvement: (1) concern for the well-being of young children, often their own; (2) fear of physical harm, incarceration, or both; (3) time to contemplate their lives, often done in detention facilities; and (4) support and modeling by helping professionals and indigenous community helpers.

The most promising reason for the transition from gang life, according to Hughes (1997), appears to be respect and concern for the safety of young children. Many gang members have fathered children and as their children begin to grow, fathers experience concern for their welfare. Additionally, ex-gang members have begun to share similar concerns with at-risk youth in their communities and mentor them away from gang involvement. Using the notion of concern for young children as a reason for transitioning from gang life, it would be very useful to find out when that concern for the safety of children begins and how human service professionals can use this information to facilitate the transition from gang involvement. It might also be useful to find out if the transition from gang involvement occurs early enough to discourage the young children related to gang members from involvement in gang-related activities.

One of the major reasons for gang involvement, according to Sechrest (2001), is the family tradition of being in the same gang as a parent or sibling. Sometimes family tradition is used in the form of a "legacy" for early recruitment into gangs, and may occur during elementary school when young recruits are given assignments to test their mettle as potential gang members. Such assignments may involve school violence and/or random violence involving the use of weapons. Dangerous as gang activity can be in schools, Schwartz (1996) writes that:

> *Gang activity at school is particularly susceptible to the "ostrich syndrome," as administrators may ignore the problem. An unfortunate consequence of such denial is that opportunities to reduce violence are lost. This creates a situation where teachers feel unsupported when they impose discipline, students do not feel protected, and the violence-prone think they will not be punished (p. 1).*

Schwartz (1996) offers some general violence reduction approaches that may help in reducing potential gang activity in schools. They include:

1. An accurate assessment of the existence of violence, and especially gang activity.
2. Use of all the resources in the community, including social service and law enforcement, and to not rely solely on school officials to deal with the problem.
3. Incorporation of family services into both community and school programs.
4. Intervention early in a child's life.
5. Inclusion of not only anti-violence strategies but also positive experiences.
6. Creation of and communication of clearly defined behavioral codes, and strict and uniform enforcement.
7. Preparation for engaging in a long-term effort (Schwartz, 1996, p. 5).

Another potential remedy for gang violence in schools is a program called "Father to Father," a national initiative supported by former Vice President Gore for the purpose of strengthening the bond between fathers and sons. Nationally, numerous programs have joined this initiative and have developed specific programs focused on fatherhood, an idea which could help gang members use their concern for the safety of children to leave gang life. While these programs have promising anecdotal rates of success, none have been studied with any degree of objectivity.

20.5. GANG VIOLENCE

There are generally thought to be four types of gangs (Wikipedia, 2008, p. 1):

1. *Schoolyard gangs* involve children who want to be gang members and probably will, but are in the initial stage of courting organized gangs through their use of intimidation and aggression generally focused on school mates.
2. *Scavenger gangs* are typically not well organized and often become involved in low-level crime committed impulsively. Leadership in scavenger gangs is very short-lived and chaotic.

3. *Territorial gangs* are better organized than scavenger gangs and use violence to defend their territories, a process which develops bonding among members and strengthens the social structure of the gang.
4. *Corporate gangs* are highly organized and are involved in marketing illegal commodities such as drugs and weapons. They have a very highly structured etiquette which is very strictly enforced and strong and the often successful leadership?

Using Office of Juvenile Justice and Delinquency Prevention data from 2004, Egley and Ritz (2006) estimate that there are approximately 760 000 gang members nationally in 24 000 active gangs in the United States. In 1995, Spergel (1995) estimated that more than 3875 youth gangs existed, with a total of more than 200 000 gang members in the 79 largest U.S. cities, a considerably smaller number than more current data.

Research suggests that there is a significant connection between gang involvement, gang violence, and firearms. Quinn and Downs (1995, p. 15) studied 835 male inmates in six juvenile correctional facilities in four states. The authors found that movement from non-gang membership to gang membership brought increases in most forms of gun-involved conduct. Forty-five percent of the sample described gun theft as a regular gang activity. Sixty-eight percent said their gang regularly bought and sold guns, and 61% described "driving around and shooting at people you don't like" as a regular gang activity involving children as young as 10.

Johnson (1999) notes that during the past two decades, the United States has seen the youth gang problem grow at an alarming rate, with gang members increasingly under the age of 12. Johnson (1999) reports that the number of cities with youth gang problems has increased from an estimated 286 with more than 2000 gangs and nearly 100 000 gang members in 1980 to about 2000 cities with more than 25 000 gangs and 650 000 members in 1995, data that are almost three times higher than Spergel's (1995) estimates. Youth gangs are present and active in nearly every state, as well as in Puerto Rico and other territories. Few large cities are gang-free and even many cities and towns with populations of less than 25 000 are reporting gang problems. Thus, the issue of youth gangs is now affecting new localities, such as small towns and rural areas.

20.6. METHODS OF DECREASING SCHOOL VIOLENCE

Peterson and Skiba (2001, p. 155) suggest four methods of decreasing school violence from an institutional point of view: (a) Parental and community involvement; (b) character education; (c) violence-prevention and conflict-resolution curricula; and (d) bullying prevention.

1. **Parental and community involvement:** Christenson (1995) and Weiss and Edwards (1992) report that parent involvement encourages a more constructive learning environment by creating goals for parents in the home and teachers in the school which work to enhance both environments and are consistent in their objectives. With parents and teachers working together, the impact on the community is positive and

goals for all three environments are consistent. Peterson and Skiba (2001) believe that increasing the involvement of parents can result in home environments which enhance student learning and increase cooperation with schools. High levels of parent–school cooperation can lead to less violent schools which respond to the potential for violence in more creative and effective ways. Epstein (1992) believes that schools can become involved in teaching parents better skills related to managing and enforcing discipline in the home. One school, for example, requires parents of students who are at risk of being expelled to attend meetings to work on solutions to their child's acting out behavior (Peterson and Skiba, 2001). Tasks that need to be done at home by children can be shared with parents so they are involved. By encouraging parents to become involved with schools, a cooperative spirit emerges that leads to faster and more effective responses to issues of violence. Parental involvement has been positively associated with student success, higher attendance rates, and lower suspension rates (Kube and Ratigan, 1991). Increased involvement by parents has been shown to provide better teacher satisfaction, improved parent understanding of school policies, better parent–child communication, and more successful and effective school programs according to Peterson and Skiba (2001).

2. **Character education:** Character education is the notion that schools have to take a direct role in teaching values to children. This should be done across the curriculum. London (1987) believes that character education focuses on civic involvement, the rules of citizenship in a just society, and in a child's personal adjustment to helping children become productive and dependable citizens. According to Lickona (1988), character education in elementary school should achieve three objectives:
   1. Promote development away from egocentrism and excessive individualism and toward cooperative relationships and mutual respect;
   2. Foster the growth of moral agency – the capacity to think, feel, and act morally; and
   3. Develop in the classroom and in the school a moral community based on fairness, caring, and participation – such a community being a moral end in itself as well as a support system for the character development of each individual student, (Lickona, 1988, p. 420)

To achieve these goals, Lickona proposes four processes in the classroom: Building self-esteem and a sense of community, learning to work together and to help others, thinking about the outcomes of one's behavior and its impact on others, and learning to make decisions which reflect group input and are participatory.

1. **Violence and conflict-resolution curricula:** These approaches teach children to use alternatives to violence when resolving interpersonal conflict. They may include programs which teach children conflict resolution strategies, actual conflict resolution teams which are headed up by students who patrol the school grounds and can provide conflict resolution as a way of reducing tension before the conflict is reported to the school authorities, and programs which teach children ways of avoiding situations in which violence might occur. Films, role-plays, and simulations may be used, or parents might become involved and conflict resolution might be extended to problems in the home. Topics covered in conflict resolution curricula include anger management, learning to identify and express feelings about others, discussing issues related to racial, ethnic and gender differences, and learning to cope with stress.

2. **Bullying prevention programs:** Bullying prevention programs are school-wide zero-tolerance polices toward bullying. The components of a successful bullying prevention program include improved adult supervision, classroom rules against bullying, positive and negative consequences for following and violating rules, interventions with the bullies and victims, meetings with parents of bullies and victims, and regular classroom meetings to discuss ways of dealing with bullying. In elementary schools, worksheets, role-plays, and related literature (stories about bullies and victims, for example) may be incorporated into the curriculum. These comprehensive programs to deal with bullying have been used in many schools in many different countries and cultures, according to Olweus and Limber (1999). Olewus (1993) reports that one program using school, classroom, and individual and family interventions reduced bullying by 50%. Other programs, reported by Peterson and Skiba (2001, p. 155), have been shown to reduce fighting, vandalism and truancy, while at the same time increasing overall student satisfaction with school. However, as a number of authors remind us, most bullying goes undetected or ignored and leads to very negative effects on victims, bullies, and the entire school system. Well-developed programs teach all students that bullying will not be acceptable behavior. Effective programs have significantly reduced the rate of bullying and have lead to much better school climates.

20.7. ADDITIONAL APPROACHES TO DECREASING SCHOOL VIOLENCE

Schwartz (1996) suggests a variety of anti-violence programs in the schools. Among those programs are a no-tolerance policy for any sort of dangerous weapon, with frequent searches for weapons in lockers and weapons detection at the school entryway. She also believes that helping children find suitable activities after school and until their parents are home is another highly effective way of reducing school violence after school lets out. She strongly supports a program to help children and adolescents have an opportunity to stay after school under supervision to improve their scholastic performance, and for older children to find work in the community through help from the school. Schwartz (1996) strongly encourages school systems to initiate anti-gang programs and to maintain dress codes that forbid the use of gang paraphernalia. Security of schools can be enhanced by monitoring halls at all time and by helping students and parents understand the dangers of violence through cooperative meetings. She also believes that anti-violence programs, with their focus on a safe school environment for everyone, require a very high degree of cooperation among teachers who must sign on to such programs because they have the majority of the responsibility for enforcing the programs. Schools with violence problems should also provide self-esteem programs for children who often suffer from low self-esteem which leads to learning delays. Finally, Schwartz (1996) believes that most school violence originates with violence in the home, and urges schools to initiate programs to provide services to the children from violent homes and their families. She rightly notes that violence in families has a way of filtering back to the school in the form of school violence.

Several factors related to the school environment have been linked with aggression in youth, including strict and inflexible classroom rules, teacher hostility, and the lack of classroom management. In addition, youth in overcrowded schools are more aggressive toward peers than are adolescents attending uncrowded schools. Within the classroom, aggressive children have been observed to be more disruptive and off-task than non-aggressive peers. Furthermore, low academic achievement, academic failure, lack of commitment to school, and school drop-out have been associated with delinquent and aggressive behavior (Sechrest, 2001).

Official school disciplinary or expulsion statistics may not accurately capture the true level of criminality, violent behavior, or gun possession problems at schools. Because most school-based crimes are customarily resolved as disciplinary offenses rather than matters that are resolved by authorities outside of the school, rates of violence and weapon possessions at schools may greatly underestimate such behavior because official tracking mechanism are inadequate. For example, students and teachers may not report violent incidents or weapon possessions because they are afraid of reprisals or because they might feel that they will incur official criticism. Schools are relatively safe places in comparison to estimates of aggregate juvenile crime and violence numbers; nevertheless, school-based levels of crime and violence are underestimated. School environments today are places where too much violence, crime, and weapons possession occur, and student fears concerning violence and crime are real and adversely impact student school attendance and learning. To reinforce the concerns students have about the safety of schools, the National Center for Education Statistics (1995) estimates that about 160 000 students are absent from school every day because they do not want to become victims of violence.

Studer (1996) suggests the use of assertiveness training to teach children that one can be assertive without being aggressive and writes:

> *Aggression is an action that enhances the aggressor while it minimizes and violates the rights of others. The intent of the aggressive behavior is to humiliate and dominate. This behavior is in contrast to passive behaviors that are self-denying and inhibiting, as a person's own rights are disregarded and he or she gives in to demands of others. Instead, Baer defined assertiveness as "win-win" behavior in which an individual can stand up for his or her own rights in such a way that the rights of others are not disregarded (Studer, 1996, p. 188).*

Huey and Rank (1984) found assertiveness training to be very helpful with disruptive, low achieving children who were referred for counseling because of their aggressive, acting-out behavior. The authors noted that after being given eight hours of assertiveness training, these children were less aggressive but were more assertive in the classroom. Mathias (1992) reports that the "DeBug" system, a training program which teaches children assertiveness, showed overwhelmingly positive results in the classroom and reduced aggressive behavior substantially.

20.8. CHARACTERISTICS OF CHILDREN WITH POTENTIAL FOR SCHOOL VIOLENCE

The FBI, in a 1999 report entitled *The School Shooter: A Threat Assessment Perspective* (Critical Incident Response Group of the National Center for the Analysis of Violent Crime, 1999), developed a profile of characteristics consistent with children who have potential to kill others at school (1999, pp. 17–21). It should be noted that this list of characteristics is meant to provide a cumulative picture of many disparate characteristics. Children may have some of these characteristics and not be considered dangerous. When a child has many of these characteristics, however, the potential for violence increases.

1. **Low frustration tolerance:** The student is easily insulted, angered and hurt by real or perceived injuries inflicted on him by others and has difficulty tolerating frustration.
2. **Poor coping skills:** The student consistently shows little if any ability to deal with frustration, criticism, disappointment, failure, rejection, or humiliation. His or her response is typically inappropriate, exaggerated, immature or disproportionate.
3. **Lack of resiliency:** The student is unable to bounce back even when some time has elapsed since a frustrating or disappointing setback or putdown.
4. **Failed love relationship:** The student feels rejected and humiliated after the end of a love relationship and cannot accept or come to terms with the rejection.
5. **Injustice collector:** The student will not forgive or forget the wrongs [others have done] or the people they believe responsible. The student may keep a "hit list" with the names of people he feels have wronged him.
6. **Signs of depression:** The student shows lethargy, physical fatigue, a morose or dark outlook on life, a sense of malaise, and a loss of interest in activities that he once enjoyed.
7. **Narcissism:** The student is self-centered, lacks insight into the needs of others, and blames others for failures and disappointments. He or she may display signs of paranoia and assumes an attitude of self-importance or grandiosity that masks feelings of unworthiness (Malmquist, 1996).
8. **Alienation:** The student consistently feels different or estranged from others. It is more than being a loner and involves feelings of isolation, sadness, loneliness, not belonging, and not fitting in.
9. **Dehumanizes others:** The student views other people as "non-persons" or objects to be thwarted. This attitude may appear in the student's artwork, writing, or conversations with others.
10. **Lack of empathy:** The student shows an inability to understand the feelings of others. When others show emotion, the student may ridicule them.
11. **Exaggerated sense of entitlement:** The student expects special treatment and reacts negatively when he does not receive it.
12. **Attitude of superiority:** The student has a sense of being superior and presents himself as smarter, more creative, more talented, more experienced, and worldlier than others.
13. **Exaggerated need for attention:** The student shows a pathological need for attention, positive or negative.

14. **Externalizes blame:** The student fails to take responsibility for his actions. Often the student seems impervious to rational arguments or to common sense.
15. **Masks low self-esteem:** Though appearing arrogant, the student's conduct veils underlying low self-esteem.
16. **Anger management problems:** The student is unable to express anger appropriately and has temper tantrums and outbursts which may be directed at people who had nothing to do with the original incident.
17. **Intolerance:** The student expresses racial or religious intolerance and displays symbols, jewelry or tattoos to express that intolerance.
18. **Inappropriate humor:** The student's humor is insulting, macabre, belittling, or mean.
19. **Manipulative:** The student constantly tries to con others and win the trust of others so that they will excuse away threatening or aberrant behavior.
20. **Lack of trust:** The lack of trust may approach a clinically paranoid state.
21. **Closed social group:** The student appears introverted or only associates with a small group and excludes others.
22. **Dramatic changes in behavior:** The student may show reckless disregard for school rules, dress codes, schedules, and other regulations.
23. **Rigid and opinionated:** The student appears rigid, judgmental, and cynical and voices strong opinions about subjects they know little about, often disregarding logic and facts.
24. **Unusual interest in sensational violence:** The student demonstrates an unusual interest in school shootings and other acts of violence. He may even admire the killers or express a desire to carry out similar acts.
25. **Fascination with violence-filled entertainment:** The student shows an unusual fascination with movies, TV shows, computer games, music videos or printed material that focus intensively on themes of violence, hatred, control, power, death and destruction.
26. **Negative role models:** The student may be drawn to inappropriate role models such as Hitler, Satan or others associated with violence and destruction.
27. **Behavior appears relevant to carrying out a threat:** The student may spend inordinate amounts of time practicing with firearms, at the expense of other activities. The behavior appears to be related to possible threats to others.

20.9. AN ALTERNATIVE PROFILE: INVISIBLE CHILDREN

Shubert et al. (1999) studied the random school shootings which took place from October 1997 to May 1998, in Pearl, Mississippi; West Paducah, Kentucky; Jonesboro, Arkansas; Edinboro, Pennsylvania; and Springfield, Oregon. The authors used various source materials from multiple press reports to develop primary reasons for the shootings. The data Shubert et al. (1999) collected suggest the following:

(1) Peers thought the shooters had serious emotional problems and a disregard for human life. (2) The shooters were almost completely estranged from family and friends. (3) All of the shooters had discussed violence and the killing of others in advance of the shootings. These discussions of violence and killings

were ignored. (4) All the shooters had average or above average intelligence. (5) On the days of the shootings, all of the perpetrators acted in organized and deliberate ways, suggesting that they had a plan and that the plan had been practiced in advance.

The authors also examined two subsequent shootings at Columbine High School in Littleton, Colorado, and Heritage High School in Conyers, Georgia. In the Georgia shootings, the student was being treated medically for depression (Skeesis, 2000), while one of the Columbine killers was described as troubled and suffering from depression and obsessive thinking. Fellow students at Columbine High School said that prior to the killings the shooters would "walk with their heads down, because if they looked up they'd get thrown into lockers and get called a 'fag"' (Bender, 1999, p. 106). The shooters at Columbine High School made a videotape before the killings showing the two boys acting out feelings of anger and revenge (Skeesis, 2000). Pressley (1999) reports that just before the killings in Georgia, the shooter had broken up with his girlfriend and spoke of suicide and of bringing a gun to school. Only a day before the killings, the student told classmates that he would "blow up the classroom" (Cloud, 1999). Skeesis (2000) reports that all of the shooters involved in the Columbine and Georgia killings had access to many weapons and had built up arsenals of guns and ammunition that they had bought at gun shows. Barnard (1999) reports that the two Columbine killers had an increasing disregard for life and bragged to friends about mutilating animals.

Bender et al. (2001) suggest that in the young adolescent children involved in the prior-mentioned incidents of school killings, the FBI profile we usually associate with violent children does not fit. Instead,

> *... [I]t becomes increasingly clear that the perpetrators are not the children who, traditionally, have been associated with violent acts within the schools; that is, they are not the school bullies or kids who have been previously identified as aggressive. [They are] the students who are easiest to ignore and they are using violence to offset and counteract their anonymity. They have internalized their aggression to such an extent that an explosion of violence is the result. Bender (1999) initially used the term "invisible kids" to identify the group of kids who were the perpetrators in the random shootings in schools. This term was selected to underscore the fact that these students were generally unknown by many school personnel prior to the shooting incidents because they were not noted for overt behavior problems. On the other hand, because these perpetrators seem to be frequently identified as "nerds" or "geeks," other students may bully and pick on them rather than ignore them. Emotionally wounded because of being shunned by other students, these students are essentially invisible to the adults in the school. Through an overtly violent act, these invisible kids seem to be demonstrating that they do have power in the school environment and that they will no longer accept a peer-imposed label of "nerd" or "geek." (Bender et al., 2001, p. 108)*

20.10. THE RELATIONSHIP BETWEEN FAMILY DETERIORATION AND SCHOOL VIOLENCE

Studer (1996) writes that the family is thought to be the most violent institution in our society (Myers, 1993). Problems within the family, she notes, are often solved using aggression. Myers (1993) reports that 17% of all homicides in the United States occur within a family situation. Studer (1996) believes that when parents use harsh physical means to discipline their children, children learn that battering and physical aggression are normal ways of expressing frustration and resolving problems. Aggressive problem-solving techniques may frequently be practiced in the school setting and are reinforced when the child successfully resolves conflict through the use of aggression and intimidation. Griffin (1987) found that children who demonstrate physically aggressive and antisocial behaviors and have developmental and academic problems before age nine display more aggressive tendencies as adults than individuals who do not demonstrate early behavioral and educational problems.

Herrenkohl and Russo (2001) suggest that child abuse and neglect reinforce a sense of distrust in children which may lead to aggressive interactions with peers and adults. The authors believe that abuse and neglect by parents model the way a child is likely to interact with others. Eriksson's (1963) "stages" of psychosocial development include the development of trust. If a child experiences harsh physical punishment and neglect by a parent, it's possible that distrust related to hostile feelings toward the parents might result. This distrust defines a child's interactions with others. Rutter (1987) believes that abuse and neglect by parents often lead to a sense of vulnerability in children which may cycle into aggression. Rutter (1987) believes that vulnerable children sometimes use aggression as a way of coping with feelings of vulnerability and fear. Schools are one of the earliest social situations where children may feel vulnerable, inadequate, angry, less intelligent, ignored and a host of other emotions that may result in early aggression.

In a study of teachers' ratings of the causes of school violence, Petersen et al. (1998) found that the top four rated causes were: Lack of rules or family structure, a lack of involvement or parental supervision, violence acted out by parents, and parental drug use. Commenting on the changing structure of American families and what they consider to be the increasing deterioration of family life, the authors write:

> *As the basic structure of the family disintegrates, violence among family members increases, and this domestic violence spills into the classroom (Lystad, 1985). A new picture of the school must emerge to provide the variety of services that are needed by families to alleviate incidents of school violence. Home, school, and community must come together in a central location (i.e., the school campus) to make possible this reorganization of schools. Schools should strive to become part of any positive community effort (Hranitz and Eddowes, 1990). The successful combination of administrators,*

> *faculty, health care practitioners, counselors, social workers, childcare workers, technological support, and community agency availability and funding is an essential component of the proactive elementary model. The family must be committed to the educational process, whereas the educational structure must be committed to the family. Because the data indicate that schools need to take on roles previously played by family members, the roles of teacher and administrator must also evolve. It may be that schools will need to fill the gap in these areas for families who are unable or unwilling to become involved. (Petersen et al., 1998, p. 353)*

The idea that schools may need to fill the gap left by violent and/or deteriorating families is one frequently expressed in the literature, but often criticized by educators. Educators complain that not enough training, time, or resources are available to teach academic subjects let alone make up for deteriorating families. However, in their study of school violence, Bender et al. (2001) write, "Educators must be proactive and demand that some of the funds spent on school safety efforts be allocated to support educators' time to reflect on the emotional well-being of each student in an effort to identify the children who need some significant adult to reach out to them" (p. 109).

Rather than doing as Bender et al. (2001) suggest, however, Murray and Myers (1998) note that all too often children who begin to act out in the classroom are placed in special education classes and are classified as "severely emotionally disturbed, following a serious offense, as the path of least resistance" (p. 48). Often these children have conduct disorders and are neither severely emotionally disturbed nor in need of special education classes which are, they note, for truly disabled children. "Mislabeling a child to obtain services, to prevent a child from being expelled, or to remove the student to a special classroom is both inappropriate and unethical" (Murray and Myers, 1998, p. 48). The authors believe that children who act out do not fare well in special education classes and can disrupt a truly disabled population of students. Schools which support inappropriate diagnoses and placements, they write, "may be creating incubators for future antisocial or even criminal behavior" (p. 48). To emphasize their point, they give an example of misdiagnosis by a group of teachers in which, "[a]t the end of the exercise, teacher groups were embarrassed to learn they had recommended severely emotionally disturbed special-education placement and little if any success for each of the fictitious students – Abraham Lincoln, Eleanor Roosevelt, Thomas Edison, Albert Einstein, and Will Rogers" (p. 53).

Petersen et al. (1998) call for a new definition of schools as "town centers" which offer a variety of services needed by deteriorating and dysfunctional families to reduce school violence. Because family life is so chaotic for many violence-prone children, the authors argue that schools must assume many of the roles previously played by family members and that the function of teachers and administrator must also change. Family disintegration, the authors argue, requires schools to take responsibility for teaching moral conduct. Education, they note, is more than "simply teaching the cognitive attributes of character development; it must also include the emotional attributes of moral maturity, such as conscience, self-respect, empathy, and self-control" (Petersen et al., 1998, p. 350).

20.11. A PROGRAM FOR VIOLENT FAMILIES

Because family violence is so often related to school violence, the Rose Elementary School in a moderately sized industrial city in the northeastern industrial belt of the country believed that reducing the amount of bullying and intimidation of children and the hidden violence that resulted would require work with children and their families in which family violence was known or suspected. The school board passed a policy that all bullying, intimidation, threats, harassment, theft or any form of physical abuse used against another child, teacher or staff member would result in mandatory counseling for the child and for his or her parents. Many of the children and parents in this cohort were involved in family violence (80%). Another 10% of the parents were abusing substances, while the remaining 10% had problems in disciplining and establishing consistent rules for the child to follow. All were brought together for counseling sessions with school social workers on a weekly basis. There were also required parenting classes. To make the point abundantly clear, a police officer was present at the meetings in case an adult became abusive. Many of the children from families known to be involved in domestic violence were being seen professionally but the extra attention was welcomed by the children. The parents were being seen in treatment on a hit-and-miss basis and many of the fathers had never been involved in treatment or parenting classes because of work or the unwillingness to cooperate.

Some of the parents were openly hostile to the need to attend and voiced their objection frequently. It was made clear to parents that early signs of violence in school were intolerable behaviors in this era of school shootings. Schools should be safe havens for children and teachers, and the learning environment should be stress-free. Children who intimidated, bullied and frightened the other children made learning difficult. Much of the reason for the child's behavior came from home situations where there was considerable violence. Violence at home was intolerable and the continued violence by children in school would be taken as a sign of the parents' inability to resolve their problems in non-violent ways. Parents would be charged with child endangerment if family violence did not stop immediately. The purpose of the classes the parents were attending was to teach parents the new skills needed to control their anger and to eliminate violence. If parents failed to attend, the matter would be turned over to the police. School violence had become an epidemic and it would stop, now.

Parents were provided individual and group therapy Saturday mornings from 8:00 a.m. to 11:00 a.m. From 11:00 a.m. to 2:00 p.m., they sat in anger management classes and parent effectiveness training classes. From 2:00 p.m. to 4:00 p.m., they provided feedback, stories of success and failure, concerns about their children, lack of awareness of the harm the parental fighting was having on their kids, and other topics that evolved as the sessions continued. There were 40 sets of parents at the beginning of the program. Three sets dropped out and were reported to the police. Eight fathers dropped out but the mothers stayed on. The fathers were reported to the police and six returned as a result. The program was planned for 12 weeks but went on for almost a year as families began to experience the giddy feeling of functioning well. The bullying behavior ceased among the children of the parents being treated. The Rose School believes that bullying is a very serious sign of dangerous aggression, one that is preventable and treatable. As bullying rates declined, the school blossomed and Rose became a model school for the district and attracted many of the district's most promising kids. Rose is a strict, no-nonsense school. Rules are taken seriously and it's not everyone's cup of tea. But as far as violence prevention, Rose is a safe school with increased state achievement scores that have placed it in the upper five percent of all schools in the state. Before the violence prevention program, the school was in the 50th percentile. Stopping violence makes a difference and the children and parents at Rose are the beneficiaries of a tough, expensive stance taken by the local school board members.

20.12. CASE STUDY: AN INNOVATIVE SCHOOL DISTRICT DEVELOPS A PROGRAM TO DECREASE SCHOOL VIOLENCE

The school district in this case study has asked that its name not be used since it is in the midst of a study to test the effectiveness of the approach described here. Undue attention might create changes in the data which would affect the findings. For this reason, the district will be called the Petofsky School District, an urban inner city school district with very high rates of school violence and gang activity.

After the beating and rape of a sixth grade teacher by one of her 12-year-old students, one of a series of violent crimes to plague the school district, the Petofsky School Board voted to adopt a no-tolerance policy on violence, but one with a heart. All incidents of violence, either committed or prevented, were to be assessed and, if possible, treated. This policy was adopted as threats were called in daily of school bombings. These threats effectively closed down all of the schools in the district, including the K-6 elementary schools. A chance break helped authorities identify the child who called in the bomb threats. He was identified as an 11-year-old male Caucasian youth with an unremarkable school record and no history of acting-out behavior. The child, whose name is Robert, is one of the invisible children who act out against classmates because they perceive themselves as being bullied and mistreated by classmates.

This is certainly the case with Robert, who has been the object of ridicule since kindergarten because of a severe cleft palate and speech problem. Many of the children have been unmerciful in their bullying and taunting of Robert, who has a deep sense of rage at the hurtful behavior he has had to endure. Robert has had his clothes taken away in the boys shower, his picture posted all over the school with derogatory statements, his hair forcibly cut Marine fashion, and an endless number of hurtful, ego-deflating and damaging acts of violence. He is full of rage and sought to take it out by disrupting the school and frightening his classmates. Robert is a very intelligent child and had been able to computer enhance his voice so that his bomb threats had a robot-like quality which frightened the secretaries and the school-aged helpers who answered the phones.

Robert's parents are very angry at the school for not controlling the bullying he has had to endure. They have done everything to protect their child but have had no help from the school. The school sympathizes with Robert's plight but says that it is too understaffed to do much about it. When the school board discovered the reason for the bomb threats, they created a policy that makes taunts and humiliating statements as serious as actual violence. Three boys and a girl in Robert's fifth grade class were suspended with mandatory treatment. Robert was also suspended for a semester, but he was provided very high-level treatment and then transferred to a charter school with a good reputation for controlling mean-spirited behavior among its students.

Since instituting the no-taunting or bullying policy, Petofsky has experienced a sharp decline in school violence. As the violence has been reduced, the level of achievement of the children has gone up significantly. Petofsky recognizes that children do badly in violent environments and has made a concerted effort to prevent violence at all costs and, when it does take place, to determine the cause, provide expert treatment, and recognize that children who act out in school do so for reasons that may be preventable and treatable. The suspended children are all in empathy-training classes and continue on in treatment. Children who force other children to the brink of violence are dangerous and need the same help as the offenders they taunt and abuse into violence.

20.13. SUMMARY

School violence is a serious American problem plaguing school systems all over the country. The increase in rates of violence and the fact that many victims of school violence may become perpetrators should give us pause as we consider the many intelligent children who are treated badly by lower functioning classmates, and who consider acts of violence as methods of pay back for the humiliation they have suffered. An FBI profile was presented giving a number of characteristics of violence-prone youth in school, but several writers advanced the notion that children who have been bullied and harassed by school mates may form a core of "invisible children" who outwardly seem non-violent but inwardly harbor strong feelings of anger which sometimes lead to violence.

20.14. QUESTIONS FROM THE CHAPTER

1. In your school experiences, did you feel that teachers and administrators ignored the bullying and harassing behavior of certain students?
2. In your school experiences, did you encounter gang activities? What were they, how young were the gang members and how dangerous did you perceive those activities to be?
3. While school shootings have resulted in few lost lives, they do underscore school violence. In your school experiences, what student behaviors do you find the most disruptive, potentially dangerous and in need of prevention?
4. Do you feel that dress codes, intolerance for violence policies and stricter codes of conduct will reduce school violence?
5. In the discussion of invisible children who end up instigating violence activities in school, why do you think the students assess them as violent and the teachers and administrators do not?

References

Barnard, N. D. (1999, November). The psychology of abuse. Retrieved November 1999 from *Physicians Committee for Responsible Medicine* (PCRM). Web site: www.perm.org.

Bender, W. N. (1999, April). *Violence prevention in the school.* An invited workshop presented at the Doylestown Public School Board of Education, Doylestown, PA.

Bender, W. N., Shubert, T. H., & McLaughlin, P. J. (2001, November). Invisible kids: Preventing school violence by identifying kids in trouble. *Intervention in School and Clinic, 37*(2), 105–111.

Bureau of Justice Statistics. (1997). *Criminal victimization, 1973–95.* Washington, DC: Government Printing Office.

Christenson, S. L. (1995). Families and schools: What is the role of the school psychologist?. *School Psychology Quarterly, 10*(2), 118–132.

Cloud, J. (1999, May). *Just a routine school shooting.* Time. Retrieved October 1999 from the World Wide Web: http://www.time.com: Just a routine school shooting.

Committee for Children. (1997). *Second step: Violence prevention curriculum.* Seattle: Committee for Children.

Critical Incident Response Group. (1999). *The school shooter: a threat assessment perspective.* National Center for the Analysis of Violent Crime. Quantico, Virginia: FBI Academy.

Crowe, T. (1991). *Habitual offenders: Guidelines for citizen action and public responses.* Washington, DC: Office of Juvenile Justice and Delinquency Prevention, U.S. Department of Justice.

Egley, A., & Ritz, C. E. (2006, April). Highlights of the 2004 National Youth Gang Survey OJJDP Fact Sheet #1. *U.S. Department of Justice Office of Justice Programs.*

Epstein, J. L. (1992). School and family partnerships: Leadership roles for school psychologists. In S. L. Christenson & J. C. Conoley (Eds.), *Home-school collaboration* (pp. 215–243). Silver Spring, MD: The National Association of School Psychologists.

Eriksson (1963).

Fitzpatrick, K. M. (1999, October). Violent victimization among America's school children. *Journal of Interpersonal Violence, 14*(10), 1055–1069.

Glicken, M., & Sechrest, D. (2003). *The role of the helping professions in treating and preventing violence*. Boston: Allyn and Bacon.

Griffin, G. (1987). Childhood predictive characteristics of aggressive adolescents. *Exceptional Children, 54*, 246–252.

Herrenkohl, R. C., & Russo, M. J. (2001). Abusive early child rearing and early childhood aggression. *Child Maltreatment, 1*, 3–16.

Hranitz, J. R., & Eddowes, E. A. (1990, Fall). Violence: A crisis in homes and schools. *Childhood Education, 67*, 4–7.

Huey, W. C., & Rank, R. C. (1984). Effects of counselor and peer-led groups' assertive training on Black adolescent aggression. *Journal of Counseling Psychology, 31*, 95–98.

Hughes, M. J. (1997, June). An exploratory study of young adult Black and Latino males and the factors facilitating their decisions to make positive behavioral changes. *Smith College Studies in Social Work, 67*(3), 401–414.

Johnson, L. (1999, August). Understanding and responding to youth violence: A juvenile corrections approach. *Corrections Today, 61*(5), 62–64.

Kauffman, J. M. (1997). *Characteristics of emotional and behavioral disorders of children and youth* (6th ed.). Upper Saddle River, NJ: Merrill.

Kube, B. A., & Ratigan, G. (1991). All present and accounted for: A no-nonsense policy on student attendance keeps kids showing up for class – and learning. *The American School Board Journal*, 22–23.

Lickona, T. (1988, February). Four strategies for fostering character development in children. *Phi Delta Kappan*, 419–423.

London, P. (1987, May). Character education and clinical intervention: A paradigm shift for US schools. *Phi Delta Kappan*, 667–673.

Lystad, M. (1985). Innovative mental health services for child disaster victims. *Children Today, 14*, 13–17.

Malmquist, C. P. (1996). *Homicide: A psychiatric perspective*. Washington, DC: American Psychiatric Press.

Mathias, C. E. (1992). Touching the lives of children: Consultative interventions that work. *Elementary School Guidance & Counseling, 26*, 190–201.

Murray, B. A., & Myers, M. A. (1998, April). Conduct disorders and the special-education trap. *The Education Digest, 63*(8), 48–53.

Myers, J. (1993). *Social psychology* (3rd ed.). New York: McGraw-Hill.

Myles, B.S, & Simpson, R. L. (1998, May). Aggression and violence by school-age children and youth: understanding the aggression cycle and prevention/intervention strategies. *Intervention in School and Clinic, 33*(5), 259–264.

National Center for Education Statistics. (1995). Annual Report 1995.

National School Safety Center. (1996, March). *National School Safety Center newsletter*. Malibu, CA: National School Safety Center.

Olweus, D. (1993). *Bullying at school: What we know and what we can do*. Malden, MA: Blackwell Publishers.

Olweus, D., & Limber, S. (1999). Bullying prevention program. In D. S. & Elliot (Ed.), *Blueprints for violence prevention*. Denver, CO: C & M Press.

Petersen, G. J., Pietrzak, D., & Speaker, K. M. (1998, September). The enemy within: a national study on school violence and prevention. *Urban Education, 33*(3), 331–359.

Peterson, R. L., & Skiba, R. (2001, January/February). Creating school climates that prevent school violence. *The Clearing House*, 74(3), 155–163, ISSN: 0009-8655.

Pressley, S. A. (1999, May). Six wounded in Georgia school shooting. *Washington Post*. Retrieved October 1999 from www.washingtonpost.com: Wounded in GA. School Shooting.

Quinn, J. F., & Downs, B. (1995). Predictors of gang violence: The impact of drugs and guns on police perceptions in nine States. *Journal of Gang Research, 2*(3), 15–27.

Rutter, M. (1987). Psychological resilience and protective mechanisms. *American Journal of Orthopsychiatry, 57*, 316–331.

Sautter, R. (1995, January). Standing up to violence [Special report]. *Phi Delta Kappan*, 76, kl–k2.

Schwartz, W. (1996, October). An overview of strategies to reduce school violence. *ERIC Clearing House on Urban Education*, No. 115, EDO-UD-96-4.

Sechrest, D. (2001). *Juvenile crime: A predictive study*. Unpublished document.

Shubert, T. H., Bressette, S., Deeken, J., & Bender, W. N. (1999). Analysis of random school shootings. In W. N. Bender, G. Clinton, & R. L. Bender (Eds.), *Violence prevention and reduction in schools* (97–101). Austin: PRO-ED.

Siegel, L. J., & Senna, J. J. (1994). *Juvenile delinquency: Theory, practice, and law* (5th ed.). St. Paul, Minn: West.

Skeesis, A. (2000, January). Monsters among us . . . The tragedy at Columbine high: The victims/the heroes, Could it have been prevented? Columbine High School Tragedy Web Ring. Retrieved June 2002 from www.angelfire.com.

Spergel, I. (1995). *The youth gang problem: A community approach*. New York, NY: Oxford University Press.

Sprague, J. R., & Walker, H. M. (2000, Spring). Early identification and intervention for youth with antisocial and violent behaviour. *Exceptional Children, 66*(3), 367–379.

Studer, J. (1996). Understanding and preventing aggressive responses in youth. *Elementary School Guidance and Counseling, 30*, 194–203.

Stevens, R., (1995, April 26). Increasing violence in schools. In W.N. Bender & R.L. Bender (Eds.), *Teachers' Safety*. (Teleconference produced by the Teacher's Workshop, Bishop, GA).

The W.M. Keck Foundation. (2007). *The challenge of school violence*. http://www.crf-usa.org/violence/school.html

Walker, H. M., Colvin, G., & Ramsey, E. (1995). *Antisocial behavior in school: Strategies and best practices*. Pacific Grove, CA: Brooks/Cole.

Weiss, H. M., & Edwards, M. E. (1992). The family-school collaboration project: Systemic interventions for school improvement. In S. L. Christenson, & J. C. Conoley (Eds.), *Home-school collaboration* (pp. 215–243). Silver Spring, MD: The National Association of School Psychologists.

Wikipedia. (2008). *Gang*. http://en.wikipedia.org/wiki/Gang.

Further reading

Office of Juvenile Justice and Delinquency Prevention, April 2006 #01 http://www.ncjrs.gov/pdffiles1/ojjdp/fs200601.pd.

21 Oppositional Defiant and Conduct Disorders Leading to Anti-Social Behavior and Violence

21.1. INTRODUCTION

In this chapter, the issue of early diagnosis of violent behavior in children will be discussed. It is important to note that although there is evidence that early onset of violent behavior in children is associated with adolescent and adult violence, we are, after all, discussing children whose behavior is not completely formed. Many factors contribute to the continuation or discontinuation of violent behavior in young children. One of the strongest reasons for discontinuance of violent behavior is early intervention. Further, while profiling children for early signs of violence may lead to needed treatment, we should be cautious about using indications of violent behavior to project into the future. Many things change in a child's life and the benefits of positive influences, including helping professionals, teachers, mentors, religious affiliations, parents, siblings and extended family, should not be discounted. Children with early signs of violent behavior should not be categorized, but an evaluation should be made to find out why the violent behavior is beginning to show itself so early in life. There are many reasons for early violent behavior. Violent behavior is often a reflection of early childhood physical and sexual abuse and neglect. Early violence may be associated with parental drug and alcohol abuse, learning difficulties, poor peer relationships, and a host of treatable conditions. If we do not show caution and humanity in working with violent children, we run the risk of so categorizing these children that they may live with stigma that only serves to exacerbate their anger.

In the following section the two most commonly used diagnoses predicting anti-social and violent behavior (ODD and CD) will be discussed. Please use caution when considering the implications for future behavioral problems in adolescence and adulthood when considering the following discussion.

21.2. OPPOSITIONAL DEFIANT DISORDER (ODD)

Oppositional defiant disorder (ODD) is a behavior disorder, usually diagnosed in childhood that is characterized by uncooperative, defiant, negativistic, irritable, and annoying behaviors toward parents, peers, teachers and other authority figures. Oppositional defiant disorder is reported to affect between 2% and 16% of children and adolescents in the general population and is more common in boys than in girls. Most symptoms seen in children and adolescents with oppositional defiant disorder also occur occasionally in children without this disorder, especially around the ages or two or three, or during the teenage years. Many children, especially when they are tired, hungry, or upset, tend to disobey, argue with parents, or defy authority. However, in children and adolescents with oppositional defiant disorder, these symptoms occur more frequently and often interfere with learning, school adjustment, and sometimes with the child's relationships with others. Symptoms of oppositional defiant disorder may include frequent temper tantrums; excessive arguments with adults; refusal to comply with adult requests; always questioning rules; refusal to follow rules; behavior intended to annoy or upset others, including adults; blaming others for his/her misbehaviors or mistakes; being easily annoyed by others; frequently having an angry attitude; speaking harshly or unkindly; and seeking revenge. The reader should note that while many of the symptoms of ODD are also found in normal children, frequency and severity of the behavior are the keys to diagnosis. (WebMD, 2005, p. 1)

The age of onset of ODD seems to be associated with the development of severe problems later in life, including aggressiveness and anti-social behavior. However, not all children with ODD have a poor prognosis. Studies suggest that less than 50% of the most severe cases become anti-social as adults. Nevertheless, the fact that this disorder continues into adulthood for many people indicates that it is a serious and life-long problem (Webster-Stratton and Dahl, 1995).

The Behavioral Neurotherapy Clinic (2007) notes that although not all ODD children develop conduct disorder, and not all conduct disorder children become anti-social adults, there are certain risk factors that have been shown to contribute to the continuation of the disorder. The risk factors identified include an early age of onset (preschool years), the spread of anti-social behaviors across settings, the frequency and intensity of anti-social behaviors, the forms that the anti-social behaviors take, having covert behaviors at an early age and also particular parent and family characteristics. However, these risk factors do not fully explain the complex interaction of variables involved in understanding the continuation of conduct disorder in any one individual.

21.3. CONDUCT DISORDER

Conduct disorder is a serious behavioral and emotional disorder that can occur in children and teens. A child with this disorder may display a pattern of disruptive and violent behavior and have problems following rules. It is not uncommon for children and teens to have behavior-related problems at some time during their development. However, the behavior is considered to be a conduct disorder when it is long-lasting and when it violates the rights of others, goes against accepted norms of behavior and disrupts the child's or family's everyday life. According to research cited in Phelps and McClintock (1994), 6% of children in the United States may have conduct disorder, but since prevalence estimates are based primarily upon referral rates, and since many children and adolescents are never referred for mental health services, the actual incidences may well be higher (Phelps and McClintock, 1994).

Symptoms vary depending on the age of the child and whether the disorder is mild, moderate or severe. In general, symptoms of conduct disorder fall into four general categories:

- **Aggressive behavior:** These are behaviors that threaten or cause physical harm and may include fighting, bullying, being cruel to others or animals, using weapons and forcing another into sexual activity.
- **Destructive behavior:** This involves intentional destruction of property such as arson (deliberate fire-setting) and vandalism (harming another person's property).
- **Deceitful behavior:** This may include repeated lying, shoplifting or breaking into homes or cars in order to steal.
- **Violation of rules:** This involves going against accepted rules of society or engaging in behavior that is not appropriate for the person's age. These behaviors may include running away, skipping school, playing pranks or being sexually active at a very young age.

In addition, many children with conduct disorder are irritable, have low self-esteem and tend to throw frequent "temper tantrums." Some may abuse drugs and alcohol. Children with conduct disorder often are unable to appreciate how their behavior can hurt others and generally have little guilt or remorse about hurting others.

The onset of conduct disorder may occur as early as age five or six, but more usually occurs in late childhood or early adolescence; onset after the age of 16 years is rare (American Psychiatric Association, 1994). The results of research into childhood aggression have indicated that externalizing problems are relatively stable over time. Richman and colleagues, for example, found that 67% of children who displayed externalizing problems at age three were still aggressive at age eight (Richman et al., 1982). Other studies have found stability rates of 50–70%. However, these stability rates may be higher due to the belief that the problems are episodic, situational, and likely to change in character (Loeber, 1991).

21.4. VIOLENCE IN CHILDREN UNDER 18

Commenting on juvenile crime, Osofsky and Osofsky (2001) write,

> *Put simply, youth violence in the United States has reached epidemic proportions (Rosenberg and Fenley 1991; Rosenberg et al., 1992). According to the FBI Uniform Crime Reports (Pellegrini et al., 2000), the homicide rate has more than doubled since 1950, with the most recently reported rate being*

> *22 per 100 000 for young people 15–24 years old. To punctuate the meaning of these numbers, it is important to compare this data with that of other similar countries. For example, the homicide rate among males 15–24 years old in the United States is 10 times higher than in Canada, 15 times higher than in Australia, and 28 times higher than in France or Germany (Lester and Yang, 1998) (p. 287).*

Herrenkohl et al. (February 2001) report that individuals involved in early onset childhood violence are at a very high risk of committing violent crimes in adolescence and adulthood. The risk for later violent behavior increases the younger the violence begins. Elliott (1994) found that 45% of the children who commit violent offenses by age 11 go on to commit violent offenses in their early 20s. The older the age at onset of violence, the less likely children are to commit violent offenses in adulthood. According to Thornberry et al. (1995), almost twice as many children committing violent acts before the age of nine commit violent acts in adulthood as compared to children between the ages of 10 and 12.

Kauffman (1997) reports that 80–90% of school-age children and youth, in self-reports, indicate that they have been involved in acts of violence and aggression. The author notes that 60% of the students from 6th through 12th grade in inner cities, suburbs, and rural areas were easily able to purchase handguns. Thirty-nine percent of the youths who were surveyed said they knew someone who had been killed or wounded by gunfire. In the same poll, over one-third of the students surveyed said that their lives would be shortened because of easy access to guns.

Myles and Simpson (1998) believe that violence among children has increased for the following reasons:

1. There is more violence in society. Children who are exposed to a great degree of violence become desensitized to the meaning and impact of violence.
2. The increased number of violent and seriously disturbed children who are being mainstreamed through regular classrooms has increased school violence at a time when there are decreasing opportunities to place children in residential placements and group homes that might offer a more appropriate experience with less harm to the remaining school-aged children.
3. Many of the violent and emotionally disturbed children currently being mainstreamed in regular classrooms are being taught by teachers who are untrained to work with children who have special social, emotional and educational needs.
4. There are more negative influences in a child's life than ever. This is a result of gang activity, child abuse, family violence, child neglect, and violent neighborhoods which offer few positive role models for children (Kauffman, 1997; Walker et al., 1995).

Wolfgang (1972, 1987) reports that 6–7% of all boys in a given birth year will become chronic offenders, meaning that they will have five or more arrests before their 18th birthdays. He also suggests that these same 6–7% will commit half of all crimes and two-thirds of all violent crimes committed by all the boys born in a given birth year by age 18. Briscoe (1997) notes that Wolfgang's studies have been found accurate by a number of other studies and that increases in the numbers of adolescent males bodes badly because it increases the number of boys in the 6–7% category who will become violent perpetrators.

Horowitz (2000) writes that as the number of high profile cases increases:

> *. . . [S]o do the thousands of less visible homicides that occur daily in inner cities and in poor, minority neighborhoods. Approximately 23 000 homicides occur each year in the United States, roughly 10% of which involve a perpetrator who is under 18 years of age. Between the mid-1980s and the mid-1990s, the number of youths committing homicides had increased by 168%. Juveniles currently account for one in six murder arrests (17%), and the age of those juveniles gets younger and younger every year. For example, in North Carolina in 1997, 70 juveniles under 18 years of age were arrested on murder charges. Thirty-five were 17, 24 were 16, seven were 15, and four were 13 or 14. In 1999, for the first time in North Carolina's history, two 11-year-old twins were charged with the premeditated murder of their father as well as the attempted murder of their mother and sister (p. 133).*

21.5. EARLY SIGNS OF AGGRESSION AND ANTI-SOCIAL BEHAVIOR

Murray and Myers (1998) report that conduct disorders in childhood are frequently predictive of later delinquency and adult criminality. By age six, family functioning is a strong indicator of delinquency. At age nine, the child's antisocial and aggressive behavior further predicts delinquent tendencies. Sprague and Walker (2000) report that:

> *Well-developed antisocial behavior patterns and high levels of aggression evidenced early in a child's life are among the best predictors of delinquent and violent behavior years later (Fagan, 1996; Hawkins and Catalano, 1992). Antisocial patterns that appear early in a child's life and are characterized by high-frequency, intense severity, and occurrence across multiple settings predicts a number of ominous outcomes later on, including victimization of others, drug and alcohol use, violence, school failure and dropout, and delinquency (Loeber and Farrington, 1998; Patterson et al., 1992). Over the developmental age span, these behavior patterns become more destructive, more aversive, and have much greater social impact as they become elaborated (p. 369).*

Dwyer et al. (1998) believe that we can diagnose potential violence as early as five, but that few at-risk youths will commit serious violent acts throughout their life span. Many at-risk youths with early diagnoses of aggression and violent behaviors, however, will display such major life problems as drug and alcohol abuse, domestic and child abuse, divorce or multiple relationships, employment problems, mental health problems, dependence on social services, and involvement in less serious crimes (Obiakor et al., 1997).

Wagner and Lane (1998) studied an 8% youth cohort ages 10–17 that had a Youth Services referral in 1997 in a large Oregon county whose arrest statistics, according to the authors, are representative of the nation as a whole. Of that 8%, 20% of the offenders committed 87% of all new crime. Sprague and Walker (2000) suggest that there is a small group of juvenile youth who commit almost all serious crimes and that these same youth, "are very likely to have begun their careers very early (i.e., before age 12)" (p. 369).

There appears to be a relationship between violence and school disciplinary problems. Disciplinary referrals in elementary and middle schools indicate that 6–9% of the referred children are responsible for more than 50% of the total disciplinary referrals and practically all of the serious offenses, including possession of weapons, fighting, assaults on other children, and assaults on teachers (Skiba et al., 1997). Early disciplinary problems in school are accurate predictors of future and more serious problems (Walker et al., 1995). According to Walker et al. (1995), students with 10 or more disciplinary referrals per year are seriously at risk for school failure and for other more serious life problems. Many of the children who are frequently referred to principals for disciplinary action are defiant and disobedient and may often be involved in bullying and intimidation of other students. They are, according to Sprague and Walker (2000), likely to move on to more serious offenses, including "physical fighting, and then ultimately rape, serious assault, or murder" (p. 370).

21.6. EARLY AND LATE STARTERS OF VIOLENCE

Moffitt (1994) believes that children who develop early aggressive tendencies are much more likely to move on to more seriously violent behaviors than children who show no violent tendencies before adolescence. He calls these two cohorts early and late starters. Late starters show signs of violent behavior in late middle school and even high school. Early starters often show signs of disobedience, bullying, intimidation and fighting when they begin kindergarten and elementary school.

According to Sprague and Walker (2000), "Early starters are likely to experience antisocial behavior and its toxic effects throughout their lives. Late starters have a far more positive long-term outcome" (p. 370). Walker and Severson (1990) suggest that diagnostic signs of "early starters" include disobedience, property damage, conduct problems, theft, the need for a great deal of attention, threats and intimidation, and fighting. While it's wise to remember that diagnostic labels can be misleading and incorrect when applied to children, labels that have been used with children that correlate with violent behavior include: (1) inattention, and impulsivity (Lynam, 1996); (2) antisocial personality disorder; (3) conduct disorder; (4) oppositional defiant disorder; and (5) serious emotional disturbance (APA, 1994). Mayer (1995) and Reid (1993) suggest that certain environmental factors may correlate with the potential for violent behavior. The most prominent environmental factors include inconsistent and harsh parenting styles as well as disorganized or badly functioning schools and the availability of drugs, alcohol, and weapons.

Herrenkohl et al. (2001) note that:

> *... Individuals who initiate violent behavior in childhood are at particularly high risk for serious violent offending in adolescence and adulthood. . . . Risk for later violent offending typically diminishes with later ages of initiation (Elliott 1994; Thornberry et al., 1995), although initiation of violence at any age into adolescence is associated with an increased probability for violence at subsequent ages (Farrington, 1998) (p. 45).*

Elliott (1994) found that 45% of the pre-adolescents who began violent behavior by age 11 went on to commit violent offenses by their early 20s, while 25% of the children who began violent behavior between the ages of 11 and 12 committed violent offenses through adolescence and into adulthood. Thornberry et al. (1995) found similar patterns. The later the onset of violence, the less likely the child is to cycle into adult violence. The earlier the violent behavior begins, the more likely it is to continue on into adulthood. Herrenkohl et al. (2001) in a study of early onset violence noted four indicators of future violent behavior in children aged 10: Hitting a teacher, picking fights, the tendency to attack other children, and a report by parents indicating that a child fights a great deal at home or in the neighborhood.

Catalano and Hawkins (1996) suggest that youth violence is the result of socialization into violent behavior that begins in early childhood and continues on through adolescence. Violent behavior in elementary school increases the risk for violence in adolescence and adulthood. By socialization into violence, the authors believe that children have early experiences in anti-social behavior that are reinforced by peers and fail to be extinguished by adults monitoring the behavior. As the anti-social behavior continues on with its particular rewards, the child seeks out others with similar behaviors who may accept, reinforce, and promote new antisocial behaviors which often lead to violence.

Longitudinal studies by Widom (1999) and by McCord (1999) support the concern about aggressive behavior at an early age, particularly its linkages to child abuse and neglect. McCord, whose study of families and child rearing spanned 30 years, found that parental response to aggressive behavior in their sons was related to later aggressive behavior (p. 169). A recent survey of self-reported delinquency found that one in seven 12-year-olds, or 14%, had engaged in assaultive behaviors, and that 7% reported carrying a handgun (Puzzanchera, 2000).

Statistics on juvenile offenders and victims found that the number of children abused, neglected, or endangered more than doubled from 1986 to 1993 (Snyder and Sickmund, 1999, p. 40). In 1993, there were almost three million "maltreated or endangered" children, up from 1.4 million in 1986. Abuse and neglect were classified as physical, sexual, or emotional. Most of these youths entered the child welfare system through child protective services. In 1997, 14.1 million juveniles lived in poverty, or one-fifth of all juveniles.

Thornberry et al. (1999) report on the impact of family disruption and its relationship to delinquency. Citing census data, they report that from 1970 to 1997, the proportion of American households having children who live with both parents declined by 64–35% for African-Americans, and from 90% to 74% for whites. Their conclusions were that, "Overall, the data reported here indicate a consistent relationship between a greater number of family transitions and a higher level of delinquency and drug abuse" (Thornberry et al., p. 4). The authors indicate that adolescents who experience family stress may be more likely to have difficulty managing anger and other negative emotions, although further research is needed.

Another factor related to the increase in delinquent behavior is the relative isolation of some neighborhoods from their larger communities. This is especially true in the case of inner city youth who are insulated from outside influences. Poor schools and weak social institutions can lead to lack of achievement and lower motivation. Economic and social discrimination and poor employment prospects can lead to participation in gangs and criminal activity that may ultimately lead to violent crimes. The *1999 National Report Series* of the Office of Juvenile Justice and Delinquency Prevention (Bilchik, 1999, p. 1) describes minority involvement in the juvenile justice system:

> *The most recent statistics available reveal significant racial and ethnic disparity in the confinement of juvenile offenders. In 1997, minorities made up one-third of the juvenile population nationwide but accounted for nearly two-thirds of the detained and committed population in secure juvenile facilities. For black juveniles, the disparities were most evident (Bilchik, 1999, p. 1).*

Juveniles aged 16–17 accounted for 48% of all juvenile arrests and 51% of the violent crimes. Black youth comprised 15% of the juvenile population in 1997, but accounted for 26% of all arrests and 44% of all juvenile arrests for violent offenses. Minorities accounted for seven in 10 youths held in custody for a violent offense (Bilchik, 1999, p. 11). The report calls for an effort to provide "all youth with an equal opportunity to learn, thrive, and achieve at every stage of their lives" (p. 1).

21.7. PESSIMISM ABOUT THE EFFECTIVENESS OF CLINICAL WORK WITH VIOLENT YOUTH

It is troubling but understandable to note the general skepticism in the literature regarding the effectiveness of clinical approaches to treating children with early onset violence. Rae-Grant et al. (1999) write, "Because exclusive individual clinical interventions for violent conduct disorders do not work, the child and adolescent psychiatrist must seek opportunities to be a leader or team member in well-organized and well-funded community prevention efforts" (p. 338). Sprague and Hill (Spring 2000) complain about poorly matched treatment approaches, which deny the severity of the problem. Elliott et al.

(1998) report that counseling has no effect on the problems of antisocial and pre-delinquent youth.

Steiner and Stone (March 1999) note the widespread pessimism among clinicians regarding effective clinical work with violent youth, but believe that this pessimism is unwarranted. The authors indicate that treating childhood violence requires clinicians to practice with flexibility and to be cognizant of the need to develop treatment approaches that permit clinicians to offer interventions in many different settings, including schools, juvenile detention centers, prisons, homes, as well as in the consulting room. Patterson and Narrett (1990) believe that there is strong evidence to support the effectiveness of family- and parent-based interventions in the elementary grades to reduce violence and related pathology. Myles and Simpson (May 1998) argue that because aggressive and violent children often experience a range of problems, that we should provide services to meet the child's academic and social needs. Those services should include counselors, psychologists, social workers and treatment interventions that meet the social and emotional needs of aggressive and violent children.

In writing about therapeutic approaches to working with gang members, a unique subset of violent children, Morales (1982) provides the following reasons clinical interventions often do not work with gang members. They are:

> *(a) The belief by many clinicians that antisocial personality disorders and/or gang members are untreatable; (b) the therapists' fear of violent people and the assumption that all gang members are violent; (c) a belief in the lack of the psychological capacity for insight of poor and uneducated people, a cohort usually associated with gang activity; (d) an over-appreciation of the value of treatment and a belief that every gang member can benefit; (e) the opposite belief that gang members can't be treated and that all gang members are manipulative and dishonest; and (f) the belief that the therapist has the power and hence will control the interview (Morales, 1982, p. 142).*

Morales (1982) also notes that gang member entering treatment may also have issues that must be understood by the therapist. They include: (a) a distrust/dislike of authority figures, often the result of prior negative experiences with parents, teachers, and police; (b) a strong resentment at being forced into treatment involuntarily as the result of legal mandate; (c) a feeling of discomfort with the therapist who might be of a different ethnic/racial group; (d) a sense of a generational, cultural, and perhaps language gap with the therapist; and (e) the anticipation of looking forward to winning yet another struggle with a social control agent or the notion of the therapist as Freudian cop (p. 143).

21.8. TREATING EARLY ONSET VIOLENCE

Carey (2007) reports that although we often think that children who show early signs of behavioral problems do badly academically, an international team of researchers analyzed measures of social and intellectual development from over 16 000 children and found that disruptive or antisocial behaviors in kindergarten did not correlate with academic results at the end of elementary school. Kindergartners who interrupted the teacher, defied instructions and even picked fights were performing as well in reading and math as well-behaved children of the same abilities when they both reached fifth grade, the study found.

Steiner and Stone (March 1999) suggest that whatever we may say about large-scale programs and the ineffectiveness of clinical work, violent clients, particularly children, almost always see a clinician at some point in the life cycle. To show the importance of early and effective intervention, the authors note that young men representing only 8% of the population commit almost half of all violence. Many of these young men could be helped in clinical work if seen early enough, according to the authors, who go on to indicate that the cost of violence to victims and to taxpayers is "staggering." Mandel and Magnusson (1993) report that the lifetime cost for all Americans aged 12 and older who were victims of violent crime was estimated to be 178 billion dollars a year, while the cost to taxpayers to incarcerate one juvenile was \$32 000 a year in California, according to Butts (1994). Steiner and Stone (March 1999) believe that juvenile delinquency is a problem that presents a high probability of multiple pathologies, all requiring well-researched treatment approaches. The authors argue that without effective interventions, we will be unsuccessful in curtailing future relapses and continued violence throughout the life cycle.

Ellickson and McGuigan (April 2000) note that because early deviance and poor grades are useful predictors of later violence, violence intervention should begin as early as elementary school and should focus on issues of self-esteem, life choices, drug and alcohol abuse, and peer choices, all issues clinicians routinely deal with when treating children and adolescents. More significantly, Steiner and Stone (March 1999) write that:

> *Our understanding of how to help these children and adolescents is far from complete, and many more studies of interventions are necessary to advance science, clinical care, and public understanding. We need better tools to mitigate the human suffering of perpetrators and victims alike. Such a recommendation is not easily brought in line with the prevailing canons of the time, where we seek to prosecute children as adults and seek the death penalty for 10-year-olds. By involving our profession, which has a long and distinguished history of standing up for those who cannot do so for themselves (p. 234).*

Studer (1996) suggests that children with behavioral problems may benefit from learning anger management techniques, assertiveness training, problem-solving techniques, and conflict mediation.

1. **Anger management:** Anger management is a cognitive therapy approach in which children learn to identify situations that lead to angry responses, recognize their physical reaction to anger (clenched fists, sweaty palms, heightened heart rate), and learn

to rationally perceive their role in the situation so that the anger can dissipate or be dealt with appropriately.
2. **Assertiveness training:** A way to help the child learn to have his needs met without violating the rights or feelings of others. Baer (1976), in distinguishing aggression from assertiveness, notes that the purpose of aggression is to have needs met by violating the rights of others. Assertiveness is an approach used to help children have their needs met without disregarding the needs of others. Huey and Rank (1984) report that a class in assertiveness training was taught to disruptive 8th grade urban male students. The class met one hour a week for four weeks for a total of eight hours. The students in the class showed decreased aggressive behavior and increased assertiveness. Mathias (1992) supports the use of assertiveness training for elementary students and notes that assertiveness training programs get overwhelmingly positive evaluations.
3. **Problem-solving training:** This is a type of training that helps children learn to think their way through difficult social situations and to increase empathy and sensitivity for others. Rundie (as cited in Goldstein and Glick, 1987) notes that when 5th grade students were allowed to process actual life situations that affect most 5th graders (issues like cheating, stealing, using drugs, lying to parents), they did much better on group tasks than children who were not involved in problem-solving discussions.
4. **Conflict mediation:** This approach helps children learn to resolve conflicts with others by actually negotiating solutions. Schrumpt et al. (1991) outlined six basic steps in the mediation process: *Step 1*: Open the session by explaining the ground rules and describing the conflict. *Step 2*: Gather information. Each person is permitted time to tell his or her story without interruption. *Step 3*: Focus on common interests: The purpose of this step is to help the people in conflict identify common goals and to find out what each person views as a suitable resolution of the problem. *Step 4*: Create options. People in dispute are permitted to think the problem through, offer solutions, list possible options, and to provide a venue for joint problem resolution. *Step 5*: Evaluate options and choose a solution. People in conflict are encouraged to agree on the list of options that come from step 4. *Step 6*: Write an agreement and close the mediation session. A written agreement is presented which all parties sign, and which spells out the conditions of the conflict resolution and each party's responsibility to abide by the agreement. As a further aspect of solidifying the agreement, the parties are asked to shake hands. Lane and McWhirter (1992) report that mediation improves potentially troubled behavior, helps children improve their listening skills, and enhances the climate of the school.

Mental health professionals have implemented a wide variety of treatment approaches in an attempt to address one or more of the many psychosocial risk factors associated with youth violence. The approaches include cognitive-behavioral skills interventions with seriously aggressive or violent youth, cognitive restructuring techniques, role-plays, therapist modeling, and behavioral assignments. All of the preceding approaches attempt to reduce violent behavior by directly addressing psychosocial risk factors within individual youths (e.g., ineffective problem solving, deficits in moral development). Unfortunately, little to no significant impact on long-term recidivism (i.e., recurrence of violent offenses) has been demonstrated with these interventions (Sechrest, 2001).

Parent training models to help parents learn effective communication skills, conflict resolution, family problem solving, contracting, positive reinforcement, mild punishment and modeling, are effective in reducing child noncompliance and aggressive behavior among pre-school and elementary school-age children. These models attempt to reduce aggressive behavior by addressing the psychosocial risk factors that occur at the family level (e.g., poor parental monitoring and discipline practices, and coercive family interactions). However, only minimal improvements in family functioning occur in families of violent youth, and again, no significant reduction in recidivism rates have been demonstrated (Sechrest, 2001).

Overall, most mental health treatments have been most effective with younger, nonviolent, or mildly aggressive youths (Sechrest, 2001). However, they have been largely ineffective in reducing or preventing further violence with more serious or chronically violent offenders. As a result, many professionals and nonprofessionals are skeptical that the juvenile justice system and the mental health profession can rehabilitate violent youth. It has been argued that the approaches previously reviewed have not been successful for two main reasons. First, they have included interventions that focus on only one or two psychosocial risk factors associated with youth violence (e.g., individual cognition, family relations) and have failed to simultaneously address the many other factors (i.e., peer, school, neighborhood) that contribute to youth violence. Second, these interventions take place in only one location, such as a mental health clinic or juvenile incarceration facility, and fail to address the other influences on violent behavior such as home life, school, or neighborhood.

Sechrest (2001) notes that one notable advance in the treatment of violent juvenile behavior is multi-systemic therapy. MST is a departure from the more traditional approaches such as residential and inpatient treatment, detention and incarceration, and outpatient or clinic-based services. MST is offered in the juvenile's home, school, and neighborhood, and the interventions are flexibly tailored to the psychosocial needs of each client and his or her family. MST targets the family system (improving family emotional bonding and parental discipline strategies), the school (increasing parent–teacher communication and child academic performance), peers (promoting involvement in extracurricular activities, structured sports, or volunteer organizations), and community agencies (eliciting help from social service agencies).

In a thorough review of treatment research for conduct disordered children and adolescents, the Ontario Department of Mental Health (2001) notes that there is preference for social learning interventions including cognitive therapy and multiple interventions at home and in the child's environment with "enough frequency and long enough to produce the desired treatment outcomes" (p. 12). The report found little evidence that brief interventions or shock treatments, including boot camps or psychiatric hospitalization work. The report mentions the use of Problem-Solving Skills Training (PSST) developed by Spivak and Shure (1974, 1976, 1978) as one possible choice because it suppresses anti-social behavior while creating "structure in a child's life that provides the security to build positive relationships as therapy progresses" (p. 12). Kazdin (1995) found that PSST helps children manage cognitive deficiencies that may contribute to anti-social behavior by improving communication skills, problem-solving skills, impulse control, and anger management.

21.9. CHILDHOOD ONSET CONDUCT DISORDER: A CASE STUDY

This case first appeared in a book the author wrote on childhood violence (Glicken, 2004, pp. 27–29). The author wishes to thank Pearson Education, Inc. for permission to reprint that material.

Johnny is a 7-year-old child who has been acting out in his first grade class. He hits, kicks, pulls hair, bullies, and steals from the other children. The problem has been escalating over the past year. Johnny has been tested for hyperactivity, minimal organic brain damage, low intelligence, learning disorders, physical problems that might trigger violent reactions, and a battery of tests to rule out medical problems that might be consistent with highly aggressive behavior. All the tests have come back negative for any particular problem. Johnny's parents are mortified by his behavior. They have two older children who do very well in school and are considered model students. The parents report that Johnny showed signs of aggression very early in life. By age one, he was terrorizing their dog. They had to give their dog away to friends because John would not let it alone. At age three, Johnny walked across the street and killed the fish in a neighbor's tank. When caught emptying the tank on the floor, he calmly denied that he done anything. Johnny lies easily and by 5 years of age he was accomplished at covering up any aggressive and anti-social acts he committed. He has set two fires in the past year that the parents know about and was caught by his father trying to burn down a garden shed in the back of the house. Johnny tends to blame others for everything. He needs a great deal of attention. When it isn't forthcoming, he physically attacks his classmates and his teachers, all of whom are frightened of him. Enough parents have complained so that John has been taken out of school and is being seen in therapy for the first time.

The clinician gave Johnny a battery of psychological tests, including several projective tests developed for children. His conclusion was that if Johnny were an adult, he would have many of the diagnostic characteristics of a Personality Disorder, Anti-Social Type (301.7) (AMA, 1994, p. 649). Because of his age, the clinician was tempted to give Johnny a diagnosis of Oppositional Defiant Disorder (313.81) (APA, 1994, p. 93). This is a less severe diagnosis and involves loss of temper, arguing, and defiant and spiteful behavior. After eight hours of testing and interviewing, however, the clinician diagnosed Johnny with a Conduct Disorder, Childhood Onset Type (312.81) (APA, 1994, p. 86). The DSM–IV defines a Childhood Onset Type Conduct Disorder in children who have at least one characteristic of a conduct disorder before the age of 10. Children with Child Onset Conduct Disorders "... frequently display physical aggression toward others, have disturbed peer relationship, may have had oppositional defiant disorder during early childhood, and usually have symptoms that meet full criteria for Conduct Disorder before puberty. These individuals are more likely to have persistent Conduct Disorder and Adult Anti-social Personality Disorder than are those with Adolescent Onset Type Conduct Disorders" (APA, 1994, p. 86).

The DSM-IV goes on to say that a diagnosis of a Conduct Disorder can be given when persistent anti-social behavior exists over the prior 12 months in which the child has met three or more of the following criteria with at least one criterion present in the past 6 months:

1. **Aggression to people and animals:** (a) The child bullies, threatens and initiates fights; (b) has used a weapon; (c) is physically cruel to people and\or animals; (d) has stolen while confronting others; and (e) has forced someone into sexual activity.
2. **Destruction of property:** The child deliberately sets fires and/or deliberately destroys property.
3. **Deceitfulness or theft:** The child has broken into someone else's property, lies or cons others, and/or is involved in shoplifting.
4. **Serious violation of rules:** (a) The child often stays out at night without parental permission before age 13; (b) has run away at least twice, and; (c) is often truant before the age of 13 (APA, 1994, p. 90).

The clinician believes that Johnny has almost all of the characteristics of a Childhood Onset Type Conduct Disorder and believes that the problem is "severe" in nature. In a severe form of a childhood Conduct Disorder, "[m]any conduct problems [exist] in excess of those required to make the diagnosis *or* the conduct problems cause considerable harm to others" (APA, 1994, p. 91). The clinician believes that Johnny is developing highly dangerous behaviors that will very likely cycle on through childhood, into adolescence, and on to adulthood. In males under 18, the diagnosis of Conduct Disorder appears to be increasingly used and rates of Conduct Disorder for males under 18 are estimated at 6–16%, while rates for females are estimated as 2–9% (APA, 1994, p. 88). Murray and Myers (1998) describe Conduct Disorders as chronic, severe antisocial behaviors that typically begin in early childhood and extend into adulthood. The authors believe that symptoms of a Conduct Disorder are consistently present at home, at school, with peers, and in the community. However, the invisible children who make up a cohort of those who commit school violence (Shubert et al., 1999) may not exhibit these exact behavioral problems and are often diagnosed as severely depressed or emotionally labile.

In describing Johnny, the clinician went on to note that, "Johnny is a robust and severely Conduct Disordered child. He acts out whenever he feels like it, has no sense of right or wrong, is driven by impulses, doesn't respect authority, is manipulative, and is able to get his way much of the time. When he doesn't get his way, he uses high levels of violent aggression with children, adolescents, and adults. Most people are frightened by his naked aggression and see in Johnny a very dangerous child capable of doing great harm. Just as there are people who are born with birth defects, mental retardation, and other infirmities, Johnny seems to have been aggressive and impulse-driven from an early age. There is nothing to suggest parental neglect or abuse. The parents are appalled by his behavior, unable to control it, and believe that Johnny needs very intensive professional help. For these reasons, I am recommending that Johnny be placed in a facility for young emotionally disturbed children. There have been some very positive results from early residential placements for children with severe Childhood Onset Conduct Disorders. Perhaps placing him as early as age seven will have a positive preventative impact."

21.10. DISCUSSION

The diagnosis of a Conduct Disorder so early in a child's life may be seen by some as overly harsh, pejorative, and even leading to a life-long label, implying that Johnny will be a dangerous person throughout his life. Clinicians sometimes use a diagnosis that is more severe than might be called for by the child's behavior to get needed help for the child before the symptoms worsen and the child does something violent leading to severe harm to others. In Johnny's case, the diagnosis seems correct. Johnny needs residential help. He needs to live in an environment where he can learn restraint, impulse control, right from wrong, and the other developmental behaviors he should have mastered at an earlier age, but has not. While it is true that almost half of the children with early onset behavioral problems move into more aggressive behavior during adolescence and adulthood, treatment is certainly worth a try. More than a few early onset behaviorally troubled children like Johnny have reduced or even eliminated their aggressive, anti-social behavior as a result of positive intervention. In Johnny's case, he was transferred to a private facility that deals exclusively with children very much like Johnny. It is a highly regimented facility with strict rules and a token economy. The better children do in obeying the rules of the facility and in their individual and group therapy, schoolwork, and personal conduct, the more benefits and privileges they receive. Johnny, as it turns out, likes the military structure of the facility. He likes knowing what is acceptable and unacceptable. He appreciates it when people know he is lying and trying to con them and when they confront him with his behavior. It is an exhilarating experience to be around others who know more about him than he does. The staff is highly professional and fair. If there are disagreements among the residents, the problem is worked out quickly, equitably, and in Johnny's view, in a way that allows everyone to save face. Johnny is thriving in the facility. His initial score on an IQ test in the low normal range has been replaced by a score in the high normal range. He was not trying on the initial test. His social behavior has improved and he has begun to think about becoming a soldier. The transformation in his behavior is startling. He sees his family often and has gone home on vacations without incident.

Johnny was re-evaluated by a clinician a year after being sent to the private facility. The clinician wrote: "Johnny is still an impulse-driven, amoral, and potentially dangerous child. The initial diagnosis was correct. The benefit of the early intervention has been to provide external controls that are fair and reasonable and that act to inhibit his more anti-social impulses. With children like Johnny who enjoy the paramilitary structure of the facility and the tightly enforced rules, they do well as long as the facility stays within their narrow definition of what they consider a healthy environment. As staff change or as the child matures, age and maturation might find the child influenced by other more powerful role models among the residents. When this happens, children like Johnny who have such good initial gain, often take a turn for the worse. A number of our residents have become participants in hate groups that utilize paramilitary organizational structures. Others have entered gang life that is, in a way, a paramilitary structure. We always hope that children like Johnny will develop a moral compass because of the treatment they receive, but robust and severe childhood onset Conduct Disorders have a poor track record and tend to cycle on to other more serious offenses once they leave the facility. Johnny will need long-term outpatient help when he returns home."

Johnny is 12 now and lives at home. He is a mediocre but compliant student who has begun entering chat rooms with adolescents who have strong feelings of hatred for certain ethnic, religious, and racial groups. Johnny believes that if these groups were eliminated, that the world would be a "cleaner" place. He has begun attending meetings of a domestic hate group organized along paramilitary lines and is learning military discipline. He has promised the group leader to stay out of trouble at school so he can help the group when it begins to rid the world of Blacks, Jews, immigrants with dark skin, and Arabs. Johnny is also developing strong fantasies of raping young girls and finds others among his peers in the hate group with similar fantasies. John thinks he has finally come home and is happy now. He thinks his special skills will be useful and that he will make a contribution to the world, something his parents preach to him everyday.

21.11. SUMMARY

Once again we caution the reader to remember that the early signs of violence in children noted in this chapter are overall signs to consider in evaluating children. They are to be used to diagnose and treat and not to label or predict long-term problems with violence. Changes in the child's life, as we will note throughout this book, can bring with it some startling changes in the child's potential for violence. The chapter noted a strong relationship between early life child abuse and violence. Further, violent children may show potential for violence through bullying, fire setting, cruelty to animals, school misconduct and poor performance, and compulsive attraction to mass media violence.

21.12. QUESTIONS FROM THE CHAPTER

1. The question of early diagnosis of violent behavior is fraught with moral issues. If we label too early and if the label is incorrect, children may be stigmatized for life. Can you think of alternatives to using DSM-IV labels with children?

2. There appears to be a fairly strong relationship between child abuse and neglect and early onset childhood violence. Should not we be putting our energies into reducing the amount of child abuse and neglect rather than punishing young children for the acts of their parents?
3. Older adolescents commit most violent behavior. Do you accept the labels noted in this chapter of early and late violence starters and the belief that late violence starters are ultimately less dangerous over the life span?
4. What might be some reasons why many fire starters are very young children?
5. The idea that a very small number of violent children do most of the violent crime throughout the life cycle suggests that we focus on that cohort of young children by preventing their violent behavior through early and perhaps long term incarceration. Do you agree?

References

American Psychiatric Association. (1994). *Diagnostic and statistical manual of mental disorders* (4th ed.). Washington, DC: APA.

Baer, J. (1976). *How to be an assertive (not aggressive) woman in life, in love, and on the job: A total guide to self-assertiveness.* New York: New American Library.

Behavioral Neurotherapy Clinic. (2007). *Disruptive behaviour disorders.* http://www.adhd.com.au/conduct.html.

Bilchik, S. (1999). Minorities in the juvenile justice system. *1999 National Report Series.* Washington, DC: Office of Juvenile Justice and Delinquency Prevention. U.S. Department of Justice.

Briscoe, J. (1997). Breaking the cycle of violence: A rational approach to at-risk youth. *Federal Probation, 61*, 3–13.

Butts, J. A. (1994). *Offenders in juvenile court,* 1992. Juvenile Justice Bulletin, OJJDP Update on Statistics.

Carey, B. (2007, November 13). Bad behavior does not doom pupils. NYTIMES.COM. http://www.nytimes.com/2007/11/13/health/13kids.html?th&emc=th.

Catalano, R. F., & Hawkins, J. D. (1996). The social development model: A theory of antisocial behavior. In J. D. & Hawkins (Ed.), *Delinquency and crime: current theories* (pp. 149–197). New York: Cambridge University Press.

Dwyer, K. P., Osher, D., & Warger, W. (1998). *Early warning, timely response: A guide to safe schools.* Washington, DC: U.S. Department of Education, (ERIC Document Reproduction Service No. ED 418 372).

Ellickson, P. L., & McGuigan, K. A. (2000). Early predictors of adolescent violent. *American Journal of Public Health, 90*(4), 566–572.

Elliott, D. S. (1994). Serious violent offenders: onset, developmental course, and termination: The American Society of Criminology 1993 Presidential Address. *Criminology,* 32, 1–21.

Elliott, D. S., Hamburg, B., & Williams, K. R. (1998). *Violence in American schools: A new perspective.* Boulder, Colo: Center for the Study and Prevention of Violence.

Fagan, J. (1996). *Recent perspectives on youth violence.* Paper presented at the Northwest Conference on Youth Violence, Seattle, Wash.

Glicken, M. D. (2004). *Violent young children.* Boston, MA: Pearson Education, Inc..

Goldstein, A. P., & Glick, B. (1987). *Aggression replacement training: A comprehensive intervention for aggressive youth.* Champaign, IL: Research Press.

Hawkins, D., & Catalano, R. (1992). *Communities that care*. San Francisco: Jossey-Bass.

Herrenkohl, T., Huang, I., Kosterman, B., Hawkins, R., David, J., et al. (2001, February). A comparison of social development processes leading to violent behavior in late adolescence for childhood initiators and adolescent initiators of violence. *Journal of Research in Crime & Delinquency, 38*(1), 45–63.

Horowitz, M. A. (2000, Summer). Kids who kill: A critique of how the American legal system deals with juveniles who commit homicide. *Law and Contemporary Problems, 63*(3), 133–177.

Huey, W. C., & Rank, R. C. (1984). Effects of counselor and peer-led groups' assertive training on Black adolescent aggression. *Journal of Counseling Psychology, 31*, 95–98.

Kauffman, J. M. (1997). *Characteristics of emotional and behavioral disorders of children and youth* (6th ed.). Upper Saddle River, NJ: Merrill.

Kazdin, A. E. (1995). *Conduct disorder in childhood and adolescence* (2nd ed.). Thousand Oaks, CA: Sage.

Lane, P. S., & McWhirter, J. J. (1992). A peer mediation model: Conflict resolution for elementary and middle school children. *Elementary School Guidance & Counseling, 27*, 15–21.

Lester, D., & Yang, B. (1998). *Suicide and homicide in the 20th century: Changes over time*. Thousand Oaks, CA: Nova Science Publishers.

Loeber, R. (1991). Antisocial behaviour: More enduring than changeable?. *Journal of the American Academy of Child and Adolescent Psychiatry, 30*, 303–397.

Loeber, R., & Farrington, D. P. (1998). *Serious and violent juvenile offenders: Risk factors and successful interventions*. Thousand Oaks, CA: Sage.

Lynam, D. (1996). Early identification of chronic offenders: Who is the fledgling psychopath?. *Psychological Bulletin, 120*, 209–234.

Mandel, M. J., & Magnusson, P. (1993, December 13). The economics of crime. *Business Week*, 72–80.

Mathias, C. E. (1992). Touching the lives of children: Consultative interventions that work. *Elementary School Guidance & Counseling*, 26, 190–201.

Mayer, G. R. (1995). Preventing antisocial behavior in the schools. *Journal of Applied Behavior Analysis, 28*, 467–478.

McCord, J. (1999). Family relationships, juvenile delinquency, and adult criminality. In F. R. Scarpitti, A. L. & Nielson (Eds.), *Crime and Criminals: Contemporary and Classic Readings* (pp. 167–176). Los Angeles: Roxbury.

Moffitt, T. E. (1994). Adolescence-limited and life-course persistent antisocial behavior: A developmental taxonomy. *Psychological Review, 100*, 674–701.

Morales, A. (1982). The Mexican American gang member: evaluation and treatment. In R. Becerra, M. Karno, & J. Escolar, (Eds.) *Mental health and Hispanic Americans: A clinical perspective*. New York: Grune and Stratton, 140–176.

Murray, B. A., & Myers, M. A. (1998). Conduct disorders and the special-education trap. *The Education Digest, 63*(8), 48–53.

Myles, B. S., & Simpson, R. L. (1998). Aggression and violence by school-age children and youth: Understanding the aggression cycle and prevention/intervention strategies. *Intervention in School and Clinic, 33*(5), 259–264.

Obiakor, F. E., Merhing, T. A., & Schwenn, J. O. (1997). *Disruption, disaster, and death: Helping students deal with crises*. Reston, VA: The Council for Exceptional Children, (ERIC Document Reproduction Service No. ED 403 709).

Ontario Department of Mental Health. (2001) Children and Adolescents with Conduct Disorder: Findings from the Literature and Clinical Consultation in Ontario http://www.kidsmentalhealth.ca/documents/EBP_conduct_disorder_findings.pdf. (Author).

Osofsky, H. J., & Osofsky, J. D. (2001, Winter). Violent and aggressive behaviors in youth: A mental health and prevention perspective. *Psychiatry, 64*(4), 285–295.

Patterson, G., & Narrett, C. (1990). The development of a reliable and valid treatment program for aggressive young children. *International Journal of Mental Health, 19*, 19–26.

Patterson, G. R., Reid, J. B., & Dishion, T. J. (1992). *A social interactional approach: Antisocial boys*. Eugene, OR: Castalia Press.

Pellegrini, R. J., Roundtree, T., Camagna, T. F., & Queirolo, S. S. (2000). On the epidemiology of violent juvenile crime in America: A total arrest-referenced approach. *Psychological Reports, 86*(3), 1171–1186.

Phelps, L., & McClintock, K. (1994, February). Conduct Disorder. *Journal of Psychopathology and Behavioural Assesment, 16*(1), 53–66.

Puzzanchera, C. (2000, February). *Self-reported delinquency by 12-year-olds, 1997*. Washington, DC: Office of Juvenile Justice and Delinquency Prevention. U.S. Department of Justice.

Rae-Grant, N., McConville, B. J., & Fleck, S. (1999). Violent behavior in children and youth: Preventative intervention from a psychiatric perspective. *Journal of the American Academy of Child and Adolescent Psychiatry, 38*(3), 235–241.

Reid, J. (1993). Prevention of conduct disorders before and after school entry: Relating interventions to developmental findings. *Development and psychopathology, 5*(1/2), 243–262.

Richman, N., Stevenson, L., & Graham, P. J. (1982). *Pre-school to school: A behavioural study*. London: Academic Press.

Rosenberg, M. L., & Fenley, M. A. (1991). *Violence in America: A public health approach*. New York: Oxford University Press.

Rosenberg, M. L., O'Carroll, P., & Powell, K. (1992). Let's be clear: Violence is a public health problem. *Journal of the American Medical Association, 267*, 3071–3072.

Schrumpt, F., Crawford, D., & Usadel, H. C. (1991). *Peer mediation: Conflict resolution in schools*. Champaign, IL: Research.

Sechrest, D. (2001). *Juvenile crime: A predictive study*. Unpublished document.

Shubert, T. H., Bressette, S., Deeken, J., & Bender, W. N. (1999). Analysis of random school shootings. In W. N. Bender, G. Clinton, R. L. & Bender (Eds.), *Violence prevention and reduction in schools* (pp. 97–101). Austin, TX: PROED.

Skiba, R. J., Peterson, R. L., & Williams, T. (1997). Office referrals and suspensions: Disciplinary intervention in middle schools. *Education and Treatment of Children, 20*, 295–315.

Snyder, H. N., & Sickmund, M. (1999). *Juvenile offenders and victims: 1999 national report*. Washington, DC: Office of Juvenile Justice and Delinquency Prevention. U.S. Department US Department of Justice, Office of Juvenile Justice and Delinquency Prevention.

Spivak, G., & Shure, M. B. (1974). *Social adjustment of young children: A cognitive approach to solving real-life problems*. San Francisco, CA: Jossey-Bass.

Spivak, G., & Shure, M. B. (1976). *The problem-solving approach to adjustment*. San Francisco, CA: Jossey-Bass.

Spivak, G., & Shure, M. B. (1978). *Problem-solving techniques in child-rearing.* San Francisco, CA: Jossey-Bass.

Sprague, J. R., & Hill, W. M. (2000, Spring). Early identification and interventions for youth with antisocial and violent behavior. *Exceptional Children, 66,* 367–379.

Sprague, J. R., & Walker, H. M. (2000, Spring). Early identification and intervention for youth with antisocial and violent behavior. *Exceptional Children, 66*(3), 367–379.

Steiner, H., & Stone, L. A. (1999). Introduction: Violence and related psychopathology. *Journal of the American Academy of Child and Adolescent Psychiatry, 38*(3), 232–234.

Studer, J. (1996, February). Understanding and preventing aggressive responses in youth. *Elementary School Guidance and Counseling, Private Practice, 30,* 194–203.

Thornberry, T. P., Huizinga, D., & Loeber, R. (1995). The prevention of serious delinquency and violence: Implications from the program of research on the causes and correlates of delinquency. In J. C. Howell, B. Krisberg, J. D. Hawkins, J. J. & Wilson (Eds.), *A sourcebook: Serious, violent, and chronic juvenile offenders* (pp. 213–237). Thousand Oaks, CA: Sage.

Thornberry, T. P., Smith, C. A., Rivera, C., Huizina, D., & Stouthamer-Loeber, M. (1999, September). *Family disruption and delinquency.* Washington, DC: Office of Juvenile Justice and Delinquency Prevention. U.S. Department of Justice.

Walker, H. M., Colvin, G., & Ramsey, E. (1995). *Antisocial behavior in school: Strategies and best practices.* Pacific Grove, CA: Brooks/Cole.

Wagner, L., & Lane, L. (1998). *Juvenile justice services: 1997 report.* Eugene, OR: Lane County Department of Youth Services.

Walker, H. M., & Severson, H. H. (1990). *Systematic screening for behavior disorders.* Longmont, CO: Sopris West.

Webmd. (2005, July) Oppositional Defiant Disorder. http://www.webmd.com/content/article/60/67118.htm?printing=true.

Webster-Stratton, C., & Dahl, R. W. (1995). Conduct disorder. In M. Hersen, R. T. & Ammerman (Eds.), *Advanced abnormal child psychology* (pp. 333–352). Hillsdale, New Jersey: Lawrence Erlbaum Associates.

Widom, C. S. (1999). The cycle of violence. In F. R. Scarpitti, A. L. & Nielson (Eds.), *Crime and criminals: Contemporary and classic readings* (pp. 332–334). Los Angeles: Roxbury.

Wolfgang, M. E. (1972). *Delinquency in a birth cohort.* Chicago: University of Chicago Press.

Wolfgang, M. E. (1987). *From boy to man, from delinquency to crime.* Chicago: University of Chicago Press.

Part Five
Evidence-Based Practice and Alternative Approaches to Helping

22 Evidence-Based Practice and the Effectiveness of Indigenous Helpers, Mentors, and Self-Help Groups with Children and Adolescent Health and Mental Health Problems

22.1. INTRODUCTION

The author wishes to thank Pearson Education, Inc. for permission to use some of the material written about self-help found in a book the author wrote on the strengths perspective (Glicken, 2004, pp. 90–102).

This chapter discusses the potential of self-help groups and mentoring in the treatment of health and mental health problems in children and adolescents. Because there is such passion for self-help groups and mentoring in the absence of supportive data, this chapter considers the available research data on the treatment effectiveness and the reasons self-help and mentoring have become so popular in America. Clearly one reason is the financial condition of the health care industry. According to Humphreys (1998):

> *Professional substance abuse treatment in the United States grew extensively through the 1970s and 1980s... In recent years, however, the professional treatment network has contracted due to the arrival of managed health care.... But there is a potential bright spot in the current gloomy addiction care picture – the possibility that self-help/mutual aid organizations can help substance abusers recover, while at the same time lowering demand for scarce formal health care resources. (Humphreys, 1998, p. 13)*

In another article urging cooperation between self-help groups and the professional community, Humphreys and Ribisl (1999) ask, "Why should public health and medical professionals be interested in collaborating with a grassroots movement of untrained citizens?" (p. 326). Their answer is that money for health care is being reduced and that "self-help groups can provide benefits that the best health care often does not: identification with other sufferers, long-term support and companionship, and a sense of competence and empowerment" (p. 326).

However, Kessler et al. (1997a) caution that self-help groups will "never be a substitute for professional care. Such groups should not be looked to as a cheap and quick fix to the health care crisis" (p. 27).

22.2. SELF-HELP GROUPS

In defining self-help groups, Wituk et al. (2000) write that "[s]elf-help groups consist of individuals who share the same problem or concern. Members provide emotional support to one another, learn ways to cope, discover strategies for improving their condition, and help others while helping themselves" (p. 157). Kessler et al. (1997a, 1997b) estimate that 25 million Americans have been involved in self-help groups at some point during their lives. Positive outcomes have been found in self-help groups treating substance abuse (Humphreys and Moos, 1996), bereavement (Caserta and Lund, 1993), care giving (McCallion and Toseland, 1995), diabetes (Gilden et al., 1992), and depression (Kurtz, 1988). Riessman (2000) reports that "[m]ore Americans try to change their health behaviors through self-help than through all other forms of professional programs combined" (p. 47).

Kessler et al. (1997b) indicate that 40% of all therapeutic sessions for psychiatric problems reported by respondents in a national survey were in the self-help sector as compared to 35.2% receiving specialized mental health services, 8.1% receiving help from the general physicians medical sector, and 16.5% receiving help from social service agencies. Wuthnow (1994) found that self-help groups are the most prevalent organized support groups in America today. The author estimated that 8–10 million Americans are members of self-help groups and that there are at least 500 000 self-help groups in America.

Fetto (2000) reports a study done by the University of Texas at Austin which found that approximately 25 million people will participate in self-help groups at some point in their lives, and that 8–11 million people participate in self-help groups each year. Men are somewhat more likely to attend groups than women and Caucasians are three times as likely to attend self-help groups as African-Americans. This number is expected to be much higher with the full use of the Internet as a tool for self-help. Participants most likely to attend self-help groups are those diagnosed with alcoholism, cancer (all types), diabetes, AIDS, depression, and chronic fatigue syndrome. Those least likely to attend suffer from ulcers, emphysema, chronic pain, and migraines, in that order (Fetto, 2000).

Riessman (1997) identifies the principles defining the function and purpose of self-help groups as follows: (1) members share a similar condition and understand each other; (2) members determine activities and policies which make self-help groups very democratic and self-determining; (3) helping others is therapeutic; (4) self-help groups build on the strengths of the individual members, the group, and the community, charge no fees, and are not commercialized; (5) self-help groups function as social support systems which help participants cope with traumas through supportive relationships between members; (6) values are projected which define the intrinsic meaning of the group to its members; (7) self-help groups use the expertise of members to help one another; (8) seeking assistance from a self-help group is not as stigmatizing as it may be when seeking help from a health or mental health provider; and (9) self-help groups focus on the use of self-determination, inner strength, self-healing, and resilience.

Wituk et al. (2000), studied the characteristics of self-help groups in a specific geographic area and report the following: (1) groups had been in existence an average of 8 years; (2) thirty percent of the groups studied met weekly with an average attendance of 13 participants; (3) twenty new members joined the group in the prior year; (4) sixty-eight percent of the participants were female; (5) minority participation was proportionately in keeping with the minority population of the regions studies; (6) group outreach was usually done by word of mouth, but some groups used newspaper ads and radio and television spot ads; (7) thirty-four percent of the groups were peer-led with some professional involvement. Professionals led groups 28% of the time. Twenty-seven percent of the groups had no professional involvement, while 86% of the groups had two or more members acting in leadership capacities; (8) the primary function of the groups was to provide emotional and social support to members (in 98% of the groups reporting), while 32% of the groups provided information and education, and 58% provided advocacy services for members and their families; (9) seventy-seven percent of the groups felt that networking with the larger community was important and accomplished this through guest speakers, buddy systems, training seminars open to the public, and social events open to the community; (10) a large majority of the groups held meetings in very easily accessible places; (11) many of the groups offered childcare during meetings, transportation, and bi-lingual meetings for non-English speaking participants; (12) over half the groups had national affiliations and reported receiving a great deal of help from these organizations through brochures, newsletters, conferences and workshops, but very little help with finances or information about advances in research; (13) seventy-five percent of the groups had local affiliations with hospitals, churches, and social service agencies; and (14) the self-help groups were all very well connected to the professional community.

In summary, self-help groups for children and adolescents are comprised of youth who share similar problems, life situations or crises. Members provide emotional support to one another, learn new ways to cope, discover strategies for improving their condition, and help others while helping themselves. In self-help groups people find individuals much like themselves who are able to share pragmatic, experience-tested insights gained from first-hand experience with the same situation. Self-help groups are generally self-governed, cost-free and readily available for major health and emotional problems, physical disabilities, eating disorders, habits or addictions, bereavement, academic difficulties and for issues pertaining to family functioning. Self-help groups often create genuine community support systems which enhance and supplement existing health and mental health care systems for children and adolescents.

22.3. INDIGENOUS HELPERS

Patterson and Marsiglia (2000) report remarkable similarities in the characteristics of two cohorts of natural (or indigenous) helpers from two very different geographic locations in the United States. Those similarities include offering assistance to family and friends before it was asked for, an attempt to reduce stress in those helped, and a desire to help people strengthen their coping skills. Lewis and Suarez (1995) identify the primary functions of indigenous helpers as buffers between individuals and sources of stress, providers of social support, information, and referral sources and lay consultants. Waller and Patterson (2002) believe that indigenous helpers strengthen the social bond-holding communities which increase the well-being of individuals and communities.

Patterson et al. (1972) found that natural helpers used one of three helping styles: (1) active listening, encouragement, emphasizing positives about the client, and suggesting alternative solutions to problems; (2) direct intervention by doing something active for the client which had an immediate impact; and (3) a combination of (1) and (2) in a way which fits the client's needs. However, Memmott (1993) found little difference between natural helpers and professionals, although natural helpers were more inclined to advocate and intervene on behalf clients than professionals, tended to think much less about causal reasons for a client's problems than professionals, and used direct methods of help which were atheoretical but often sound.

Bly (1986) suggests that we seek out others in the community for advice and support. He calls these natural helpers "People of Wisdom" because they listen well, are empathic and sensitive, and are known for their expertise in solving certain types of problems. We gravitate to these people because they help us in unobtrusive and informal ways which are often profoundly subtle, since the lack of formal training by natural helpers is offset by their kindness, patience, common sense, and good judgment.

22.4. EVIDENCE OF THE EFFECTIVENESS OF SELF-HELP GROUPS WITH CHILDREN AND ADOLESCENTS

Recognizing the methodological limitations of research effectiveness reports on self-help groups is important for the reader to understand because self-help groups are not under the same obligation to test for effectiveness as their professional counterparts. For that reason alone, there are a number of explanations for methodological limitations in determining best evidence of the effectiveness of non-professionally led self-help groups, including the following: (1) self-help groups pride themselves on confidentiality and sometimes discourage research because it can be intrusive; (2) most self-help groups do not think of themselves as competing with professional helpers. Trying to prove their effectiveness is not seen as part of their mission; (3) there is no real way to force people to accept research responsibilities when services are led by volunteers, are free to the public, and make no claims to be alternatives to professional help; (4) the research process sets up barriers to the functioning of self-help groups and may subtly or overtly change the way a group operates; (5) many people attend self-help groups to avoid the way professional treatment sometimes compromises individuality. Adding a research component may make people feel as if they have lost their uniqueness; (6) self-help groups are loosely organized and run. People come and go as they please. It is difficult to make research effective in an atmosphere in which the experimental group has only a very loose attendance pattern; and (7) as Kessler et al. (1997a) report, more than half of the people attending self-help groups also receive professional help, making it difficult to determine whether self-help causes improvement, the professional help, or a combination of both.

The following discussion summarizes studies found in the literature on self-help groups with children and families. The literature is not large, and of 500 self-help articles consulted, only a few were found on self-help groups with children and adolescents. Also, most of the authors cautioned that methodologies were weak and that the reader should not take the few studies reported as an objective indication of the effectiveness of self-help with youth. With that in mind, here are a few outcome studies of self-help groups with children and adolescents.

Anderson et al. (1989) found that young diabetics who learn self-care techniques and participate in member-run support groups after 2 years were less depressed, less stressed, gained more knowledge about their diabetes, and rated the quality of their lives higher than those who were not involved in a self-help group. Anderson also found that group leaders do not need to be experienced to be effective leaders. Hughes (1977) found that children of parents with drinking problems who participated in Alateen, a self-help group sponsored by Alcoholics Anonymous, suffered less emotional and social disturbance than peers who did not belong.

Potasznik and Nelson (1984) found that participating in a self-help group for families of psychiatric patients reduced the family's sense of burden. Members found the group helpful because it provided them with information about schizophrenia and coping strategies, which professionals didn't provide. Participation also helped parents to develop supportive social bonds with others who were experiencing similar problems. Becu et al. (1993) reported on a 4-month longitudinal study of 67 epileptic patients, a fourth of whom were youth, who participated in weekly self-help group meetings. Epileptic patients trained by psychologists led the groups. Group participants had decreased depression and other psychological problems over the course of the study.

Nash and Kramer (1993) studied 57 young African-Americans who had been members of self-help groups for sickle-cell anemia. The members who had been involved the longest reported the fewest psychological symptoms and the fewest psychosocial interferences from the disease, particularly in work, school, and relationship areas. Sibthorpe and Fleming (1994) studied young injection drug users ($N = 234$) who had shared a dirty needle in the previous 30 days and were followed over 6 months. Those who attended self-help groups (mostly Narcotics

Anonymous and Alcoholics Anonymous) during that time were almost twice as likely to report reducing or eliminating their risk of exposure to HIV compared to those who did not attend such groups.

Goh et al. (2007) found support groups composed of children with disfiguring dermatological processes to be helpful in increasing self-esteem and in providing family understanding and support of the child's disease. Barak and Dolev-Cohen (2006) found that active involvement in an online support group by adolescents experiencing distressing emotional problems as indicated by the number of messages posted and responses to those messages resulted in lower levels of distress, and write:

> *[T]here are people who find the group to be a relieving vehicle, indeed: these are the people who take an active part in them (writing messages and receiving replies). The main implication of this finding is that appropriate instructions should be delivered to participants in order to encourage their active involvement in the group, which will consequently promote their emotional relief. Likewise, online support-group facilitators should be instructed and trained accordingly and, they should also play a major role in encouraging participants' active involvement. (p. 188)*

Dadich (2006) interviewed 28 adolescent males who had experienced a mental health issue. The author indicated that self-help support groups offered participants emotional and practical support, information on mental health matters, the opportunity to relate to the mental health experiences of others, inspiration and hope, strong social networks, and a reminder of the importance of self-care in the management of mental health issues. Dadich adds, "Reflecting on the benefits of group participation, the research participants said that the groups provided a strong sense of support. They spoke of feeling nurtured and comforted by a collective of individuals who shared a similar experience" (p. 38).

Weidle et al. (2006) studied three self-help groups for youth diagnosed with Asperger's syndrome and found the great majority of the participants completed the course of the group. In a consumer satisfaction survey, 76.5% of the group members and nearly all of their parents (95%) rated satisfaction with the group meetings as good or very good. Of the participating adolescents, 86% completed the group sessions, with an attendance rate of 93%. Feedback from adolescents and parents was very positive.

22.5. MENTORING

The objective of mentoring programs is to provide individual or group interventions in the lives of children and adolescents at risk for the purpose of improving protective factors that might lead to improved social functioning. Larose and Tarabulsy (2005) describe a socio-motivational mentoring program in which the mentor can use the time together with a child to help regulate negative emotions, intervene in negative environments, mobilize social supports, encourage autonomy and independent thinking and affirm the uniqueness of the mentored child. In many ways mentoring is the provision of a substitute parent to offer support, advice and modeling to help children develop positive ties to the community and enhance self-righting skills. Several studies regarding the effectiveness of mentoring at-risk children are provided here. It should be noted, however, that in evaluating the research to date on a number of mentoring programs, Britner et al. (2006) caution that too little well-constructed research has been done on the impact of mentoring in at-risk children to make judgments other than anecdotal ones on the effectiveness of mentoring. While mentoring appears to help, it awaits more thorough evaluation.

Regarding the strength of the matches between a mentor and a child, Britner and Kraimer-Rickaby (2005) found that matches which ended prematurely were marked by poor or inconsistent contact and by mentors who did not "feel a connection" to the child. Intact matches included consistent and stable contact, and mentors and children who enjoyed each other's company. Children who had experienced maltreatment or foster care were more likely to be disrupted within a month than matches with children who had not experienced abuse (Rhodes, 2002). Grossman and Rhodes (2002) studied 487 mentored youth and 472 control youth in an urban Big Brothers/Big Sisters program at baseline and at an 18-month follow-up. Youth who had experienced emotional, sexual, or physical abuse were more likely than other youth to have had their mentor relationship end. However, using the same dataset, Rhodes et al. (1999) studied 90 mentored foster youth (78 in relative care, 12 in non-relative care) in comparison to control foster youth. Over a period of 18 months, mentored foster youth reported significant improvements in prosocial support and self-esteem, whereas those without mentors reported declines.

McCord (1992) reports that the Cambridge–Somerville Youth Study (CSYS) recruited boys younger than 12 years old from a low-income, high-crime area. Boys were matched on age, family environment, and delinquency-prone histories and then randomized to either an untreated control or an experimental condition. In the experimental condition, "a social worker... tried to build a close personal relationship with the boy and assist both the boy and his family in a number of ways" (McCord, 1992, p. 198). At the program's end, boys in the experimental condition had been visited, on average, two times a month for 5.5 years. When the men were about 47 years old, three objectively-defined adverse outcomes were measured: conviction of a Federal Bureau of Investigation (FBI) index crime, death before age 35, and an alcoholic, schizophrenic, or manic-depressive diagnosis. The experimental group fared significantly worse than the untreated control group on all outcomes. No added benefit resulted from more frequent help, longer duration of help, or better rapport.

Rhodes et al. (2000) studied academic mentoring through the Big Brothers/Big Sisters Program and found grade improvements and reductions in truancies. Larose and Tarabulsy (2005) found that mentoring of new high-risk college-age students resulted in improved relationships with teachers, better social adjustment and improved feelings of attachment to school. Blinn-Pike et al. (1998)

studied mentoring of 100 pregnant and parenting youth over a 3-year period and found that at 1-year postpartum, (1) the mentored group fared more positively on a measure of child abuse potential, (2) had taken their infants to the hospital less frequently, (3) breast-fed longer, and (4) felt less depressed and socially isolated than the non-mentored group.

Powers et al. (1995) studied the effects of mentoring on self-efficacy and community-based knowledge of adolescents with severe physical disabilities. The youth who had mentors had more knowledge of strategies for overcoming barriers to independence, and their parents had more knowledge about how to promote the independence and the abilities of their children than those without mentors. Watkins et al. (1998) developed a program with deaf mentors to help deaf children and their families improve their communication skills and increase the parent's understanding and appreciation of deaf culture. The results suggested that the experimental group made quicker and stronger gains in communication skills.

In determining where mentoring should take place, however, DuBois et al. (2002) found that the impact of mentoring programs held within the school structure was substantially lower than programs set up within the community, suggesting perhaps that each setting must develop its own unique approach to mentoring at-risk children.

22.6. Q AND A WITH THE AUTHOR ABOUT THE MEANING OF THESE STUDIES

The following mock question-and-answer exercise is offered to help the reader better understand the benefits, limitations, meaning, and practical use of reported findings on the efficacy of self-help groups.

Question (Q): Do these studies prove anything?

Answer (A): Probably not. What they *do* show is that people in self-help, mentoring situations and support groups report better functioning and a higher level of life satisfaction. Whether that's the case remains to be seen. Self-reports are notoriously susceptible to social desirability. People say positive things about self-help groups when there may be no empirical evidence that change in social functioning has actually taken place. The Halo Effect is also likely to influence responses. People in any type of treatment often report better results than may be the case because, in the short run, they may actually feel better and because, in the case of self-help groups, they may feel a sense of loyalty to the group which encourages them to report better social functioning than may be the case. Whether better functioning has actually occurred in the studies cited in this chapter requires evidence that only an empirical study can provide. *Saying* that you feel better is not the same as actually *being* better when social functioning is considered. Methodological problems are considerable in the measurement of self-help group effectiveness. Ouimette et al. (1997) compared 12-step programs such as AA with cognitive-behavioral programs and programs which combined both approaches. One year after completion of treatment, all three types of programs had similar improvements rates when alcohol consumption was measured. Participants in the 12-step program had more "sustained abstinence" and better employment rates than the other two programs, but Ouimette et al. (1997) cautioned the reader not to make more of these findings than were warranted because of non-random assignment of patients to the different types of treatment. A careful look at many other substance abuse treatment studies using self-help groups suggests similar methodological concerns. Clifford et al. (2000) reinforce concerns about research methodologies used to study substance abuse programs when they point out that "[i]t is recommended that treatment outcome studies be interpreted cautiously, particularly when the research protocols involve frequent and intensive follow-up interviews conducted across extended periods of time" (p. 741), because many external variables can confound the results and suggest improved functioning as a result of treatment when other factors may be more suggestive of the reasons the client has improved.

Q: Shouldn't we feel elated by studies that people live longer or use substances less as a result of self-help groups?

A: Not until the evidence is substantiated by empirical studies using random selection and very scientific methodology. Certainly one should not say that self-help groups are more effective than professional help given the weakness of self-help research to date. Statements such as the following are not supported with data: "The emergence of self-help groups may reflect a societal response to failures within the mental health community. Self-help groups have developed where society has fallen short in meeting the needs of its members" (Felix-Ortiz et al., 2000, p. 339).

Q: But aren't we being too harsh? Isn't it likely that self-help groups, through support and affiliation, help people feel more accepted, appreciated, and cared for, and isn't that important for positive mental health?

A: Certainly, but it's possible that self-help groups may have short-term benefits that, in the long run, aren't likely to continue, or may actually cause harm. T-Groups and the encounter movement come to mind as negative examples.

Q: But what's wrong with short-term results if they're positive? Can't we say the same thing about professional treatment?

A: There's nothing wrong with short-term results and professional treatment may have the same limited results as self-help groups, but the studies cited here don't permit us to make predictions about efficacy because they don't show cause–effect relationships between self-help groups and improvement rates. A belief that self-help groups can replace professional help, without appropriate data, is troubling, since it gives people confidence in a treatment that may not actually help and may, in some cases, do harm. During the current health care crisis, suggesting that self-help groups may replace professional help because someone thinks they work better may leave a large number of clients who desperately need professional help without that option because managed care might increasingly rely on self-help groups to treat a number of serious social, emotional, and medical problems.

Q: So what's the answer?

A: Much more research but, in the meantime, a sense of optimism that perhaps self-help groups might be an alternative answer or, at least, an adjunct to professional help.

Q: Why feel optimistic in view of the weak research data to support the benefits of self-help groups?

A: A preponderance of positive results tends to suggest that something works. It may not prove that something works, but the weight of the evidence suggests that many self-help groups *do* help. This should make us optimistic without making us true believers. EBP is a conservative and cautious paradigm. It doesn't accept best evidence until it's been proven. At the same time, the evidence thus far would suggest that we cautiously use the findings. A case study is presented in this chapter that might be instructive about how best to use self-help groups when professional services are also being provided.

Q: Would the author refer a client to self-help group?

A: Yes, but only after meeting with the group leader and evaluating the group objectives to make certain that they were consistent with the needs of the client. And even then, I would suggest that the client use high standards and caution before joining the group. I would also want to be involved in a discussion with the client about what was taking place in the group and the client's feelings about the worth of the group. Perhaps contacting current and former group members would also help.

Q: Aren't you being overly cautious?

A: Yes, but self-help groups, just like professional help, has the potential for doing harm. It's my responsibility to see that this doesn't happen since I'm the referring source.

Q: Really? What harm could they do?

A: Some self-help groups have been likened to cults. The tendency to make people accept a philosophy through group pressure which may be contrary to their own belief systems or to a process that might not be right for them, may actually cause harm. Similarly, groups that are badly run may inhibit client progress. Relationships develop among group members that may be harmful. An example might be the case of substance abusers developing romantic or sexual attachments to one another that lead to more substance abuse. Granfield and Cloud (1996) studied middle class alcoholics who used self-healing approaches alone with neither professional help nor self-help group intervention. Many of the participants felt that the "ideological" base of some self-help groups were in conflict with their own philosophies of life. Concerns were raised that some groups were overly religious, or that groups saw alcoholism as a lifelong struggle. The subjects in the Granfield and Cloud study also felt that some self-help groups encouraged dependence and that associating with other alcoholics would probably make recovery more difficult. In summarizing their findings, the authors concluded:

> *Many [research subjects] expressed strong opposition to the suggestion that they were powerless over their addictions. Such an ideology, they explained, not only was counterproductive but was also extremely demeaning. These respondents saw themselves as efficacious people who often prided themselves on their past accomplishments. They viewed themselves as being individualists and strong-willed. (Granfield and Cloud, 1996, p. 51)*

Q: But couldn't the same thing happen in a professionally-led group?

A: Yes, but professionals are all bound by codes of ethics and, in a number of states, licensure laws that provide certain protections for clients against extreme behavior by professionals. Non-professional leaders may be less sensitive to inappropriate relationships among group members, or they may not see the harm in developing their own relationship with a group member. Professionals are also guided by a belief that they should respect the rights of clients. That would hopefully eliminate religious proselytizing or other behaviors in conflict with a client's belief system.

Q: Doesn't the fact that self-help groups are usually free of cost and non-discriminating suggest, at the very least, that they may provide a helping intervention that is an alternative to professional help?

A: Yes, but is this a financial argument or an argument about best evidence of effectiveness? Shouldn't clients in need be offered the best help available rather than the help that's cheapest?

Q: Yes, of course, but you can't argue that professional help is always excellent help or that it works, can you?

A: No, I certainly can't, and that's what makes this entire discussion so troubling. When professional help isn't effective, it means that something is fundamentally wrong with our system of treatment. An analogy would be finding that folk healers are more effective than medical doctors. If that's the case, we really would need to reexamine what we believe and whether it's worth maintaining that belief.

Q: Don't a lot of people get better on their own? Is it always necessary to compare self-help groups against professional services?

A: Good point. Waldorf et al. (1991) found that many addicted people with supportive elements in their lives (a job, family, and other close emotional supports) were able to "walk away" from their very heavy use of cocaine. The authors suggest that the "social context" of a drug user's life may positively influence their ability to discontinue drug use. Granfield and Cloud (1996) add to the social context notion of recovery by indicating that many of the respondents in their study had fairly stable lives with social and family supports, college credentials, and a great deal to lose if they continued their substance abuse. "Having much to lose," they write, "gave our respondents incentives to transform their lives. However, when there is little to lose from heavy alcohol or drug use, there may be little to gain by quitting" (p. 55).

Q: So do you feel positively or negatively about self-help groups? You sound awfully negative.

A: Actually, I feel very positively about self-help and I think the research makes a compelling argument that self-help groups may be very effective with a number of health and mental health problems. And I confess that my heart is in the notion of people helping one another, but in a book on best evidence, I think the jury is still out until we have a substantial body of knowledge to show a relationship between self-help and it's level of effectiveness with a range of problems experienced by a cross section of people across gender, age, ethnicity, and socio-economic class. In other words, I hope self-help groups develop the same body of research data to show effectiveness that I expect, but often don't find, for services provided by professionals. When that happens, we'll have a basis for comparison. Until then, I'm hopeful and optimistic while still being cautious. I don't believe, however, that self-help is a substitute for professional help and I worry that a health care system in crisis will turn to self-help as a last resort before needed services are withdrawn completely.

22.7. CASE STUDY: REFERRAL OF AN ADOLESCENT CLIENT TO A SELF-HELP GROUP FOR SEVERE DEPRESSION

Curtis is a 16-year-old client suffering from chronic depression lasting since first onset at 12. Curtis is being seen by a psychiatrist to monitor his anti-depression medication and has been in therapy with a clinical psychologist for almost 5 years. The medication and therapy have a negligible impact, and he still suffers from very severe depression that interferes with school, social activities, relationships, and has, of late, begun to cause weight gain and high blood pressure. Curtis is too depressed to exercise and has become a compulsive eater, having gained almost 100 pounds above his ideal weight. His therapist suggested a self-help group for youth with chronic depression as an adjunct to therapy and medication, but Curtis has been unwilling to attend meetings, believing that the group will be as unsuccessful as his current treatments. The therapist arranged for Curtis to meet with the group leader, a young adult like Curtis who suffers from chronic depression but has successfully learned to cope with it.

The leader invited Curtis to attend a meeting and asked participants to stay after so they could honestly discuss their feelings about the group and to answer questions Curtis might have about the group's effectiveness. The group leader also shared effectiveness research that the national chapter of the group had accumulated on the effectiveness of the self-help group that, while subjective and not terribly sound methodologically, still suggested positive results. Over 2000 former participants of group chapters around the country returned questionnaires. Five thousand questionnaires representing a 10% sample of the 50 000 former national participants in the organization were sent out. Over 70% of the participants who stayed in the group for more than 2 years reported fewer missed days at work, fewer doctor visits, less frequent use of anti-depressants, and fewer days of depression. The average length of depression before the respondents began their group participation was more than 5 years. Participants who stayed with the group 2 years or longer had better results than those who discontinued participation before completing a full year of group participation. Those who dropped out of the group early cited personality clashes with the group leader and differences of opinion about the purpose of the group as the major reasons for attrition.

Since Curtis was unwilling to attend the meeting alone, the therapist met him at the group meeting and sat with him. After the group, people spoke about how the group had helped them. Following the meeting, Curtis shared his positive sense of the group with the therapist and his surprise at how strongly the members felt the experience had helped them. He decided to give it a try and began attending sessions on a regular basis while also seeing his therapist weekly and continuing with his anti-depression medication. After 6 months as a participant, Curtis summarized the experience: "It's pretty nice to be in the group. Everyone there is like me. They're all dealing with depression. The difference is that they get on with their lives. That's what I've begun doing. I've been assigned a girl my age as a mentor who I call when I feel real down. We take walks together and talk, and it's helped me lose weight. I feel a lot of support from the other people, and that helps a lot. We have speakers who talk about depression and who tell us about the latest research. I've been assigned as a mentor to a new member, and I'm sort of surprised but he seems to get a lot of help from our contacts. I still feel really depressed, but while it used to be every day, now I have good and bad days. I think I'm less depressed than I was before I started the group. Mainly, I think the support, the way people don't judge each other, and the feeling that we're all experts on depression and have something to say worth listening to about how to handle depression, are what helps the most. I've made a couple of good friends from the group and instead of staying home and being lonely and down, I go out to movies or have breakfast with my friends. It helps keep me from feeling lonely, which is one of the things depressed people often experience. Do I feel better than I did six months ago? Yes. Is it because of the group? I think some of it is but I have to admit that because of the group, I'm using therapy better. So, yes, it's helping. I'll stay with it and maybe, in time, I'll be able to get by without any help at all. That's my goal, for sure."

22.8. THE CES-D: A MEASURE OF DEPRESSION

The reader might be interested in a simple measure of depression used in the research noted in the case study on the effectiveness of his self-help group. The CES-D (Radloff, 1977) is a widely-used instrument to measure depression with good reliability and validity. Scores of 16–30 indicate the presence of depression requiring intervention. Scores over 30 suggest concern for suicide and would require very serious interventions.

Directions: I am going to read you some statements about the ways people act and feel. On how many of the last 7 days did the following statements apply to you?

22.9. SUMMARY

This chapter on self-help groups offers some hopeful evidence that self-help may provide assistance to a variety of clients experiencing problems with addictions, health, mental health, and other social and emotional problems. A large

	None or 1 day	2 or 3 days	4 or 5 days	5 or more days
1. I was bothered by things which usually don't bother me	0	1	2	3
2. I did not feel like eating. My appetite was poor	0	1	2	3
3. I felt that I could not shake off the blues even with help from friends and family	0	1	2	3
4. I felt I was just not as good as others	0	1	2	3
5. I had trouble keeping my mind on what I was doing	0	1	2	3
6. I felt depressed	0	1	2	3
7. I felt that every-thing I did was an effort	0	1	2	3
8. I felt hopeful about the future.	0	1	2	3
9. I thought my life was a failure	0	1	2	3
10. I felt fearful	0	1	2	3
11. My sleep was restless	0	1	2	3
12. I was happy	0	1	2	3
13. I talked less than usual	0	1	2	3
14. I felt lonely	0	1	2	3
15. People were unfriendly	0	1	2	3
16. I enjoyed life	0	1	2	3
17. I had crying spells	0	1	2	3
18. I felt sad	0	1	2	3
19. I felt people disliked me	0	1	2	3
20. I could not get going	0	1	2	3

number of Americans use self-help but questions remain about the validity of findings indicating that self-help may be an effective alternative to professional assistance. Most of these questions relate to research issues that may be difficult to resolve, given the fact that self-help groups do not have the same expectations as professional help to prove effectiveness. Self-help is generally supportive in nature and usually provides an affirming and positive approach to problem-solving. Some concern is raised that self-help groups may not be effective for everyone because they sometimes have an unacceptable religious ideology or encourage people to believe that recovery is a life-long struggle. Still, the weight of findings provides a reason for optimism until empirically-based research, with strong methodologies provide more compelling evidence of effectiveness.

22.10. QUESTIONS FROM THE CHAPTER

1. Do you agree that treatment provided in self-help groups can harm people? If so, under what circumstances might that be the case?
2. What possible harm is there in a group of people with the same problems getting together and offering support and encouragement? Why must we think of this as treatment and why should we even consider researching the effectiveness of this type of benign helping process?
3. If self-help groups turn out to be more effective than professional help, how would professionals justify their existence? What might they do to improve the effectiveness of their services?
4. Leaders of self-help groups can sometimes be officious or power hungry. Do you think either, in pursuit of honest help to people in need, would be an inhibitor to good treatment? If so, why might this be the case?
5. The research seems to suggest that the most effective self-help groups are the ones in which people attend regularly and stay in the group for two or more years. Could not people get better as a result of other factors during that time? What might be some of the reasons for improvement other than the self-help received by the client?

References

Anderson, B., et al. (1989, March). Effects of peer-group intervention on metabolic control of adolescents with IDDM. *Diabetes Care, 12*(3), 179–183.

Barak, A., & Dolev-Cohen, M. (2006, September). *Counseling & Psychotherapy Research, 6*(3), 86–190.

Becu, M., Becu, N., Manzur, G., & Kochen, S. (1993). Self-help epilepsy groups: An evaluation of effect on depression and schizophrenia. *Epilepsia, 34*(5), 841–845.

Blinn-Pike, L., Kuschel, D., McDaniel, A., Mingus, S., & Poole-Mutti, M. (1998). The process of mentoring pregnant adolescents: An exploratory study. *Family Relations, 47*, 119–127.

Bly, R. (1986, April–May). Men of wisdom. *Utne Reader*, 37–41.

Britner, P. A., Bacazar, F. E., Blechman, E. A., & Blinn-Pike, S. (2006). Mentoring special youth populations. *Journal of Community Psychology, 34*(6), 747–764.

Britner, P. A., & Kraimer-Rickaby, L. (2005). Abused and neglected youth. In D. L. DuBois, & M. J. Karcher (Eds.), *Handbook of youth mentoring* (pp. 482–492). Thousand Oaks, CA: Sage.

Caserta, M. S., & Lund, D. A. (1993). Intrapersonal resources and the effectiveness of self-help groups for bereaved older adults. *Gerontologist, 33*(5), 619–629.

Clifford, P. R., Maisto, S. A., & Franzke, L. H. (2000). Alcohol treatment research follow-up and drinking behaviors. *Journal of Studies on Alcohol, 61*(5), 736–743.

Dadich, A. (2006). Self-help support groups: Adding to the tool box of mental health care options for young men. *Youth Studies Australia, 25*(1), 33–41.

DuBois, D. L., Neville, H. A., Parra, G. R., & Pugh-Lilly, A. O. (2002). Testing a new model of mentoring. *New Directions for Youth Development, 93*, 21–57.

Felix-Ortiz, M., Salazar, M. R., Gonzalez, J. R., Sorensen, J. L., & Plock, D. (2000). Addictions services: A qualitative evaluation of an assisted self-help group for drug-addicted clients in a structured outpatient treatment setting. *Community Mental Health Journal, 36*(4), 339–350.

Fetto, J. (2000). Lean on me. *American Demographics, 22*(12), 16.

Gilden, J. L., Hendryx, A. S., Clar, S., Casia, S., & Singh, S. P. (1992). Diabetes support groups improve health care of older diabetic patients. *Journal of the American Geriatrics Society, 40*, 147–150.

Glicken, M. D. (2004). *Using the strengths perspective in social work practice*. Boston, MA: Pearson Education, Inc.

Goh, C., Lane, A. T., & Bruckner, A. L. (2007). Support groups for children and their families. *Pediatric Dermatology, 24*(3), 302–305.

Granfield, R., & Cloud, W. (1996, Winter). The elephant that no one sees: Natural recovery among middle-class addicts. *Journal of Drug Issues, 26*, 45–61.

Grossman, J. B., & Rhodes, J. E. (2002). The test of time: Predictors and effects of duration in youth mentoring relationships. *American Journal of Community Psychology, 30*, 199–219.

Hughes, J. M. (1977). Adolescent children of alcoholic parents and the relationship of Alateen to these children. *Journal of Consulting and Clinical Psychology, 45*(5), 946–947.

Humphreys, K., & Moos, R. H. (1996). Reduced substance-abuse-related health care costs among voluntary participants in Alcoholics Anonymous. *Psychiatric Services, 47*, 709–713.

Humphreys, K. (1998). Can addiction-related self-help/mutual aid groups lower demand for professional substance abuse treatment? *Social Policy, 29*(2), 13–17.

Humphreys, K., & Ribisl, K. M. (1999). The case for partnership with self-help groups. *Public Health Reports, 114*(4), 322–329.

Kessler, R. C., Mickelson, K. D., & Zhao, S. (1997a). Patterns and correlates of self-help group membership in the United States. *Social Policy, 27*, 27–46.

Kessler, R. C., Frank, R. G., Edlund, M., Katz, S. J., Lin, E., & Leaf, P. (1997b). Differences in the use of psychiatric outpatient services between the United States and Ontario. *New England Journal of Medicine, 336*, 551–557.

Kurtz, L. F. (1988). Mutual aid for affective disorders: The manic depressive and depressive associations in the United States. *Social Policy, 27*, 27–46.

Larose, S., & Tarabulsy, G. M. (2005). Mentoring academically at-risk students: Processes, outcomes, and conditions for success. In D. L. DuBois, & M. J. Karcher (Eds.), *Handbook of youth mentoring* (pp. 440–453). Thousand Oaks, CA: Sage.

Lewis, E. A. & Suarez, Z. E. (1995). Natural helping networks. *Encyclopedia of Social Work*, 19th ed. (pp. 1765–1772). Silver Spring, MD: National Association of Social Workers.

McCallion, P., & Toseland, R. W. (1995). Supportive group interventions with caregivers of frail older adults. *Social Work with Groups, 18*(1), 11–25.

McCord, J. (1992). The Cambridge–Somerville study: A pioneering longitudinal experimental study of delinquency prevention. In J. McCord, & R. E. Tremblay (Eds.), *Preventing antisocial behavior: Interventions from birth through adolescence* (pp. 196–206). New York: Guilford.

Memmott, J. L. (1993). Models of helping and coping: A field experiment with natural and professional helpers. *Social Work Research & Abstracts, 29*, 11–22.

Nash, K. B., & Kramer, K. D. (1993). Self-help for sickle cell disease in African American communities. *Journal of Applied Behavioral Science, 29*(2), 202–215.

Ouimette, P. C., Finney, J. W., & Moos, R. H. (1997). Twelve-step and cognitive-behavioral treatment for substance abuse: A comparison of treatment effectiveness. *Journal of Consulting and Clinical Psychology, 65*(2), 230–240.

Patterson, S. L., Holzhuter, J. L., Struble, V. E., & Quadagno, J. S. (1972). *Final report, utilization of human resources for mental health* (Grant No. MH 16618). Unpublished report, National Institute of Mental Health, Washington, DC.

Patterson, S. L., & Marsiglia, F. F. (2000). Mi casa es su casa: Beginning exploration of Mexican Americans' natural helping. *Families in Society, 81*(1), 22–31.

Potasznik, H., & Nelson, G. (1984). Stress and social support: The burden experienced by the family of a mentally ill person. *American Journal of Community Psychology, 12*(5).

Powers, L. E., Sowers, J., & Stevens, T. (1995). An exploratory, randomized study of the impact of mentoring in the self-efficacy and community-based knowledge of adolescents with severe physical challenges. *Journal of Rehabilitation, 61*, 33–41.

Radloff, L. S. (1977). The CES-D scale: A self-report depression scale for research in the general population. *Applied Psychological Measurements, 1*, 385–407.

Rhodes, J. E. (2002). *Stand by me: The risks and rewards of mentoring today's youth.* Cambridge, MA: Harvard University Press.

Rhodes, J. E., Haight, W. L., & Briggs, E. C. (1999). The influence of mentoring on the peer relationships of foster youth in relative and nonrelative care. *Journal of Research on Adolescence, 9*, 185–201.

Rhodes, J. E., Grossman, J. B., & Resch, N. L. (2000). Agents of change: Pathways through which mentoring relationships influence adolescents' academic adjustment. *Child Development, 71*, 1662–1671.

Riessman, F. (1997). Ten self-help principles. *Social Policy, 27*, 6–11.

Riessman, F. (2000). Self-help comes of age. *Social Policy, 30*(4), 47–49.

Sibthorpe, B., & Fleming, D. (1994). Self-help groups: A key to HIV risk reduction for high-risk injection drug users? *Journal of Acquired Immune Deficiency Syndromes, 7*(6), 592–598.

Waldorf, D., Reinarman, C., & Murphy, S. (1991). *Cocaine changes: The experience of using and quitting.* Philadelphia: Temple University Press.

Waller, M. A., & Patterson, S. (2002). Natural helping and resilience in a Dine (Navajo) community. *Society, 81*(1), 73–84.

Watkins, S., Pittman, P., & Walden, B. (1998). The deaf mentor experimental project for young children who are deaf and their families. *American Annals of the Deaf, 143*, 29–34.

Weidle, B., Bolme, B., & Hoeyland, A. L. (2006). Are peer groups for adolescents with Asperberg's syndrome helpful? *Clinical Child Psychology and Psychiatry, 11*(1), 45–62, Sage Publications.

Wituk, S., Shepherd, M. D., Slavich, S., Warren, M. L., & Meissen, G. (2000). A topography of self-help groups: An empirical analysis. *Social Work, 45*(2), 157–165.

Wuthnow, R. (1994). *Sharing the journey: Support groups and America's quest for community.* New York: Free Press.

Part Six
Evidence Based Practice and Future Trends, Social Involvement, and Final Words

23 Evidence-Based Practice and Resilient Children and Adolescents

23.1. INTRODUCTION: UNDERSTANDING RESILIENCE

Walsh (2003) defines resilience as "the ability to withstand and rebound from disruptive life challenges. Resilience involves key processes over time that foster the ability to 'struggle well,' surmount obstacles, and go on to live and love fully" (p. 1). Gordon (1996) defines resilience as "the ability to thrive, mature, and increase competence in the face of adverse circumstances" (p. 1). Glick (1994) writes,

> *"Resilience is the ability to 'bounce back' from adversity, to overcome the negative influences that often block achievement. Resilience research focuses on the traits and coping skills and supports that help kids survive, or even thrive, in a challenging environment." (p. 1)*

Henry (1999) suggests that the notion of resilience was created to help explain why some children do well under very troubled circumstances. Resilience describes children who grow up in highly unfavorable conditions without showing negative consequences. Henry (1999) defines resilience as "the capacity for successful adaptation, positive functioning, or competence despite high risk, chronic stress, or prolonged or severe trauma" (p. 521). In a further definition of resilience, Abrams (2001) indicates that resilience may be seen as the ability to readily recover from illness, depression, and adversity. Walsh (2003) says that,

> *The concept of family resilience extends our understanding of healthy family functioning to situations of adversity. Although some families are shattered by crisis or chronic stresses, what is remarkable is that many others emerge strengthened and more resourceful. (p. 1)*

Anderson (1997) says that resilient people have been described as being,

> *Socially, behaviorally, and academically competent despite living in adverse circumstances and environments as a result of poverty (Werner and Smith, 1992), parental mental illness (Beardslee and Podorefsky, 1988), interparental conflict (Neighbors et al., 1993), inner-city living (Luthar, 1993), and child abuse and neglect (Farber and Egeland, 1987). Resilient children who are functioning well despite enduring hardships often do not receive treatment*

services because they find ways to be successful despite their troubled environments. (p. 594)

Mandleco and Peery (2000) are concerned about the inconsistent meaning of the term resilience and wonder if it has begun to mean whatever the author wishes it to. For example, resilience has been described as a personality characteristic not related to stress; a characteristic of some *children* from at-risk environments; the absence of psychopathology in a child whose parents have serious emotional problems; success in meeting societal expectations or developmental tasks; characteristics which help *children* to succeed contrary to predictions; the ability to restore equilibrium and adapt to life situations. The authors note that Polk (1997) tried to synthesize a model of resilience suggesting that "*resilience* is a midrange theory with a four-dimensional construct, where dispositional, relational, situational, and philosophical patterns intermingle with the environment to form *resilience*" (Mandleco and Peery, 2000, p. 100). The result of these various definitions of resilience is that while a "commonsense" universal definition is assumed, when one attempts to identify specifics affecting *resilience*, these definitions are inadequate and confusing (Mandleco and Peery, 2000, p. 100).

23.2. ATTRIBUTES OF RESILIENT CHILDREN

A consistent finding over the last 20 years of resilience research is that most children from highly dysfunctional families or very poor communities do well as adults. This finding applies to almost all populations of children found to be at risk for later life problems, including children who experience divorce; children who live with step-parents; children who have lost a sibling; children who have attention deficit disorder or suffer from developmental delays; and children who become delinquent or run away. More of these children make it than do not. Furstenberg (1998) reviewed the research and found that 70–75% of children at risk do well in later life, including children born to teen-aged mothers, children who were sexually abused (Wilkes, 2002), children who grew up in substance abusing or mentally ill families (Werner and Smith, 2001), and children who grew up in poverty (Vaillant, 1993). Even when children have experienced multiple risks, Werner & Smith (2001) found that half of them overcame adversity and achieved good emotional and social development.

Masten (2001) believes that resilience is part of the genetic makeup of humans and that it is the norm rather than the exception.

What began as a quest to understand the extraordinary has revealed the power of the ordinary. Resilience does not come from rare and special qualities, but from the everyday magic of ordinary, normative human resources in the minds, brains, and bodies of children, in their families and relationships, and in their communities. (Masten, 2001, p. 9)

We tend to think that traumas will generally lead to malfunctioning behavior in children and adults, but often this is not the case. A good example of how well people actually cope with trauma may be seen in the response to the World Trade Center Bombings. Gist and Devilly (2002) report that the estimates of PTSD after the 9/11 bombing dropped by almost two-thirds within 4 months of the tragedy and concluded that,

> *These findings underscore the counterproductive nature of offering a [treatment] with no demonstrable effect, but demonstrated potential to complicate natural resolution, in a population in which limited case-conversion can be anticipated, strong natural supports exist, and spontaneous resolution is prevalent. (p. 742)*

In other words, resilience to severe traumas exists when we accept the possibility that people will heal on their own and when strong social and emotional supports exist. Introducing treatment too early in the process may actually interfere with resilience.

Mandleco and Peery (2000) describe one effort to understand resilience by focusing on the self-righting tendencies that propel children toward normal development under adverse circumstances. This work has identified common dispositions and situations that describe resilient behavior in children and seem crucial in their ability to respond to stress and adversity while still maintaining control and competence in their lives even when challenged by physical handicaps, a pathological family environment, or the adverse effects of poverty, war, or dislocation. "These commonalities generally have been organized into three categories: personal predispositions of the child, characteristics of the family environment, and the presence of extra familial support sources" (Mandleco and Peery, 2000, p. 101).

Werner and Smith (1982, 1992) identified protective factors that tend to counteract the risk of stress. They categorize these protective factors as genetic (e.g., an easygoing disposition) strong self-esteem and a sense of identity, intelligence, physical attractiveness, and supportive caregivers. Garmezy et al. (1964) note three protective factors in resilient children: dispositional attributes of the child, family cohesion and warmth, and availability and use of external support systems by parents and children. Seligman (1992) says that resilience exists when people are optimistic, have a sense of adventure, courage, and self-understanding, use humor in their lives, have a capacity for hard work, and possess the ability to cope with and find outlets for emotions. Luthar and Zigler (1991) found that resilient children are active, humorous, confident, competent, prepared to take risks, flexible, and, as a result of repeated successful coping experiences, confident in both their inner and outer resources. Luthar (1993) suggests that resilient children have considerable intellectual maturity.

Other factors associated with resilience include the finding by Arend et al. (1979) that very curious children are more resilient than less curious children. Radke-Yarrow and Brown (1993) associate resilience with children who have more positive self-perceptions. Egeland et al. (1993) and Baldwin et al. (1993) found a relationship between resilience and assertiveness, independence, and a support network of neighbors, peers, family, and elders. In their 32-year longitudinal study, Werner and Smith (1982) found a strong relationship between problem-solving abilities, communication skills, and an internal locus of control in resilient children. As Henry (1999) notes, "Resilient children often acquire faith that their lives have meaning and that they have control over their own fates" (p. 522). Tiet et al. (1998) add that resilient children also have higher educational aspiration, better physical health, and healthier mothers or female caretakers than less resilient children.

In her work on resilient infants and toddlers and the relationship between early signs of resilience and resilience in later life, Gordon (1996) reports the following:

1. Resilient infants and toddlers are energetic, socially responsive, autonomous, demonstrative, tolerant of frustration, cooperative, and androgynous, among other characteristics.
2. Their environments are nurturing, responsive, and indicate a strong bond between the caregiver and the child.
3. Early signs of resilience relate directly to later life resilience and are strongly tied to early signs of an internal locus of control, social skills, and the social support of mothers including self-confidence and positive coping skills.
4. Resilience may be enhanced in very young children through social policies and practices that provide "social support for the family (such as on-site day care, flexible leave-time, and volunteer efforts), fostering an internal locus of control and sense of autonomy, modeling androgyny, and improving caregiver education" (Gordon, 1996, 2004, p. 5).

Resiliency research originally tried to discover the characteristics of at-risk children who coped well with stress (Werner, 1989). Over time, however, resiliency research has focused less on the attributes of resilient children and more on the processes of resilience. As the research has attempted to understand the processes associated with resilience, one important finding suggests that rather than avoiding risks, resilient children take substantial risks to cope with stressors leading to what Cohler (1987) calls adaptation and competence.

In a review of the factors associated with resilience to stressful life events, Tiet et al. (1998) found that: (a) higher IQ; (b) quality of parenting; (c) connection to other competent adults; (d) an internal locus of control; and (e) excellent social skills have been identified as protective factors that allow children to cope with stressful events. Protective factors, according to Tiet et al. (1998), are primary buffers between the traumatic event and the child's response. When a child's response to stress has a positive effect on the resilient child, whether the risk to the child is low or high, the author's term this a resource factor but the literature also uses the terms asset or compensatory factors (Tiet et al., 1998). The authors believe that both protective and resource factors are crucial in understanding the way resilience protects people. However, certain situations may make resilience inoperable in even the most resilient people and current research efforts are attempting to find connections between the types of adverse events (whether they are controllable or uncontrollable) and the risk factors to resilient people. Tiet et al. (1998) write,

> *To understand resilience, it is essential to identify protective factors that buffer the detrimental effects of risk factors. However, it is also important to identify resource factors because they predict good adjustment at both high and low risk and therefore become critical in the design of preventive efforts. (p. 1191)*

Tiet et al. (1998) indicate that even resilient children respond inconsistently to stressful events and that another way to look at resilience is to show the relationship between the specific traumatic event and the response. For example, in many of the maltreated children studied for resilience, school-based outcomes have been used that include grades, deportment, and the degree of involvement in school activities. Luthar (1991) notes that while resilient children do well on many school-based activities, many of these children suffer from depression. Interestingly, however, even though many of the maltreated children studied show signs of depression, they still did well on behavioral outcomes measures, such as grades and school conduct (Luthar, 1991). Tiet et al. (1998) believe that the key reason resilient children cope well with adversity is that they tend

> *to live in higher-functioning families and receive more guidance and supervision by their parents and other adults in the family. Other adults in the family may complement the parents in providing guidance and support to the youth and in enhancing youth adjustment. Higher educational aspiration may also provide high-risk youth with a sense of direction and hope. (p. 1198)*

In conversations with survivors of the Holocaust, Tech (2003) found characteristics of those who survived to include a desire for mutual cooperation in order to cope with survival. This included caring for ill concentration camp inmates, sharing rations that were minute to begin with, and forming "bonding groups" which kept inmates optimistic and positive. Tech also points out that inmates who were emotionally flexible were more likely to survive. Inmates who were very traditional in their outlook on life or who felt that they had lost a considerable amount of status were often unable to cope and frequently perished before other less healthy inmates died. However, many terribly unhealthy inmates who had a positive view of their lives survived against all medical odds. Tech reports that survivors she interviewed were filled with compassion and sadness and that "[c]onspicuously absent were expressions of hatred or hostility" (p. 345) toward their captors. Even though conditions in the camps were dreadful, "[m]any inmates created for themselves make-believe worlds – a blend of dreams, fantasies, friendships and resistance – as an antidote" (p. 351). Prisoners found these fantasies very gratifying and "such escapes into fantasy may have improved the prisoners hold on life ... Prisoners created bonding groups which, however illusory, forged links with the past and the future" (p. 351).

There are many similarities between the recollections of the survivors Tech interviewed and more scientific studies of survivors of the Holocaust. Baron et al. (1996) report that many clinicians who first interviewed survivors of the Holocaust believed that they would be very troubled parents and that their children would suffer from a range of emotional difficulties. Children of survivors, however, have shown no pattern of maladjustment or psychopathology in most research studies, other than the normal problems one might expect in any population of children. Children who have maintained the traditional religious beliefs of their parents have done particularly well socially, financially, and emotionally (Last, 1989).

In studies of the development of symptoms of PTSD following a traumatic event, Ozer et al. (2003) report that those most likely to develop PTSD have a lack of psychological resilience which can be seen as a cluster of prior social and emotional problems that include prior loss, depression, poor support from others, prior traumas, and a family history of pathology. The authors write,

> *It is tempting to make an analogy to the flu or infectious disease: Those whose immune systems are compromised are at greater risk of contracting a subsequent illness. Similarly, this cluster of variables may all be pointing to a single source of vulnerability for the development of PTSD or enduring symptoms of PTSD – a lack of psychological resilience. (p. 71)*

What the authors fail to answer is why some people who have had all of the earlier signs of coping poorly with a new trauma, in fact, cope surprisingly well. Most resilient people have had prior traumas and loss, an absence of family support, and episodes of depression but still cope well enough with new traumas to avoid serious social and emotional malfunction.

Perhaps Tiet et al. (1998) help answer this question by pointing out that in their research on resilience, resilient children and adolescents live in better functioning families, receive supervision and guidance from parents or other adults, have higher educational aspirations, and have higher IQs. The authors believe such attributes help in problem-solving and in seeking unique solutions to difficult social and emotional problems. However, resilience is often more than just individual attributes, but includes external processes or buffers that help increase resilience.

One of the continuing beliefs in the helping professions is that the higher the social and emotional risk to an individual, the more likely we are to see pathology. But resilience research suggests that risk factors are predictive of some types of dysfunction for only about 20–49% of a given high-risk population, suggesting high levels of resilience in the majority of those at risk (Werner and Smith 2001). In contrast, "protective factors," the supports and opportunities that buffer the effect of adversity and enable development to proceed, appear to predict positive outcomes in anywhere from 50% to 80% of a high-risk population. According to Werner and Smith,

> *Our findings and those by other American and European investigators with a life-span perspective suggest that these buffers [i.e., protective factors]*

> *make a more profound impact on the life course of children who grow up under adverse conditions than do specific risk factors or stressful life events. They [also] appear to transcend ethnic, social class, geographical, and historical boundaries. Most of all, they offer us a more optimistic outlook than the perspective that can be gleaned from the literature on the negative consequences of perinatal trauma, care giving deficits, and chronic poverty. (1992, p. 202)*

In summarizing our understanding of resilience, Mandleco and Peery (2000) argue that we still do not know which attribute of resilience is most significant for a particular child. "In addition, there is often marked variation in an individual's responses to stress, suggesting the presence of any specific factor does not always produce *resilience* if the person is particularly vulnerable or the adversity too great to overcome" (Mandleco and Peery, 2000, p. 101). The authors continue by noting the confusion over the factors affecting resilience. While some researchers have taken a theoretical perspective, others have summarized the research literature. There is, however, confusion over the following factors: (a) the age domain covered by the construct, (b) the circumstances where it occurs, (c) its definition, (d) its boundaries, or (e) the adaptive behaviors described (Mandleco and Peery, 2000, p. 102). One of the problems with resilience research is that it is not all inclusive of a broad population of people. Some studies consider certain age groups, most notably childhood and adolescence, and from those age groups project resilience to older populations. Another type of research considers specific problems, such as mental illness or alcoholism, and generalizes these findings to broader populations. The definition of resilience, according to Mandleco and Peery, is still vague and continues to affect research results.

23.3. COPING WITH STRESS AS AN ADDITIONAL ASPECT OF RESILIENCE

Courbasson et al. (2002) define coping as "one's efforts to reduce the impact of a difficult or stressful situation. This transactional process involves both cognition and behavior" (p. 35). The authors indicate that there are three primary styles of coping with stress: task-oriented, emotion-oriented, and avoidance-oriented *coping* (Endler and Parker, 1999). Task-oriented *coping* attempts to solve or limit the impact of the stressful situation. Emotion-oriented *coping* tries to limit the emotional impact of stress rather than resolve the stressful situation. Avoidance-oriented *coping* uses distraction and diversion unrelated to the stressful situation to reduce stress. The authors find that research in *coping with stress* suggest that a task-oriented approach benefits people under great stress more than the use of other *coping* strategies. "That is, task-oriented *coping* is associated *with* problem resolution or amelioration more often than the use of other *coping* strategies. Alternatively, both emotion and avoidance-oriented *coping* strategies may exacerbate the problematic situation" (Courbasson et al., 2002, p. 37).

Miller and Smith (2005) suggest that there are different types of stress, each with its own attributes, symptoms, duration and treatment. (1) Acute stress is the common type of stress we all feel when something goes badly or makes life temporarily more complicated. This is time limited stress and goes away when the situation rectifies itself. (2) Episodic stress is frequently experienced by some people because they often place themselves in stressful situations by being late or being in one crisis or another. These people are crisis prone and appear to lack the ability to order problems in logical ways or to deal with them in pragmatic and rational ways, allowing the crisis to be constant. Chronic stress "is the grinding stress that wears people away day after day, year after year. Chronic stress destroys bodies, minds and lives. It wreaks havoc through long-term attrition. It is the stress of poverty, of dysfunctional families, of being trapped in an unhappy marriage or in a despised job or career" (Miller and Smith, 2005, p. 1). The authors go on to say, "Chronic stress kills through suicide, violence, heart attack, stroke, and, perhaps, even cancer. People wear down to a final, fatal breakdown" (p. 1).

Coping with stress has been thought to be a dimension of resilience, although there is disagreement in the literature about the definition of coping. Some researchers see coping as a dynamic process but measure its existence by considering a person's disposition or by viewing it as something triggered by a life situation (Parkes, 1984). In this definition of coping, it is a fluctuating or transitory state. Other researchers see the ability to cope with stress as a permanent and enduring personality trait (Carver et al., 1989; McCrae, 1984; Parkes, 1984), a definition that sounds much like the definition of resilience. Still other researchers view coping as a set of positive and negative modes of behavior. People with positive coping skills are described as using "more mature, flexible, purposive, future-oriented, reality-based, and metered approaches to combating stressful and anxiety-provoking situations, whereas those with negative coping skills are viewed as rigid, past-propelled, reality-distorting, and lack real time adaptive processes" (Liveneh et al., 1996, p. 503).

Lazarus (1966) believes that coping: (a) serves to reduce the impact of harmful events and to maintain a positive self-concept; (b) includes situational factors such as the availability of resources coupled with individual factors including one's belief system and other physical and emotional skills; (c) includes an appraisal of a situation and how that situation may affect one's well-being, including the options and limitations of alternative approaches to the situation; and (d) includes very basic options such as seeking more information, asking others how they might resolve a stressful situation, and direct action.

In a slightly different vein, Billings and Moos (1981, 1984) and Pearlin and Schooler (1978) believe that there are three alternative strategies which individuals use to cope with stressful situations: (a) they may attempt to control the negative effect of the situation; (b) they may try to modify the seriousness and the meaning of the stressful event; or, (c) they may respond directly by trying to change the stressful event through the use of strategies that may have worked in the past.

Liveneh et al. (1996) found three active styles of coping that resemble notions of resilience: (a) one that utilizes planning and seeking help from others; (b) one that seeks a support group to help with the stressor rather than passively putting it in the hands of fate; and, (c) a one that utilizes direct techniques to deal with the stressor rather than such indirect techniques as denial or using other activities to temporarily try to forget about the stressor. Interestingly, the authors found that placing a problem in the hands of God or using prayer almost exclusively as a way of resolving a stressful situation was not a particularly effective way of coping, and suggested an external locus of control. The more active the coping approach, the better subjects in their study were able to cope.

In determining whether treatment with substance abusing patients would improve the type of coping approach used, Courbasson et al. (2002) treated 71 substance abusing clients in an outpatient setting for three full days a week using anger management, relaxation, *stress* management, nutrition, leisure activities, assertiveness training, loss, drug education, goal setting, relationships and intimacy, and group psychotherapy (a client-centered orientation). The authors found that therapy had the following impact: (a) following treatment, task-oriented coping increased significantly, and with it, a large decrease in anxiety and other stress-related symptoms; (b) the use of emotion-oriented coping also decreased; (c) the use of avoidance-oriented coping did not change with treatment; and (d) although the purpose of the treatment was to stop the substance abuse, better coping skills (those that tried to resolve stressful situations) resulted in sustained improvement in psychological distress.

23.4. FACTORS PREDICTING RESILIENCE IN ABUSED AND TRAUMATIZED CHILDREN AND ADOLESCENTS

Mandleco and Peery (2000, p. 101) have organized the internal and external factors supported by the research literature to affect resilience in children. The authors note that **internal factors** include biological and psychological factors, cognitive abilities, personality traits, the ability to relate to others, and health and genetic factors. **External factors** are described by family life, parenting, community resources and factors outside the person which help the person acquire resilience. Using the notion of internal and external factors influencing resilience, the following summarize the attributes we associate with resilient children.

23.5. BIOLOGICAL FACTORS

Resilient children are often healthy, have few childhood illnesses, have better than average energy, and are frequently physically strong, coordinated, and have good endurance. Family histories of resilient children note very limited occurrences of hereditary or chronic illness. An infant's easy-going temperament may predispose the child to develop resilience. Once developed, temperament is a positive factor in mediating stress. Males are more vulnerable to risk of physical and emotional problems during and after infancy than females, and suffer more chronic problems than females throughout the life cycle.

23.6. PSYCHOLOGICAL FACTORS

Cognitive capacity includes intelligence and the way in which people problem-solve, or what has been referred to as emotional intelligence. Resilient *children* score higher on educational achievement and scholastic aptitude tests and have better reading, communication, and reasoning skills than at-risk *children* who developed problems. Emotional intelligence includes introspection and impulse control. As Mandleco and Peery (2000) suggest, "these *children* carefully think about and phrase their answers before responding, instead of immediately replying" (p. 102).

Coping ability is a process rather than an attribute that includes positive responses to frustration, challenge, or stressors and may include "curiosity, perseverance, seeking comfort from another person, or protesting, and perhaps is the best external manifestation of resilience" (Mandleco and Peery, 2000, p. 103).

Personality characteristics consistently associated with resilient children include positive descriptions of self and others. Such attributes as good self-esteem, self-awareness, self-understanding and an internal locus of control, optimism, motivation, and curiosity have been associated with resilient children. Many resilient children use religion and spirituality to maintain a positive approach to life since faith provides a sense of coherence. Curiosity is another internal characteristic of resilient children. Radke-Yarrow and Brown (1993) report that resilient children living in a number of high-risk situations often found considerable information about their situation to increase their understanding of stress-producing situations and events. Resilient children also appear to be more empathic, sensitive to others, well-liked by peers, respectful and have a positive response to authority and adults.

23.7. WITHIN THE FAMILY

While this may not describe the homes of abused children, organized and structured home environments seem to be related to resilience. By extension, parental practices that are consistent and equitable are also associated with resilience. Brooks (1994) indicates that parents of resilient children provide nurturing, confidence-building, and emotionally healthy relationships with their children. Resilient children often have a strong relationship with at least one family member who acts as a stable role model. This parent is often identified by resilient children as their mother. Relationships with siblings characterized by mutual warmth and protectiveness are especially helpful.

23.8. OUTSIDE OF THE FAMILY

Supportive peers and adults outside of the family may provide at-risk children with friendship and direction and help the child view the future in a positive way. Supportive adults may include teachers, family friends, religious leaders and therapists. Schools, churches, synagogues, youth organizations and after-school programs are important for resilient children and adolescents. Schools may provide caring adults and an environment where abused children can succeed. Relationships between family life and a rich outside life may result in resilient children who respond positively to their communities and are caring and involved citizens.

In determining which of these characteristics of resilient people are most significant, Mandleco and Peery (2000, p. 103) caution that the influence of a specific component may "vary, interact differently and operate directly or indirectly over time in a particular child's situation. However, little empirical evidence suggests a significant percentage of the variance in predicting resilience can be accounted for by any one variable alone" (p. 110)

23.9. CASE STUDY: A RESILIENT CHILD COPES WITH ABUSIVE PARENTS

The following story first appeared in a book written by the author on resilience in Glicken (2004, pp. 115–117). The author wishes to thank Sage Publications for permission to reprint Jake's story.

23.10. JAKE'S STORY

You talked to me two years ago when you were writing another book but you never asked me to write anything about myself. I was 13 when you talked to me. I am 15 now. I still live with this great family since I left home, but I see my folks a lot and they're doing much better now. My dad has stopped drinking but every once in a while he goes on a binge and then the case manager won't let me see him. My mom is still pretty mad about life and she can be – you know – sarcastic a lot. She thinks I caused them a lot of trouble because I wrote a story about what they were doing to me and it got them into trouble with the police and the welfare people. I feel sorry about that but maybe I should tell my story like it happened in some kind of order. That's what my foster father says and he's an English teacher and the father of my best friend.

My parents drank a lot, and when they drank, they could be very mean. Maybe when I was four or five, I knew when they were going to be mean and I'd try and hide or I'd go to a friend's house. My dad was an accountant then and I think he was one of the smartest people I ever knew. But when he drinks, he gets really angry and mean. My granddad (his father) was the same way as my dad. He could be really nice, but when he drank, he was mean and he'd swear at me and sometimes he'd hit me. I never could figure it out. I thought drinking was supposed to make you happy or silly. I got to be good at knowing when my dad was drinking too much and I'd get out of the way as fast as I could. If I didn't, I'd get hit or punched. I guess I was able to believe that he loved me even when he hurt me because I could see how nice he was when he wasn't drinking. I figured if he'd just stop drinking, then he'd be the nice guy I sometimes saw.

My mom was different. She was always mean, even when she wasn't drinking. She was abused as a girl because she'd tell me the stories pretty often, and then she'd say how much better my life was and then she'd hit me, or pinch me, or put my hands in really hot water. I still have some scars from the things she did to me. The drinking just made her madder, and when she wasn't hitting me or calling me names like "stupid" and "dip shit" and stuff like that, she'd hit my dad and they'd have these bad fights.

A lot of the time when they were drinking and I knew I was going to get hit, I used to hide in the basement until they fell asleep. While I was down there, and maybe I started hiding from them when I was four or five, I found these books with stories. I watched the T.V. programs that helped you learn about your letters and I could even read some by then. There were hundreds of stories and I started to read them. I was pretty slow at first, but then when my reading got better, I could read pretty fast for a kid. Reading was wonderful. The stories made me forget all the fighting and I could see a whole different world than the one I lived in at home. One of my friend's dads was an English teacher. When he found out I was reading, he gave me more books to read, and we'd talk about them. I think he knew about my parents from his son and I think he was trying to make up for what was going on in my home. He was a very smart man and when we'd talk, I'd just want to read more stories. He asked me if I ever wrote things and I said no, that I never did. So he encouraged me to write and I began to write stories about my parents and the fighting and all. I guess they were pretty awful stories because after reading one (maybe I was about 11), he called the welfare office and now I'm living with my friend and his mom and dad.

It's wonderful at their house. They're really good to me. I see my mom and dad a lot and they still love me in their own way. I know I won't be able to live with them, but they're my parents and I still love them. My dad has pretty much stopped drinking and lives by himself. Sometimes he still goes on binges, but I know he's trying. There's some chance that I might live with him, but the welfare lady said that we had to be sure that he'd stopped drinking for at least a year before we could consider that. But we do a lot together, and he's a very smart man, and he knows lots of interesting things. The last time I saw him he started to cry about how bad he was as a dad. I don't know, to me he always seemed like he was trying to be nice but he had a lot of crazy stuff inside of him because of what his dad did to him. And being an alcoholic, from the stuff I've read, is a tough thing to change. At least that's what I think.

I never felt too close to my mom, and I still don't. But I've learned from her that if you blame other people for your problems, you never do anything to change them. She hasn't learned anything from my leaving the home. She thinks it's my fault and still believes that she was a great mom. She doesn't remember any hitting, or putting my hands in hot water, or any of the stuff she did to me. I guess I love her but I don't really like her much.

You asked me how I turned out so well. I don't know. I do really well in school. I like sports and I think I'm pretty popular, but I have my days when I don't like myself much. My foster dad says I get the "blues" and he lets me listen to these old blues singers from the south and boy, one of them, Robert Johnson, he must have had the blues really bad because he sounds like I feel sometimes. I think my dad was a good guy when he wasn't drinking. He helped me feel loved and I could forgive him for drinking. My granddad, even though he could be mean, the summers I spent with him and my grandma were pretty great. Books and reading saved my life. I learned that you could escape from the things that were happening at home and into another world. My friend's family helped too and I spent a lot of time at their house even before I went to live with them.

I've never believed much in God. If there was a God, he wouldn't let stuff like I went through or what happened to my mom ever happen to little kids. I do believe in being a good person, though, and I try to help other people. I volunteer at the hospital on the ward that takes care of kids who've been abused so bad they have to be in the hospital to mend, and I go to a couple of groups for kids like me who have been abused. I tried counseling once but the counselor wasn't very good and she kept insisting that I should be a lot sicker than I was and that, sooner or later, all the things that happened to me would end up hurting me, making me depressed, or a drunk or something. I think she sucked, and she was wrong. The groups I go to think just the opposite; that we're special because we took so much abuse and turned out so well. And I guess I'm proud that I turned out so well. Maybe the counselor was right and sometime, when I'm an adult, I'll be screwy, but I don't think so. What do you think?

23.11. UNDERSTANDING JAKE'S RESILIENCE

Very early on, Jake learned to protect himself from his parent's abusive behavior while still feeling loyalty to his parents. This is what Tiet et al. (1998) call protective factors and what Henry (1999) sees as an example of how children can make themselves invisible to their abusers while still being loyal to them.

Jake sees the dysfunctional behavior of his parents in a rational way by noting the early harm done to both parents by their families, and he is forgiving. It has probably helped him see how his grandfather's drinking affected his father and that his father grew up in an abusive environment. Henry (1999) points out that children are willing to give parents many opportunities to correct their abusive behavior.

Jake understands that it is unlikely that either parent has the emotional capacity to allow him to live with them, but he sees them often and has begun to have a good relationship with his father. He is endlessly optimistic while maintaining a realistic view of his family. He hopes for a great deal, but expects little.

Jake does well in school and has goals for himself that provide a positive view of his abilities and the way they might be used in the future. These coping skills and the rational way he views his family may exist because of significant intellectual and emotional intelligence.

Jake has a negative view of the counseling he received but a positive view of the support groups he has attended. Anderson (1997) suggests that instead of focusing on pathology or the harm done to the child by the abuse, we should focus instead on the strengths of the child. She also believes that in looking for strengths, that we find themes of resilience in the "survival stories" abused children tell us and that we should help them recognize the positive role they played in surviving their abuse. Anderson (1997) writes, "The psychological scars will never disappear completely; however, focusing on the child's strengths and resiliency can help limit the power of sexual abuse over the child" (p. 597). Henry (1999) reports that practitioners often miss an essential point by always looking for pathology and that the way the child copes with his or her abuse is actually "the strength that enables them to survive in an unsafe environment" (p. 519).

Jake had the good fortune, or the wisdom, to choose an exceptional foster family to live with. If he chose them, it shows a significant ability to recognize a nurturing and positive environment in someone so young. Jake's early escape into reading gave him a healthy outlet for his maltreatment. While some might argue that losing himself in reading might have resulted in a very introverted child and adult, this does not seem to be the case at all. The positive response for reading that he received from his foster father may be partly responsible.

Jake recognizes that he has bad days. His foster father has helped him see that many other people suffer from the "blues." By listening to someone who suffered from the blues sing so powerfully about the way he felt, he has a model of how one can feel down but hopeful, and even use sadness for extraordinary creative purposes. He certainly does not romanticize depression but sees it as a possible result of his maltreatment.

Jake recognizes his anger at his mother, tries to interact with her, but believes that she has not changed. This grounded understanding of his mother helps him deal with her without letting her behavior affect him too badly. One might suggest, however, that as he begins to date and develop intimate relationships, a negative view of the parent of the opposite sex might result in difficulties and could suggest the need for help.

Jake does not believe in God but he does helpful things for others and lives a caring life. Ambivalence about God is not terribly difficult to understand in a child who has been badly abused. The more important issue is his active role in helping others and living a socially responsible life. Some would suggest that his behavior indicates the existence of strong spiritual feelings and beliefs.

23.12. SUMMARY

This chapter on resilience discusses the many factors that define resilience. The chapter gives definitions of the term resilience and the attributes of resilient people. It also discusses the relationship between coping with stress and resilience. A discussion of resilience by youth in crisis provides a way of understanding how resilient youth who are traumatized understand their unique ways of coping with life stressors.

23.13. QUESTIONS FROM THE CHAPTER

1. Do you believe that resilient youth are resilient in every situation? What may limit resilience in otherwise well functioning children and adolescents who have experienced a trauma?
2. Why would one child in a family be resilient and another not be resilient?
3. Do not you think that resilience can be explained by just two factor? Superior intelligence and superior biology.
4. Do you believe that childhood resilience continues on throughout the life cycle into old age or does it ebb and flow with the situation?
5. If most people are emotionally OK by 18 and the rest who are not OK at 18 are mostly OK by 30, why even bother to help people? Will not they just get better on their own, anyway?

References

Abrams, M. S. (2001). Resilience in ambiguous loss. *American Journal of Psychotherapy, 2*, 283–291.

Anderson, K. M. (1997, November). Uncovering survival abilities in children who have been sexually abused. *Families in society: The Journal of Contemporary Human Services, 78*(6), 592–599.

Arend, R., Gove, F., & Sroufe, L. (1979). Continuity of individual adaptation from infancy to kindergarten: A predictive study of ego-resiliency and curiosity in preschoolers. *Child Development, 50*, 950–959.

Baldwin, A., Baldwin, C., Kasser, T., Zax, M., Sameroff, A., & Seifer, R. (1993). Contextual risk and resiliency during adolescence. *Development and Psychopathology, 5*, 741–761.

Baron, L., Eisman, H., Scuello, M., Veyzer, A., & Lieberman, M. (1996, September). Stress resilience, locus of control, and religion in children of Holocaust victims. *Journal of Psychology, 130*(5), 513–525.

Beardslee, W. R., & Podorefsky, D. (1988). Resilient adolescents whose parents have serious affective and other psychiatric disorders: Importance of self understanding and relationships. *American Journal of Psychiatry, 145*, 63–69.

Billings, A. G., & Moos, R. H. (1981). The role of coping responses and social resources in attenuating the stress of life events. *Journal of Behavioral Medicine, 4*, 139–157.

Billings, A. G., & Moos, R. H. (1984). Coping, stress and social resources among adults with unipolar depression. *Journal of personality and social psychology, 46*, 877–891.

Brooks, R. (1994). Children at risk: Fostering resilience and hope. *American Journal of Orthopsychiatry, 64*, 545–553.

Carver, C. S., Scheier, M. F., & Weintraub, J. K. (1989). Assessing coping strategies: A theoretically based approach. *Journal of Personality and Social Psychology, 56*, 267–283.

Cohler, B. (1987). Adversity, resilience, and the study of lives. In E. J. Anthony, & B. J. Cohler (Eds.), *The invulnerable child* (pp. 363–424). New York: Guilford.

Courbasson, C., Endler, M. A., Kocovski, N. S., & Kocovski, N. L. (2002, Spring). Coping and psychological distress for men with substance use disorders. *Current Psychology, 21*(1), 35–50, (p. 15).

Egeland, E., Carlson, E., & Sroufe, L. (1993). Resilience as process. *Development and Psychopathology, 5*, 517–528.

Endler, N. S. & Parker, J. D. A. (1999). *Coping inventory for stressful situations (CISS): Manual* (Rev. ed.). Toronto: Multihealth Systems.

Farber, E., & Egeland, B. (1987). Invulnerability among abused and neglected children. In E. J. Anthony, & B. J. Cohler (Eds.), *The invulnerable child* (pp. 289–314). New York: Guilford.

Furstenberg, F. F. (1998). Paternal involvement with adolescence in intact families: The influence of fathers over the life course. *Demography, 35*(2), 201–216.

Garmezy, N., Masten, A., & Tellegen, A. (1964). The study of stress and competence in children: A building block for developmental psychopathology. *Child Development, 55*, 97–111.

Gist, R., & Devilly, G. J. (2002). Post-trauma debriefing: The road too frequently traveled. *Lancet, 360*(9335), 741–743.

Glick, H. A. (1994). *Resilience research: How can it help city schools?* Found on the Internet August 1, 2004 at: http://www.ncrel.org/sdrs/cityschl/city1_1b.htm NCRAL.

Glicken, M. D. (2004). *Using the strengths perspective in social work practice*. Boston: Allyn and Bacon/Longman.

Gordon, K. A. (1996). *Infant and toddler resilience: Knowledge, predictions, policy, and practice*. Paper presented at the Head Start National Research Conference. 3rd, Washington, DC, June 20–23, 1996.

Henry, D. L. (1999, September). Resilience in maltreated children: Implications for special needs adoptions. *Child Welfare, 78*(5), 519–540.

Last, U. (1989). The transgenerational impact of Holocaust trauma: Current state of the evidence. *International Journal of Mental Health, 17*(4), 72–89.

Lazarus, R. S. (1966). *Psychological stress and the coping process*. New York: McGraw Hill.

Liveneh, H., Livneh, C. L., Maron, S., & Kaplan, J. (1996, September). A multidimensional approach to the study of the structure of coping with stress. *Journal of Psychology, 130*(5), 501–513.

Luthar, S. (1991). Vulnerability and resilience: A study of high risk adolescents. *Child Development, 62*, 599–616.

Luthar, S. (1993). Annotation: Methodology and conceptual issues in research on childhood resilience. *Journal of Child Psychology and Psychiatry, 34*, 441–453.

Luthar, S., & Zigler, E. (1991). Vulnerability and competence: A review of research on resilience in childhood. *American Journal of Orthopsychiatry, 6*, 6–22.

Mandleco, B. L., & Peery, J. C. (2000, July–August). An organizational framework for conceptualizing resilience in children. *Journal of Child & Adolescent Psychiatric Nursing, 13*(3), 99–112.

Masten, A. S. (2001). Ordinary Magic: Resilience processes in development. *American Psychologist, 56*, 227–238.

McCrae, R. R. (1984). Situational determinants of coping responses: Loss, threat, and challenge. *Journal of Personality and Social Psychology, 46*, 919–928.

Miller, L. H. & Smith, A. D. (2005). *The different kinds of stress*. American Psychological Association Help Line. Found on the Internet May 13, 2005 at http://www.apahelpcenter.org/articles/article.php?id=21

Neighbors, B., Forehand, R., & McVicar, D. (1993). Resilient adolescents and interparental conflict. *American Journal of Orthopsychiatry, 63*, 462–471.

Ozer, E. J., Best, S. R., Lipsey, T. L., & Weiss, D. S. (2003). Predictors of posttraumatic stress disorder and symptoms in adults: A meta-analysis. *Psychological Bulletin, 129*(1), 52–73.

Parkes, K. R. (1984). Locus of control, cognitive appraisal, and coping in stressful episodes. *Journal of Personality and Social Psychology, 46*(3), 655–668.

Pearlin, L. I., & Schooler, C. (1978). The structure of coping. *Journal of Health and Social Behavior, 19*, 2–21.

Polk, L. V. (1997). Toward a middle range theory of resilience. *Advances in Nursing Science, 1*(3), 1–13.

Radke-Yarrow, M., & Brown, E. (1993). Resilience and vulnerability in children of multiple-risk families. *Development and Psychopathology, 5*, 581–592.

Seligman, M. (1992). *Learned optimism: How to change your mind and your life*. New York: Pocket Books.

Tech, N. (2003). *Resilience and courage: Women, men, and the holocaust*. New Haven, CT: Yale University Press.

Tiet, Q. Q., Bird, H., & Davies, M. R. (1998, November). Adverse life events and resilience. *Journal of the American Academy of Child and Adolescent Psychiatry, 37*(11), 1191–1200.

Vaillant, G. E. (1993). *The wisdom of the ego*. Cambridge, MA: Harvard University Press.

Walsh, F. (2003). Family resilience: A framework for clinical practice – theory and practice. *Family Processes, 42*, 1–18.

Werner, E. (1989). High-risk children in young adulthood: A longitudinal study from birth to 32 years. *American Orthopsychiatric Association, 59*, 72–81.

Werner, E., & Smith, R. S. (1982). *Vulnerable but invincible*. New York: Adams, Bannister & Cox.

Werner, E., & Smith, R. S. (1992). *Overcoming the odds: High risk children from birth to adulthood*. Ithaca, NY: Cornell University Press.

Werner, E., & Smith, R. S. (2001). *Journey from childhood to midlife: Risk, resilience, and recovery*. Ithica, NY: Cornell University Press.

Wilkes, G. (2002). Abused child to non-abused parent: Resilience and conceptual change. *Journal of Clinical Psychology, 58*(3), 229–232.

24 Needed Changes to Improve the Lives of Children

In the following discussion, some of the major issues confronting Americans and their children will be discussed with suggestions made for ways to improve the lives of children.

24.1. STOP TREATING CHILDREN AS IF THEY ARE ADULTS

We live in a time of easy fixes to complicated problems in which medications are the answer to most health problems and talking therapy is considered a luxury, or perhaps even irrelevant. This approach has put us into quite a quandary when it comes to working with children. Not only have we begun using medications with little evidence of their efficacy, but we use adult diagnostic categories to fit the medications we use with very young children. It is heartbreaking to think of a 3- or 4-year-old diagnosed with bi-polar disorder or chronic depression, or even worse, childhood schizophrenia, simply because a clinician or physician knows so little about children that he or she immediately thinks of an adult diagnosis and the adult medications for unformed and developing children whose childhoods will now be changed for, perhaps, a lifetime. To add to this tragedy, we have little evidence that adult medications actually work with children, and growing evidence that they often do harm.

24.2. MORE HELP AND LESS MEDICATIONS FOR CHILDREN

If this book has done nothing else, hopefully it has helped clinicians realize that before psychotropic medications are ever used with children, we should do everything in our power to work with them in ways that do not interfere with their physical and emotional development, but instead use their innate strengths and those of their parents and the community to help them. The scores of children incorrectly diagnosed with ADHD is simply a national tragedy and needs to be rectified immediately. A national registry much like that used in the treatment of cancer should to be established so that we can track the treatment of children and adolescents and limit the use of psychotropic medications to those cases where there is very strong evidence that they will work. One hopes that the need to justify medication will limit its use and provide better research data on effective psychosocial treatment approaches.

24.3. MORE RESEARCH

It is difficult to see how children will be helped without a considerable increase in the amount of research on effective treatment approaches. The use of best evidence should help clinicians train in approaches that actually work rather than assuming that children are simply miniature adults and therefore should be treated using the same treatment approaches as adults. Some of us shine when we work with children. We should commit ourselves to sharing with our colleagues the practice wisdom as well as the hard evidence that what we do works. It is our responsibility to do the small and large pieces of research that help develop practice wisdom for training workers in the human services. We can also use our knowledge of children to share our observations of published research studies that may be incorrectly reported in the media. And when necessary, we can use our knowledge of research on children as a "bully pulpit," to use Teddy Roosevelt's famous saying, so that we enter into the debates that rage in this country around issues of abortion, crime, educational standards, and a host of social problems for which most of us who understand research and the problems of children say virtually nothing. It is shameful how passive we have become in the human services.

24.4. REDUCE CHILD ABUSE

The incredible numbers of abused and neglected children in our communities is a disgrace. I cannot help but believe that our child protective services have become inadequate organizations more interested in political survival than in actual reductions in abuse and neglect. Not a day goes by in my state that one does not read reports of children in foster care who are beaten or killed, and that multiple reports of child abuse go uninvestigated. Worker turnover rates in these agencies suggest that the strong practitioners do not stay because, yes! the work is stressful and not for everyone, but really because their work is so little recognized and rewarded. It is our job to reduce abuse and neglect and to make a pledge that we will put our hearts and souls into the difficult task of educating the community on the damage done to children when their spirits are broken by the harmful behavior of adults.

24.5. IMPROVE THE STATUS AND SALARIES OF HUMAN SERVICE PROFESSIONALS

We should put our feet down in unison whenever politicians or policy analysts and insurance companies say we do not need therapists or that the work we do is irrelevant. The salaries we get are an indication that the community cares too little about what we do, and it is no fabrication that salaries dictate who will come into the field to do the frontline work that often needs to be done for children in desperate straits. The fact that graduating MSWs still earn less on average than what the National Association of Social Workers said they should earn in 1964 is evidence that human service education is doing too little to advocate for new social workers, and that professional organizations are doing even less. It is no wonder that students choose fields that pay well, often leaving some of the best and brightest students who really want a career in the human services to seek degrees that assure good salaries. And while we are on the subject of education, let us be clear that a profession dominated by one gender is not serving the needs of clients. Less than 10% of graduating MSWs are male, and fewer than that of either gender are professionals of color. We need diversity in our profession because we serve an increasingly diverse client population.

24.6. REDUCE POVERTY

The number of children in poverty is a national tragedy. Poverty is a killer of educational achievement, physical health and mental health, and if you have been poor, you know better than to romanticize poverty or to suggest that children should pull themselves up by their bootstraps and better themselves. The plain truth is that the chances of doing well in life significantly diminish as one moves down the economic ladder and into poverty. Our ability to help children who are malnourished, who live in dangerous neighborhoods and substandard housing, and who attend low-achieving and violent schools is just not very great, and we should challenge our political class to do much more to provide decent jobs with decent income for parents, safe and affordable housing, and the best education possible for our most vulnerable and at risk children and their families.

24.7. IMPROVE HEALTH CARE

For the first time in our history, life expectancy has become stagnant. For 25% of our population, life expectancy is decreasing, largely because of poor health choices, but more specifically because of poverty and lack of access to health care (Science Daily, 2008). This bodes badly for the health of children in poverty and should tell us that a more inclusive health care system is needed to ensure that children have the best possible health and are educated to make the best possible health care decisions. Even though low income children are often covered by Medicaid, that does not mean that parents necessarily use health care wisely or know the signs of illness that require a child to be seen by a health care provider. Human service professionals should be knowledgeable about medication for a variety of illnesses and should be a source of information to low income clients about accessing health care and the proper use of medication.

When I was a school social worker, one of the things that surprised me most was how many parents did not know how to use a thermometer, what a serious temperature reading was and what to do about it, or to distinguish non-threatening illnesses from serious problems. I found out quickly that simple bits of information to well-meaning parents made the difference between children going to school or staying home and losing valuable information to keep pace with a class. My wise supervisor told me that several simple rules could make all the difference in a child's school attendance record. She advised me to tell parents to send children to school if their temperature was below 101, they were not vomiting when they stood up, and they did not have an illness that would make others ill. That advice was something concrete that parents could use with children that allowed them to set rules about the definition of an illness that determined whether a child stayed home or went to school. I used the same rule with my 8-year-old daughter who, we discovered after a long year and a half of being bewildered by her symptoms and 15 doctor's visits, had juvenile onset diabetes and was feeling very fragile at school. After a few calls from the school that she was ill, I instituted the same rule about illness and staying home from school I had used when I was a school social worker. Within a few weeks, it worked.

24.8. REDUCE ADULT PRESSURE ON YOUNG CHILDREN

I wonder about parents today who over-schedule their children with every activity under the sun and run them ragged with activities. Who, I wonder, is getting the benefit of all this activity? Surely not the children who do not need or want to be in dance class, music class, gymnastics, soccer, acting class, and ballet (at 4 years of age), but can play nicely by themselves or with friends. I went to a birthday party for a 4-year-old recently, and these were just a few of the activities parents had their children enrolled in. I was mortified. Why so many activities? I asked the mothers. Because, they said, how will you know your child's hidden abilities if you do not test them out early and anyway, everyone is doing it. Everyone? Well everyone in our social circle. Is not it tiring and expensive? Yes, but that is the responsibility of having children.

It is a bit depressing to see what used to be a fun time to grow up, with few organized activities because it was the child's responsibility to stay active, to now see such wasteful and unnecessary activity. Parents must feel a great deal of competition with one another to drive their children and themselves around the community occupying their children in activities, which often end up boring their kids in a short period of time. Parents need some wise guidance from their own parents and the professionals in the community to give their children some leeway and free time.

Much of this pressure placed on children by parents ends in a type of mass spoiling we associate with the worst aspects of what we call Generation Y. Writing about Generation Y, Jayson (2007) says that the entire time children are growing up they have someone nearby to record every irrelevant life event and to fill them with false adulation. This leads to a sense of importance that is not shared by others. She worries that the Generation Y obsession with fame and money will end, as they age and as they experience the realities of life without parents to make sure their self-esteem is as strong as humanly possible, with many of them experiencing a sense of emptiness and depression.

24.9. EMPHASIZE GOOD CITIZENSHIP, POSITIVE VALUES, AND CIVIC INVOLVEMENT

When I was growing up in the 1940s there was a strong emphasis on becoming a good citizen, knowing our history, and appreciating our democratic institutions. We had just fought a defining world war and the civil rights movement made it clear that for all of our strengths, bigotry and discrimination were serious failures that just had to be rectified. It almost feels corny to say this, given how detached children have become from our nation's history, but healthy people understand a country's problems, become part of the solution, and want to be active in those aspects of good citizenship that define civic mindedness. I do not see strong concern for the nation, for voting, or for civic involvement in our nation's youth. It is a direction that spells trouble for the future. When few people are involved, democracy has a tendency to slip away from us. For that reason I urge readers to take a strong position on teaching children our history and their civic role in shaping the future. There is not anything corny about love of country or recognizing problems that need creative solutions and hard civic work. Children need a sense of identity and mission that provide meaning in life.

A criticism of the human services is that we fail to stress, through the work we do with our clients, a society that functions with shared values and a sense of civic cooperation. Ryff and Singer (1998) suggest that modern psychology has failed to develop a view of the client beyond the absence of dysfunctional behavior. Sandage and Hill (2001) suggest that modern psychology has no model of the "good life" or the virtues that promote healthy individual and community behavior. In fact, they suggest that much of psychology, and perhaps much of the helping professions, has no model of the positive values that we should stress with our clients. Creating positive values and civic responsibility is something all of us should be involved in if we want to create a dynamic and vital society.

24.10. IMPROVE THE WELL-BEING OF CHILDREN

A recent report (St. George, 2008) notes that children have made great strides in the past 10 years in a number of important areas. The report brings together data from a number of federal agencies and includes the following high points: Mortality rates in children aged one to four have declined by one-third from 43 per 100 000 children in 1994–28 per 100 000 because of safer communities and better health care. The number of children who feared being harmed or attacked at school declined from 14% in 1995 to 9% in 2006. The number of mothers who smoke during pregnancy declined from 15% in 1995 to 9% in 2006. More children attend full-day kindergarten than ever before, with enrollments up 48% since 1994. Problems reported by the studies noted that the incidence of low birth weight babies increased and there was a substantial increase in obesity.

You read these data and, of course, you feel proud that we are doing so well. But if only 70% of our children attend full-day kindergarten, what about the other 30%? And how do these data compare to other countries? The answer is that they compare badly. Using United Nations and International Health data, Crabtree (2008) compared 30 modern countries across a number of indicators of health and well-being. The life expectancy of Americans ranked 29th, or just above Cuba, largely because of poorer health care for racial minorities and more deaths from illnesses that seem preventable or at least treatable for most Americans. Those illnesses in which race plays a role in life expectancy include asthma, diabetes and high blood pressure. America was ranked 13th for quality of life. The factors contributing to quality of life include many issues of concern to human service professionals who work with children, such as health, freedom, unemployment, climate, political stability and security, gender equality, and family and community life. Compared to Japan, where under 2% of the population is obese, over 30% of Americans are considered to be obese. US infant mortality rates of 6.9 per 1000 live births compare unfavorably to industrial nations (such as England, Japan, Germany, France and Sweden) whose combined number of infant mortality rates were 5.7 per 1000. Japan and the Nordic countries had substantially lower infant mortality rates of 3.5 per 1000 live births. When compared to other western countries, we have a ways to go before we can say that the quality of life is very good for our children.

24.11. SAFE AND HEALTHY COMMUNITIES

Although national crime data suggest that juvenile violence has declined dramatically, there is evidence that it is on the rise. Writing about the increase in juvenile homicides in Chicago, Saulny (2008) reports that since the beginning of 2008, 24 public school children have been murdered. Most of the deaths were related to increased gang violence of the sort reported in a number of other urban communities. According to Saulny, 85% of Chicago's public school-age children live in poverty and are much more likely to experience violence in their schools, neighborhoods and homes than the remaining 15% of Chicago's public school population. In Los Angeles, where gang violence had been declining for the past 15 years, there were 256 gang-related homicides from January to August 2002. This is a 22% increase from the same time period in 2001, and a 47% increase from the 5-year average for those months (Saulny, 2008). Other large cities cite increasing gang homicides and violence. In 2002, Houston noted an increase in gang homicides by 100%, while gang violence has increased nationally by 50% over 1999. Although overall levels of violence may be down nationally, juvenile gang violence continues to increase in America's urban areas, a potential precursor to increasing levels of crime among all youth groups.

To cope with crime and other issues that affect us all, Saleebey (1996) believes we must become a cooperative and dynamic community, and writes:

> *Membership [in a community] means that people need to be citizens – responsible and valued members in a viable group or community. To be without membership is to be alienated, and to be at risk of marginalization and oppression, the enemies of civic and moral strength (Walzer, 1983). As people begin to realize and use their assets and abilities, collectively and individually, as they begin to discover the pride in having survived and overcome their difficulties, more and more of their capacities come into the work and play of daily life. These build on each other exponentially, reflecting a kind of synergy. The same synergistic phenomenon seems true of communities and groups as well. In both instances, one might suggest that there are no known limits to individual and collective capacities. (Saleebey, 1996, p. 297)*

Kesler (2000) suggests seven core beliefs that define healthy communities: (1) "The healthy community movement involves a sophisticated, integrative, and interconnected vision of flourishing of the individual and the human collective in an environmental setting" (Kesler, 2000, p. 272); (2) the healthy communities movement must involve all sectors of society, including the disenfranchised; (3) the healthy communities movement is about people connecting intimately with one another and becoming aware of special issues that need to be addressed sensitively and creatively; (4) healthy communities require a dialogue among people to help formulate public policy agendas; (5) the healthy communities movement must seek consensus and mutual ground among all community groups and political persuasions; (6) the healthy communities movement must function from a broad level of caring, maturity, and awareness; and (7) the healthy communities movement seeks to form alliances with other community-based movements. Kesler (2000) writes that the ultimate goal of the healthy communities movement is to "encourage all concerned to rise to higher integrative levels of thinking, discourse, research, policies, programs, institutions, and processes, so that they might truly begin to transform their lives, their communities, and the greater society" (p. 271).

24.12. IMPROVE AMERICAN EDUCATION

Commenting on the 25th anniversary report on the nations schools, (*A Nation at Risk, 1985*), Finn (2008) writes:

> *...[S]chool results haven't appreciably improved, whether one looks at test scores or graduation rates. Sure, there are up and down blips in the data, but no big and lasting changes in performance, even though we're also spending tons more money. (In constant dollars, per-pupil spending in 1983 was 56% of*

> *today's.) And just as "A Nation at Risk" warned, other countries are beginning to eat our education lunch. While our outcomes remain flat, theirs rise. Half a dozen nations now surpass our high school and college graduation rates. International tests find young Americans scoring in the middle of the pack. (p. 1)*

That should come as no surprise to the readers who teach in departments of higher education in the human services. Simple writing assignments are very difficult for a number of students in the human services, suggesting that something is lacking in their prior education. In their study of graduate level writing in social work, Alter and Atkins (2001) found that 60% of the graduate social work students in their sample wrote at less than graduate school level. Of the 60% of the students who wrote badly in their sample, only 20% sought help from writing centers or took tutorials or special writing classes. Something fundamental is not working when students cannot or would not write well. In the human services, children are taken from parents, elderly people have their savings placed in receivership, and people go to jail based upon the reports we write. If the writing is poor, then imagine the harm we can do?

I find this true of other areas of educational preparation. Few of my graduate students read the paper, watch the news, are aware of relevant films or TV programs that might help their practice, or know much about the political lives of the communities they live in. A graduate class I taught in Arizona on advanced social policy had not watched a single debate in the 2008 presidential primaries, even though we had had at least 10 debates by then. A graduate class I taught in Idaho was very surprised to know that much of the country viewed Idaho as a refuge for the Aryan Brotherhood, even though there were hate crimes committed in several of the larger Idaho communities while I taught there (swastikas on a Jewish synagogue, for example). When I suggested that students in a graduate class I taught in Arizona watch a television series on our work called *In Treatment*, a 9-week series about the work of a therapist that included some brilliant work with a 16-year-old, not a single student watched it or showed much interested in seeing it. A film about child abandonment called the *Martian Child* that I thought would help students planning to work with children went unwatched, and no one seemed very interested in seeing it even though it was out on DVD.

I get many e-mails from graduate students I am teaching telling me that they have never written an essay and that they are unprepared to write a research proposal. These students' lack of writing experience required me and the writing centers to do remedial work that should not be necessary by the time students reach graduate school. The educational and cultural preparation of our students makes me think that we expect too little of them, and that we are continuing the tradition of educating functionaries for agency work rather than leaders who will move our work with children forward. It is a sad commentary on education in the human services, and it is one we can change if we put our hearts and minds into the work that needs to be done.

24.13. A RETURN TO NORMALCY

In the preface to this book I wrote that rather than giving children room to grow and develop in their own unique ways, we were restricting normal development by making the word "normal" increasingly limited and narrow. I should add that the growing numbers of diagnostic categories for children only increases my concern. Children develop normally with serious and attentive parents, good educational institutions, safe communities, attention to health and poverty, and a national optimism that everyone can succeed with hard work. Increasing diagnostic categories tells many otherwise OK children that they will have trouble succeeding in life. Let us keep diagnoses of children to the relatively few children who really are not doing well, and let us work to reset our desire to pathologize the entire population of children and adolescents. It boggles the mind that we estimate that 20% of our youth are in need of treatment. I do not believe that, and I hope you do not either.

24.14. END DISCRIMINATION

I must tell you that as the child of immigrants and as a Jewish American, discrimination makes me angry beyond words. We are too good a country to have the type of discrimination I see in America during an election in which a wonderful and talented Black American has to defend himself against every type of accusation because, and only because, he is Black. It is a disgrace. I have lived in Mexico and never once have I spoken to anyone who really wanted to come to America illegally. As a people, they are the salt of the earth and their hard work and dedication to helping build this country is just another example of how immigrants help, not hurt America. That they are often treated so badly and that the political class talks about rounding up 15 million or 20 million people and deporting them makes me think of the Holocaust and what we did to native people in America. It is time we embrace our immigrants, and our people of color, and understand that diversity built America and will continue to build it and keep it strong. No child should grow up being hated and denied opportunity because of his or her color, ethnicity, gender or religion. It is an indignity to the spirit to place children in harms way because of who they are, and it just has to end.

24.15. FINAL WORDS

Thank you for reading this book on evidence-based practice with children and adolescents. Those of you who work on the frontlines with America's children are the best and the brightest. That you do your work with salaries so low it makes one want to cry out against the injustice is only further evidence that, at their core, the human services are the best thing going in a country that otherwise often seems intent on trivializing our work and that of our fellow professionals in education and community youth work. Keep up the fight, hold your ground against misinformation about children, advocate for the things we know children and their parents need to lead healthy lives, and keep the dream alive of a country of optimism and opportunity for every single child. For all of our flaws, we are a wonderful country and it would be wrong of me not to stress my optimism for the future and to leave you with a bit of my sense of America.

24.16. AMERICA

This story first appeared in a book the author wrote on research (Glicken, 2003, pp. 256–257). Thanks to Pearson Education, Inc. for permission to reprint this material.

My father came from a small rural town in Russia. Because he was coming of age when the Communists would have forced him into the military – an indignity for any Jew denied Russian citizenship – he, my aunt and my grandmother left Russia in the middle of the night. Perhaps he was 14. It took them 3 years of walking across Europe to earn enough money for their passage to America. When he saw the Statue of Liberty, he and a thousand poor Europeans came from the steerage class at the bottom of the ship, stood on the deck, and wept.

America. My father could hardly say the word without tears welling up in his eyes. America. "Give me your tired, your poor, your huddled masses yearning to breathe free." He knew the words on the statue of liberty by heart and he would say them to me until I knew the words as well as he did.

My father had a way of avoiding the downside of the country. I guess his immigrant's love of America forced him into a sort of selective perception. When we could not move from our slum house across from the railroad tracks because no one would sell us a house in a better part of town – being Jewish meant that you were something akin to having leprosy – my father said, "So, who wants to live with the bastards anyway? Better we should live among our own people where nobody makes jokes about us."

Which, of course, completely begged the question. While it was true that we lived in a small Jewish ghetto, Jewish children went to public schools and the living, as they say, was not easy. I did not know until I went to public school that we Jews drank the blood of our dead or, as my non-Jewish classmates were so ready to inform me, that we buried our dead standing on top of one another to save money. I had not heard the word "jewed" until second grade and then, I did not understand what it meant. I thought we were the chosen people and that the Jewish men and women in my community were the best and smartest and most wonderful people I could ever know. It was a mystery to me how people could say such wrong-headed and malicious things about us. I guess it still is.

And yet, America was a wonderful place for me. I could spell swear words on the bridge of my mouth with my tongue and still look decently happy whenever any anti-Semitic person would try and remind me of the failings of the Jewish people. I could co-exist because I had bigger fish to fry. America offered me opportunity and it did not matter to me what other people thought about Jews.

But ultimately, of course, it *did* matter, because they thought the same way about a lot of other people I found pretty admirable. They disliked Blacks and Hispanics and Asians for reasons I could not begin to understand. If someone Black came to my hometown, they were asked to leave by the police. Politely, of course. Hispanic farm workers could not sit in the same section of the theater as we did. And this, I want to remind you, was in North Dakota, a place so cold and isolated that you should be *paid* to be there.

I am older now and a little more cynical, but in a place deep within my heart, I still love America. To be sure, the country is full of regrettable social problems that beg for solutions. But the underlying belief system, the sense I have when I leave this country and return is that this place, this America, is full of wonders and riches. Had I lived in Europe, had my parents not left, I would be lying in a mass grave, the victim of another forgotten atrocity to Jewish people.

For my parents, for my brother and sister, for my people who lived to survive the Holocaust because America offered us a safe haven, God Bless America! May she live to offer generation after generation of immigrants a sanctuary against the barbarism and the killing fields of the world.

References

Alter, C., & Atkins, C. (2001). Improving writing skills of social work students. *Journal of Social Work Education, 3*(7), 493–505.

Finn, C. E. (2008, April 26). Twenty-five years later, a nation still at risk. *The Wall Street Journal,* A7. http://online.wsj.com/article/SB120916804732546311.html?mod=googlenews_wsj

Glicken, M. D. (2003). *Social research: A simple guide*. Boston, MA: Pearson Education, Inc..

Jayson. S. (2007). Generation Y's goal? Wealth and fame. *USA Today*. http://www.usatoday.com/news/nation/2007-01-09-gen-y-cover_x.htm

Kesler, J. T. (2000). The healthy communities movement: Seven counterintuitive next steps. *National Civic Review, 89*(3), 271–284.

Ryff, C. D., & Singer, B. (1998). The contours of positive human health. *Psychological Inquiry, 9*, 1–28.

Saleebey, D. (1996). The strengths perspective in social work practice: Extensions and cautions. *Social Work, 41*(3), 296–305.

Sandage, S. T., & Hill, P. C. (2001). The virtue of positive psychology: The rapprochement and challenge of an affirmative postmodern perspective. *Journal of the Theory of Social Behavior, 31*(3), 241–260.

Saulny, S. (2008, April 27). After killings, escorts for Chicago students. *Violence Prevention Coalition of Greater Los Angeles*. NYTIMES.COM. http://www.vpcla.org/factGang.htm

Science Daily (2008, April 23). *Life expectancy worsening or stagnating for large segment of U.S. population.* http://www.sciencedaily.com/releases/2008/04/080422103952.htm

St. George, D. (2008, April 24). Children's well-being increasing, study says. *Arizona Republic*, A12.

Walzer, M. (1983). *Spheres of justice*. New York: Basic Books.

Further reading

Crabtree, V. (2005). *Which countries set the best examples?* http://www.vexen.co.uk/countries/best.html

Index

L

M

N

O

P

Q

R

S

T

U

V

W

X

Printed and bound by CPI Group (UK) Ltd, Croydon, CR0 4YY

08/06/2025

01896873-0006